PROCEEDINGS OF THE 2018 INTERNATIONAL CONFERENCE ON HEALTH INFORMATICS & MEDICAL SYSTEMS

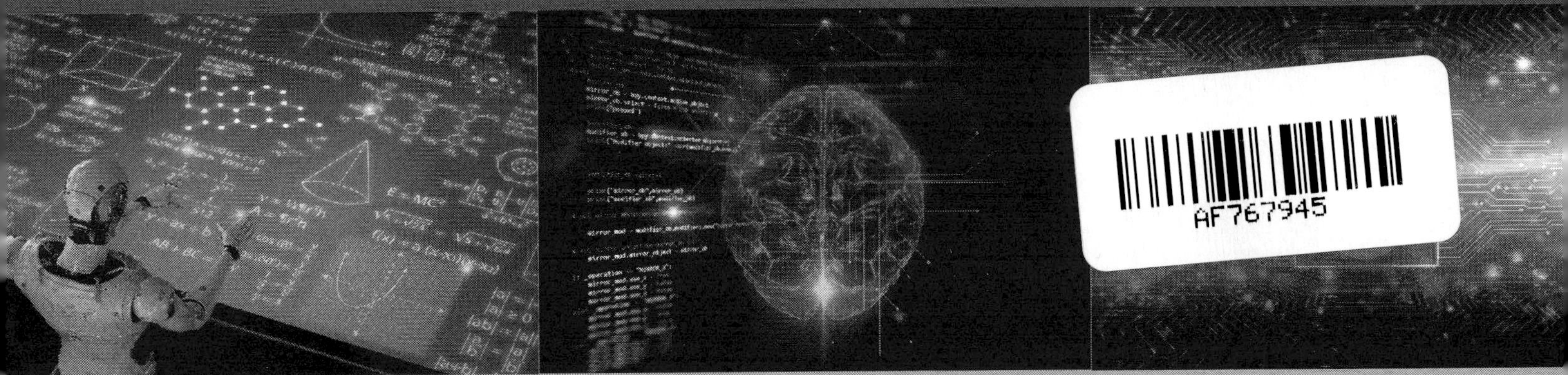

HIMS'18

Editors

Hamid R. Arabnia

Leonidas Deligiannidis, Fernando G. Tinetti

Quoc-Nam Tran

Publication of the 2018 World Congress in Computer Science, Computer Engineering, & Applied Computing (CSCE'18)
July 30 - August 02, 2018 | Las Vegas, Nevada, USA
https://americancse.org/events/csce2018

American Council on Science and Education (ACSE)

ISBN: 1-60132-479-0
Printed in the United States of America
https://americancse.org/events/csce2018/proceedings

Foreword

It gives us great pleasure to introduce this collection of papers to be presented at the 2018 International Conference on Health Informatics and Medical Systems (HIMS'18), July 30 – August 2, 2018, at Luxor Hotel (a property of MGM Resorts International), Las Vegas, USA.

An important mission of the World Congress in Computer Science, Computer Engineering, and Applied Computing, CSCE (a federated congress to which this conference is affiliated with) includes *"Providing a unique platform for a diverse community of constituents composed of scholars, researchers, developers, educators, and practitioners. The Congress makes concerted effort to reach out to participants affiliated with diverse entities (such as: universities, institutions, corporations, government agencies, and research centers/labs) from all over the world. The congress also attempts to connect participants from institutions that have teaching as their main mission with those who are affiliated with institutions that have research as their main mission. The congress uses a quota system to achieve its institution and geography diversity objectives."* By any definition of diversity, this congress is among the most diverse scientific meeting in USA. We are proud to report that this federated congress has authors and participants from 67 different nations representing variety of personal and scientific experiences that arise from differences in culture and values. As can be seen (see below), the program committee of this conference as well as the program committee of all other tracks of the federated congress are as diverse as its authors and participants.

The program committee would like to thank all those who submitted papers for consideration. About 60% of the submissions were from outside the United States. Each submitted paper was peer-reviewed by two experts in the field for originality, significance, clarity, impact, and soundness. In cases of contradictory recommendations, a member of the conference program committee was charged to make the final decision; often, this involved seeking help from additional referees. In addition, papers whose authors included a member of the conference program committee were evaluated using the double-blinded review process. One exception to the above evaluation process was for papers that were submitted directly to chairs/organizers of pre-approved sessions/workshops; in these cases, the chairs/organizers were responsible for the evaluation of such submissions. The overall paper acceptance rate for regular papers was 19%; 20% of the remaining papers were accepted as poster papers (at the time of this writing, we had not yet received the acceptance rate for a couple of individual tracks.)

We are very grateful to the many colleagues who offered their services in organizing the conference. In particular, we would like to thank the members of Program Committee of HIMS'18, members of the congress Steering Committee, and members of the committees of federated congress tracks that have topics within the scope of HIMS. Many individuals listed below, will be requested after the conference to provide their expertise and services for selecting papers for publication (extended versions) in journal special issues as well as for publication in a set of research books (to be prepared for publishers including: Springer, Elsevier, BMC journals, and others).

- *Prof. Abbas M. Al-Bakry (Congress Steering Committee); University President, University of IT and Communications, Baghdad, Iraq*
- *Prof. Nizar Al-Holou (Congress Steering Committee); Professor and Chair, Electrical and Computer Engineering Department; Vice Chair, IEEE/SEM-Computer Chapter; University of Detroit Mercy, Detroit, Michigan, USA*
- *Prof. Hamid R. Arabnia (Congress Steering Committee); Graduate Program Director (PhD, MS, MAMS); The University of Georgia, USA; Editor-in-Chief, Journal of Supercomputing (Springer); Fellow, Center of Excellence in Terrorism, Resilience, Intelligence & Organized Crime Research (CENTRIC).*
- *Prof. Dr. Juan-Vicente Capella-Hernandez; Universitat Politecnica de Valencia (UPV), Department of Computer Engineering (DISCA), Valencia, Spain*
- *Prof. Juan Jose Martinez Castillo; Director, The Acantelys Alan Turing Nikola Tesla Research Group and GIPEB, Universidad Nacional Abierta, Venezuela*
- *Prof. Kevin Daimi (Congress Steering Committee); Director, Computer Science and Software Engineering Programs, Department of Mathematics, Computer Science and Software Engineering, University of Detroit Mercy, Detroit, Michigan, USA*

- *Prof. Zhangisina Gulnur Davletzhanovna; Vice-rector of the Science, Central-Asian University, Kazakhstan, Almaty, Republic of Kazakhstan; Vice President of International Academy of Informatization, Kazskhstan, Almaty, Republic of Kazakhstan*
- *Prof. Leonidas Deligiannidis (Congress Steering Committee); Department of Computer Information Systems, Wentworth Institute of Technology, Boston, Massachusetts, USA; Visiting Professor, MIT, USA*
- *Mojtaba Sedigh Fazli; Department of Computer Science, University of Georgia, Athens, Georgia, USA*
- *Hindenburgo Elvas Goncalves de Sa; Robertshaw Controls (Multi-National Company), System Analyst, Brazil; Information Technology Coordinator and Manager, Brazil*
- *Prof. Byung-Gyu Kim (Congress Steering Committee); Multimedia Processing Communications Lab.(MPCL), Department of Computer Science and Engineering, College of Engineering, SunMoon University, South Korea*
- *Prof. Louie Lolong Lacatan; Chairperson, Computer Engineerig Department, College of Engineering, Adamson University, Manila, Philippines; Senior Member, International Association of Computer Science and Information Technology (IACSIT), Singapore; Member, International Association of Online Engineering (IAOE), Austria*
- *Prof. Dr. Guoming Lai; Computer Science and Technology, Sun Yat-Sen University, Guangzhou, P. R. China*
- *Prof. Hyo Jong Lee; Director, Center for Advanced Image and Information Technology, Division of Computer Science and Engineering, Chonbuk National University, South Korea*
- *Dr. Muhammad Naufal Bin Mansor; Faculty of Engineering Technology, Department of Electrical, Universiti Malaysia Perlis (UniMAP), Perlis, Malaysia*
- *Dr. Andrew Marsh (Congress Steering Committee); CEO, HoIP Telecom Ltd (Healthcare over Internet Protocol), UK; Secretary General of World Academy of BioMedical Sciences and Technologies (WABT) a UNESCO NGO, The United Nations*
- *Michael B. O'Hara (Vice Chair and Editor, HIMS); CEO, KB Computing, LLC, USA; Certified Information System Security Professional (CISSP); Certified Cybersecurity Architect (CCSA); Certified HIPAA Professional (CHP); Certified Security Compliance Specialist (CSCS)*
- *Prof. Dr., Eng. Robert Ehimen Okonigene (Congress Steering Committee); Department of Electrical & Electronics Engineering, Faculty of Engineering and Technology, Ambrose Alli University, Nigeria*
- *Dr. Akash Singh (Congress Steering Committee); IBM Corporation, Sacramento, California, USA; Chartered Scientist, Science Council, UK; Fellow, British Computer Society; Member, Senior IEEE, AACR, AAAS, and AAAI; IBM Corporation, USA*
- *Ashu M. G. Solo (Publicity), Fellow of British Computer Society, Principal/R&D Engineer, Maverick Technologies America Inc.*
- *Prof. Dr. Ir. Sim Kok Swee; Fellow, IEM; Senior Member, IEEE; Faculty of Engineering and Technology, Multimedia University, Melaka, Malaysia*
- *Dr. Ahmad P. Tafti; Associate Research Scientist, Biomedical Informatics Research Center, Marshfield Clinic Research Institute, Marshfield, WI, USA*
- *Prof. Fernando G. Tinetti (Congress Steering Committee); School of CS, Universidad Nacional de La Plata, La Plata, Argentina; also at Comision Investigaciones Cientificas de la Prov. de Bs. As., Argentina*
- *Prof. Hahanov Vladimir (Congress Steering Committee); Vice Rector, and Dean of the Computer Engineering Faculty, Kharkov National University of Radio Electronics, Ukraine and Professor of Design Automation Department, Computer Engineering Faculty, Kharkov; IEEE Computer Society Golden Core Member; National University of Radio Electronics, Ukraine*
- *Prof. Shiuh-Jeng Wang (Congress Steering Committee); Director of Information Cryptology and Construction Laboratory (ICCL) and Director of Chinese Cryptology and Information Security Association (CCISA); Department of Information Management, Central Police University, Taoyuan, Taiwan; Guest Ed., IEEE Journal on Selected Areas in Communications.*
- *Dr. Yunlong Wang; Advanced Analytics at QuintilesIMS, Pennsylvania, USA*
- *Prof. Layne T. Watson (Congress Steering Committee); Fellow of IEEE; Fellow of The National Institute of Aerospace; Professor of Computer Science, Mathematics, and Aerospace and Ocean Engineering, Virginia Polytechnic Institute & State University, Blacksburg, Virginia, USA*
- *Prof. Jane You (Congress Steering Committee); Associate Head, Department of Computing, The Hong Kong Polytechnic University, Kowloon, Hong Kong*
- *Dr. Farhana H. Zulkernine; Coordinator of the Cognitive Science Program, School of Computing, Queen's University, Kingston, ON, Canada*

We would like to extend our appreciation to the referees, the members of the program committees of individual sessions, tracks, and workshops; their names do not appear in this document; they are listed on the web sites of individual tracks.

As Sponsors-at-large, partners, and/or organizers each of the followings (separated by semicolons) provided help for at least one track of the Congress: Computer Science Research, Education, and Applications Press (CSREA); US Chapter of World Academy of Science; American Council on Science & Education & Federated Research Council (http://www.americancse.org/). In addition, a number of university faculty members and their staff (names appear on the cover of the set of proceedings), several publishers of computer science and computer engineering books and journals, chapters and/or task forces of computer science associations/organizations from 3 regions, and developers of high-performance machines and systems provided significant help in organizing the conference as well as providing some resources. We are grateful to them all.

We express our gratitude to keynote, invited, and individual conference/tracks and tutorial speakers - the list of speakers appears on the conference web site. We would also like to thank the followings: UCMSS (Universal Conference Management Systems & Support, California, USA) for managing all aspects of the conference; Dr. Tim Field of APC for coordinating and managing the printing of the proceedings; and the staff of Luxor Hotel (Convention department) at Las Vegas for the professional service they provided. Last but not least, we would like to thank the Co-Editors of HIMS'18: Prof. Hamid R. Arabnia, Prof. Leonidas Deligiannidis, Prof. Fernando G. Tinetti, and Prof. Quoc-Nam Tran.

We present the proceedings of HIMS'18.

Steering Committee, 2018
http://americancse.org/

Contents

SESSION: HEALTH INFORMATICS, HEALTHCARE AND PUBLIC HEALTH RELATED SYSTEMS

SESSION: MEDICAL SYSTEMS, DEVICES AND SERVICES + MONITORING SYSTEMS + TOOLS FOR REHABILITATION

SESSION: TOOLS AND MODELS FOR DECISION MAKING, SUPPORT SYSTEMS AND DIAGNOSTICS

SESSION: POSTER PAPERS

SESSION: LATE BREAKING PAPERS

SESSION

HEALTH INFORMATICS, HEALTHCARE AND PUBLIC HEALTH RELATED SYSTEMS

Chair(s)

TBA

ISBN: 1-60132-479-0, CSREA Press ©

An Automated Approach for Rating the Content Quality of Web Healthcare Information: A Case Study on Depression Treatment Web Pages

Y. Zhang[1], **J. Burkell**[1], **H. Cui**[2], **R. E. Mercer**[3]
[1]Faculty of Information and Media Studies, The University of Western Ontario, London, Ontario, Canada
[2]School of Information Resources/Library Science, University of Arizona, Tucson, Arizona, USA
[3]Department of Computer Science, The University of Western Ontario, London, Ontario, Canada

Abstract— *This study proposes an automated semantics-based approach for assessing the quality of web healthcare information by comparing the web text content with an evidence-based healthcare practice guideline. To achieve this goal, our approach utilizes semantic analysis and text classification to identify the presentation of evidence-based recommendations in web documents. As a result, the quality score of a web page reflects the number of uniquely identified guidelines. The performance of this approach is evaluated by comparing the automated quality rating results with human rating results on the same set of depression treatment web pages. The testing results show that quality rating scores generated by our automated semantics-based approach has a significantly high correlation with human rating scores.*

Keywords: Health Care Information Quality on the Web, Information Quality Assessment, Evidence-based Healthcare practice, Automated Quality Rating, Semantic Analysis

1. Introduction

The last decade has witnessed a dramatic use of web health care information. Recent national surveys in the United States show that 80% of online users look for advice or information about health or health care [1]. In fact, this percentage has been consistently above 80% since 2003 [2]. Moreover, survey results show that younger generations are increasingly turning to the Internet for health care information and it appears that the use of the web to look for health care information will become even more popular among future generations.

Although online health care information is widely used, the quality of health care information on the web is extremely variable in terms of accuracy, coverage and currency [3], [4], [5]. Since the World Wide Web provides an open platform for publishing information, any information provider, including pharmaceutical industry-sponsored organizations, medical experts, and patients, can freely post health care information for different purposes such as advertising, education, or simply the narration of personal experiences. In addition, the maintenance of website health content varies with respect to when it was "last updated" or "last reviewed". Given these factors, the uneven quality of the health care information available on the web is not surprising. Since inaccurate or biased health care information can be widely disseminated through the web to anyone, including caregivers and patients, misinformation on the web could cause and indeed has caused life-threatening accidents [6], [7]. According to a recent survey by the Pew Internet and American Life Project [1], for example, although 30% of adults in the U.S. said they or someone they know has been helped by following medical advice or health care information found online, there are also 3% of respondents who indicated that they or someone they know has been harmed by doing so. Because of the potential harm caused by inaccurate information, the quality assessment of health care information on the web has become a common interest of various health care information stakeholders, including e-health policy makers, information providers/consumers, information search service providers, etc.

Despite the great range in the quality of health care information on the web, information consumers themselves make surprisingly little effort to ensure that the information found on the web is of high quality [9]. Studies indicate that consumers rarely verify information sources or read disclaimers on the websites they use [8]. Instead of accessing health care information exclusively from credible web sources, most consumers are accustomed to querying web search engines like Google and just reading the top URLs in the retrieved item list [9], [10]. Moreover, over 50% of consumers access information from unfamiliar websites [8].

This rapid growth of publicly available healthcare information on the Web and its extreme variability of content quality has caused a great demand for the development of effective quality evaluation approaches. Measurements that rate the quality of the web health care information content could assist online consumers to access a higher grade of health care information. The extremely large amount of health care information on the web, however, easily overwhelms the capacity of any manual evaluation system. Therefore, in order to address the large-scale problem of online health care information content quality, we require automated quality assessment instruments that ideally can perform as well as a human rater in evaluating health care information quality. Much research has been done in related areas, including efforts to develop the definition of high quality online health care information (e.g., [11]), establish quality rating codes and indicators (e.g., [3], [12], [13]), and explore rating automation (e.g., [14], [15], [16]).

Because manual rating approaches that require human reading of content can be easily overwhelmed by the huge data volume, we propose a new automated approach for assessing the quality of web healthcare information by comparing the web text content with evidence-based healthcare practice guidelines and rating the quality based on the degree of concordance and the coverage of the best evidence.

Instead of using indirect quality indicators such as authorship, sponsorship, etc., this new approach is semantics-based and it aims to rate quality by relying on information content more than the approaches in previous studies. To achieve this goal, our approach uses semantic analysis and text classification to identify the presentation of evidence-based recommendations in web documents. The quality score of a web page reflects the number of identified guidelines. As the rating relies on content, the approach has an advantage over previous automated approaches in that it could provide healthcare consumers with information that is more instructive than just a quality score

This approach is designed particularly for dealing with text-based online documents. Other web document types such as multi-media web pages are not in the scope of this study.

The structure of this paper is as follows. Section 2 describes the research methodology. Section 3 provides a description of the design and development of the automated quality assessment system. Additionally, the quality rating results are presented and compared to the human rating results. Finally, Section 4 presents the conclusions.

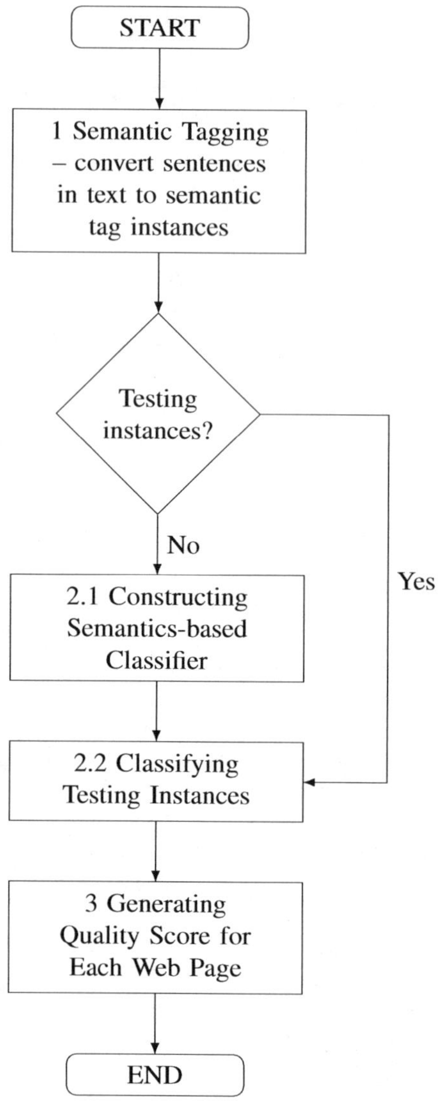

Fig. 1: Flowchart of the semantics-based quality rating

2. Methodology

This study proposes an automated semantics-based approach for rating the content quality, i.e., accuracy and comprehensiveness, of healthcare information on web pages. Depression treatment is the subject selected for study and evidence-based depression treatment guidelines edited by Griffiths and Christensen [5] are used as rating criteria.

The automated rating approach in this study uses a three-step procedure, similar to a human rating process. Given a web page, the computer, instead of a human rater, 1) reads through the text content, sentence by sentence. Sentence text in English natural language is converted to a semantic representation in a defined form. 2) The computer identifies whether a sentence has content in concordance with any predefined treatment guideline. Each sentence in a web page is considered as either a match (i.e., "positive") or non-match (i.e., "negative") with reference to a guideline. 3) The quality score of a web page is set equal to the number of unique treatment guidelines presented in the page. Fig. 1 illustrates the above processing flow.

In the first step, shallow semantic analysis is used to generate the semantic representation of a sentence. By using a semantic parsing tool called MetaMap API, published by the National Library of Medicine, healthcare concepts and terminologies are discovered and converted into semantic concepts defined in the UMLS Metathesaurus [17]. That is, synonyms and their text variants (e.g., plural variant) linking to a unique semantic concept, for example *depression*, *depressive episode* and *depressive illness*, can all be labeled as *Depressive disorder*. Thus, although biomedical terms in web text could have rich variations due to natural language expression, they are converted into unique semantic concepts.

In addition to MetaMap, NLP tools including Lexical

Original sentence:

The side effects vary depending on the type of antidepressant you take.

Semantic representation:

[effect side,95,106,1,noun] | [vary,108,111,2,verb] | [depend, 113,121,3,verb] | [type,130,133,6,noun] | [Antidepressive Agents,138,151,8,1000] | [take,157,160,10,verb]

Fig. 2: An example of the semantic representation for a sentence

Variant Generator (LVG) [18] and TaggerClient, published by NLM, are used to take care of lemmatization processing and part of speech (POS) tagging on remaining English terms in a sentence. The purpose is to convert the lexical variants in English natural language into a single normalized form. Lexical variations which can be handled by LVG include inflections and conjugations, word order in multi-word terms, alphabetic case, punctuation, and possessives. For instance, *ceases*, *ceased*, *stopping*, and *stops* can be transformed to the preferred synonym *stop*, which is one of the key semantic components for identifying sentences in concordance with guideline #12-A, i.e., *Antidepressants should not be stopped suddenly*.

In this study, semantic tags are labeled on verbs, adjectives, adverbs and nouns in a sentence, whereas articles, prepositions, etc. are considered relatively less useful for shallow semantic analysis purposes and hence are not labeled. After the above semantic tagging process, each sentence is transformed to a form of semantic representation (i.e., a vector of semantic tags) as shown in Fig. 2. Each semantic tag is enclosed by a pair of square brackets, in which three types of metadata are included: semantic concept, position information (i.e., position of the starting character, position of the ending character, sequence number of the corresponding term or phrase in the sentence), and the POS of the corresponding string. Semantic representations are the input for Step 2.

Step 2 in Fig. 1 is for identifying sentences which have content in concordance with healthcare guidelines. In this study, this task is modeled as a binary classification problem, determining whether a given sentence is a positive or negative instance of a pre-defined guideline. Therefore, a classifier is built for each guideline based on sentences in the training web pages. The training sentences have a class label manually assigned by human raters, being either positive or negative with reference to a specific guideline. Semantic representation of training sentences, rather than their original text, was studied in order to identify factors which would likely be effective in distinguishing positive cases from negative cases. In this study, a rule-based classifier was built for each guideline. The rules, i.e., classification patterns, were manually extracted based on observing and summarizing common features from training instances. Features considered for describing classification patterns include semantic tags in a sentence, their POS roles, and positioning relationship between each other. These three types of information are available from the semantic representation.

In parallel with the rule-based system, a prototype machine learning system was also developed to construct classifiers, but only for guidelines #1, #6, and #12-B since their volume of positive training cases (at minimum 50) were reasonably large for machine learning. In the testing phase, both types of learned classifiers were used to label a sentence as either a positive or negative case of a specific guideline.

In the third step of Fig. 1, the classification results are utilized to rate the content quality of a web page. A common practice is to give a quality score that is equal to the number of identified guidelines presented in the web page. If one or more sentences are classified as positive regarding a single guideline, the quality score is incremented by one. If a single sentence is considered to contain multiple pieces of content which are respectively in concordance with multiple guidelines, the quality score is incremented by the number of guidelines that are matched.

Table 1: Sources for Constructing the Corpus

General Web	Medical Search	Health Care
Search Engines	Engines	Web Portals
Google	OmniMedicalSearch	Medline Plus in US
Yahoo!	HealthFinder	HealthlinkBC in Canada
Microsoft Bing	HealthLine	HealthInsite in Australia
Ask.com	MedNar	National Health Service (NHS) in UK
WebMD	AOL	

3. Quality Rating Test

3.1 Data

This study demonstrates the semantics-based automated quality rating approach using depression treatment web pages. The whole corpus includes 201 depression treatment web pages (see Appendix B of [19]) collected from three types of sources given in Table 1. Previous studies on online health care information-seeking behavior [8], [20] show that web users typically access health web pages directly from web-based search engines and consumer health sites or portals. We use these search engines sources as they are the most popular ones [21], [22], [23]. Against each of these ten search engines, a two term search query [q = depression treatment] was submitted to retrieve web pages. URL candidates were collected from the first 30 returned pages. The four health portals are reputable health portals in four English speaking countries, hosted by government or governmental agency. These sites are committed to high editorial and ethical standards in the provision of content and related services [24], [25], [26], [27]. Candidate pages were examined manually to remove duplicate pages and pages that were deemed inappropriate for the following reasons:

- pages which focus on other diseases instead of depression, or pages that address depression, but discuss only non-treatment topics such as diagnosis; — *determination was based on document heading and sub-heading.*
- pages protected by password.
- pages not in text format (e.g., video/audio clips, PPT slides).
- pages with tables or spread sheets as a major part of page content.
- portal pages which do not have their own content, but just hyperlinks referring to other relevant pages. (e.g., URL menus/categories, list of search returns from search engines).
- pages which have article titles or bibliographic information only.
- home pages of businesses or organizations (e.g., medical centers or depression clinics).
- pages too long for human rating (e.g., online books or chapters) — *considering the expense of human rating, they were filtered out.*
- advertisement pages which do not really provide depression treatment content (e.g., Amazon book advertisements).
- academic articles which are targeted to a professional audience instead of public online users; — *due to academic complexity, some very specific research questions and terminologies can make the articles not quite understandable for most common users and human raters to conduct a rating.*

In the end, 201 web pages were selected for the corpus.

3.2 Training and Testing

The quality of the 201 web pages was rated by two human raters, one, a pharmacology instructor, the other had rating experience working in the Google Quality Rating program.

The human raters had a five-hour rating workshop to exercise quality rating using the evidence-based depression treatment guidelines as the rating criteria. The appendix lists these guidelines. Then, given the 201 pages, they were required to label each sentence with reference to the treatment guidelines. They also highlighted for the positive sentences the key phrases that led them to a positive identification. The intra-class correlation coefficient, i.e., ICC(3,1), between the webpage quality scores assigned by the two raters across all guidelines was .990. The discrepancies were later resolved through discussion between the raters. The final labeling results were the standard for evaluating the performance of the automated quality rating.

The human rated quality scores ranged between 0 and 8. The 201 web pages were divided into 5 bins (i.e., those with a quality score of 0, 1-2, 3-4, 5-6 or 7-8). Stratified random sampling was used to select 31 test web pages. The remaining 170 web pages were grouped into a training set.

3.3 Automated Quality Rating Results

In this section, we report the automated quality rating performance. Table 2 lists the quality scores generated by the automated rating approach. The automatically assigned quality scores range from 0 to 7 (i.e., a page may match 0 to 7 guidelines), and a total of 91 occurrences of the guidelines were identified from the 31 test pages.

As shown in Table 2, in 14 out of the 31 pages (45.2%) the automatically generated scores and the human rating quality scores were identical. In 10 pages (32.3%) the automatically rated scores were one lower than the human rating quality scores, and in another 6 out of 31 pages (19.4%) the rule-based quality scores were higher by one. For only one page (3.2%) was the difference between the rule-based and human scores greater than one (testing page no. 15, rule-based score was higher by 3).

The automatically generated quality rating results were very close to the human rating results not only in terms of quality score (i.e., the total number of unique rating criteria identified in each web page), but also in the specific criteria identified in the pages. The large majority of the criteria identified by the human raters was also identified using the rule-based approach (83.7% of true criteria, or 77 out of 92), and only 16.3% (i.e., 15 out of 92) of the criteria identified by the human raters was missed by the rule-based approach. Among the 91 criteria identified by the rule-based approach, 14 (or 15.3%) were "false positives" in that they were not identified by or accepted by the human raters.

The linear correlation, evaluated using Pearson correlation, between the rule-based quality scores and the evidence-based human rating quality scores was high and statistically significant ($r = 0.909$, or $r^2 = 0.827$, $p < .001$, see Fig. 3). $r^2 = 0.827$ means that 82.7% of the variance of the quality scores generated by the rule-based approach is associated with the variance in the quality scores generated by the human raters.

4. Conclusions

In the Griffiths et al. study [14], the Pearson correlation between the quality scores resulting from the keyword approach and the human rating results was also high (r=0.850, p < .001, n = 30). The semantics-based content analysis proposed in this study appears to be competitive with, if not slightly better than, the keyword approach.

As mentioned in Section 2, a prototype system using machine learning based classification was implemented on guidelines #1, #6, and #12-B. The automatically generated quality scores were also compared with the human rating scores. Strong and positive Pearson correlation was also found ($r = 0.841$, $r^2 = 0.707$, $p < .001$) between the machine learning based rating and the human rating results.

Table 2: Quality scores assigned to testing web pages by the rule-based approach

Testing Page ID	Quality Score via Human Rating	Quality Score via Rule-Based Rating	Quality Score Difference
1	7	7	0
2	7	6	-1
3	8	7	-1
4	6	5	-1
5	6	6	0
6	5	5	0
7	5	4	-1
8	4	5	1
9	3	4	1
10	4	3	-1
11	3	4	1
12	3	4	1
13	4	4	0
14	3	2	-1
15	2	5	3
16	2	3	1
17	2	2	0
18	2	2	0
19	2	2	0
20	3	2	-1
21	2	2	0
22	2	1	-1
23	2	1	-1
24	1	2	1
25	1	1	0
26	1	1	0
27	1	1	0
28	1	0	-1
29	0	0	0
30	0	0	0
31	0	0	0
Total	92	91	Not Applicable

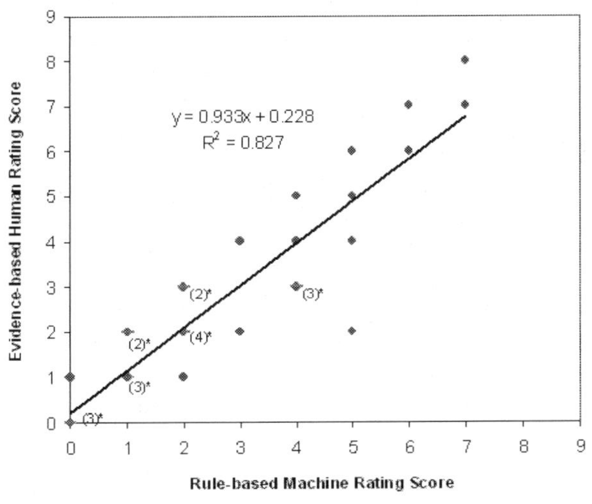

Fig. 3: Relationship between rule-based quality scores and human rating quality scores

References

[1] (2011). Pew Internet and American Life Project. — The social life of health care information. [Online] Available: http://pewinternet.org/Reports/2011/Social-Life-of-Health-Info.aspx

[2] (2003). Pew Internet and American Life Project. — Internet health resources. [Online] Available: http://www.pewinternet.org/~/media//Files/Reports/2003/PIP_Health_Report_July_2003.pdf

[3] G. Eysenbach, J. Powell, O. Kuss, and E. Sa, "Empirical studies assessing the quality of health care information for consumers on the World Wide Web," *Journal of the American Medical Association*, vol. 287, no. 20, pp. 2691–2700, 2002.

[4] H. Kunst, D. Groot, P. Latthe, M. Latthe, and K. S. Khan, "Accuracy of information on apparently credible websites: Survey of five common health topics," *British Medical Journal*, vol. 321, no. 7337, pp. 581–582, 2002.

[5] K. M. Griffiths and H. Christensen. (2005). "Website quality indicators for consumers", *Journal of Medical Internet Research*, 7(5):e55. [Online]. Available: http://www.jmir.org/2005/5/e55/

[6] A. G. Crocco, M. Villasis-Keever, and A. R. Jadad, "Analysis of cases of harm associated with use of health care information on the Internet," *Journal of the American Medical Association*, vol. 287, no. 21, pp. 2869–2871, 2002.

[7] R. Kiley, "Does the Internet harm health? Some evidence does exist that the Internet harms health," *British Medical Journal*, vol. 323, no. 7331, 328–329, 2002.

[8] (2006). Pew Internet and American Life Project. — Online health search 2006. [Online]. Available: http://www.pewinternet.org/~/media/Files/Reports/2006/PIP_Online_Health_2006.pdf

[9] G. Eysenbach and C. Köhler, "Health-related searches on the Internet," *Journal of the American Medical Association*, vol. 291, no. 24, p. 2946, 2004.

[10] G. Peterson, P. Aslani, and K. A. Williams, (2003). "How do consumers search for and appraise information on medicines on the Internet? A qualitative study using focus groups". *Journal of Medical Internet Research*, 5(4), e33. [Online]. Available: http://www.jmir.org/2003/4/e33/index.htm

[11] R. C. Bopp and L. E. Smith. "*Reference and Information Services: An Introduction*," Libraries Unlimited, 3Rev Ed edition, 2000.

[12] K. M. Griffiths and H. Christensen, "The quality and accessibility of Australian depression sites on the World Wide Web," *The Medical Journal of Australia*, vol. 160, pp. 97–104, 2002).

[13] (2007). URAC promoting quality health care. [Online] Available: http://www.urac.org/

[14] K. M. Griffiths, T. T. Tang, D. Hawking, and H. Christensen. (2005). "Automated assessment of the quality of depression websites", *Journal of Medical Internet Research*, 7(5):e59. [Online]. Available: http://www.jmir.org/2005/5/e59/

[15] D. Hawking, T. Tang, R. Sankaranaravana, K. Griffiths, N. Craswell, and P. Bailey, "Towards higher quality health search results: Automated quality rating of depression websites," In *Proceedings of Medinfo 2007 Workshop on Models of Trust for Health Websites*, August, 2007.

[16] Y. Wang and Z. Liu, "Automatic detecting indicators for quality of health care information on the Web," *International Journal of Medical Informatics*, vol. 76, pp. 575-582, 2007.

[17] (2009). UMLS – Metathesaurus release statistics. [Online]. Available: http://web.archive.org/web/20090925122534/: http://www.nlm.nih.gov/research/umls/knowledge_sources/metathesaurus/release/statistics.html

[18] (2013). Lexical Variant Generation (LVG). [Online]. Available: http://www.nlm.nih.gov/research/umls/new_users/online_learning/LEX_004.html

[19] Y. Zhang, "Semantics-based automated quality assessment of depression treatment web documents", PhD thesis, The University of Western Ontario. Available at https://ir.lib.uwo.ca/etd/1131, 2012

[20] L. Graham, T. Tse, and A. Keselman, "Exploring user navigation during online health care information seeking," *AMIA Annual Symposium Proceedings*, pp. 299–303, 2006.

G. Eysenbach, C. Köhler, G. Yihune, K. Lampe, P. Cross, and D. Brickley, "A framework for improving the quality of health care information on the World-Wide-Web and bettering public (e-)health: the MedCERTAIN approach," *Medical Information*, vol. 10 (Pt 2), pp. 1450–1454, 2001.

[21] Nielsen, (2010). "Top U.S. search stes for May 2010". [Online]. Available: http://blog.nielsen.com/nielsenwire/online_mobile/top-u-s-search-sites-for-may-2010/
[22] Leman, H. (2008). "The Top 10 Health Search Engines of 2008". [Online]. Available: http://www.altsearchengines.com/2008/12/29/the-top-10-health-search-engines-of-2008/
[23] (2009), Medical search engines. Retrieved from http://websearch.about.com/od/enginesanddirectories/tp/medical.htm
[24] (2011). Medline plus guide to healthy web surfing. [Online]. Available: http://www.nlm.nih.gov/medlineplus/healthywebsurfing.html
[25] (2011). About HealthLink BC. [Online]. Available: http://www.healthlinkbc.ca/aboutprogram.stm/
[26] (2011). The HealthInsite concept. [Online]. Available: http://www.healthinsite.gov.au/content/internal/page.cfm?ObjID=0001AC1D-0806-1D2D-81CF83032BFA006D
[27] (2011). NHS choices about us — Editorial policy. [Online]. Available: http://www.nhs.uk/aboutNHSChoices/aboutnhschoices/Aboutus/Pages/Editorialpolicy.aspx

Appendix

Evidence-based Depression Treatment Guidelines Used in [5]

Evidence-Based Rating Scale for Human Raters (Copied from [5])

The evidence-based rating scale was developed from statements in the treatment section of *A systematic guide for the management of depression in primary care* published by the Centre for Evidence-based mental health, Oxford (CEBMH, 1998).

1. Antidepressant medication is an effective treatment for major depressive disorder.
2. Antidepressants are all equally effective.
3. The effectiveness of antidepressants is around 50 to 60%.
4. Full psychosocial recovery can take several months.
5. Drop out rate is the same for different antidepressants.
6. The side effect profile varies for different antidepressants.
7. The choice of antidepressant should depend on individual patient factors (e.g., presence of co-morbid psychiatric or medical conditions, previous response to a particular drug, patient preference regarding the desirability of specific side-effects, concurrent drug therapy, suicidal risk).
8. Antidepressants are not addictive.
9. A trial of 6 weeks at full dose is needed before a drug can be considered to have failed and another tried.
10. A second-line drug should probably be from a different class of antidepressant.
11. Once improved continuation treatment at the same dose for at least 4–6 months should be considered.
12. Discontinuation syndrome may occur with abrupt cessation of any antidepressant so antidepressants should not be stopped suddenly. Where possible antidepressants should be withdrawn over a 4 week period, unless there are urgent medical reasons to stop the drug more rapidly. [To score 1, need to make general points that abrupt cessation can cause discontinuation syndrome and that antidepressants should not be stopped suddenly.]*
13. St John's Wort appears to be as effective as tricyclic antidepressants and causes fewer side effects, but little is known about any long term adverse effects.**
14. Cognitive therapy can be an effective treatment for depression.
15. Cognitive behaviour therapy is at least as effective as drug treatment in mild-to-moderate depression.
16. Cognitive behaviour therapy may be valuable for people who respond to the concept of Cognitive behaviour therapy, prefer psychological to antidepressant treatment, have not responded to antidepressant therapy. [Score 1 if mention at least one of these.]
17. Problem-solving may be effective for depression.
18. [Generic] counselling is probably no more effective than treatment as usual from the GP for depression.
19. Written information (usually based on a cognitive model of depression) can improve mild-to-moderate depression. [Score 1 if cognitive model.]
20. Exercise can be effective – alone or as an adjunct to other treatments.

For each item, score 1 if the site information is consistent with the statement. Cumulate item scores across the scale to yield a total evidence-based score for the site.

Notes regarding our modification to these guidelines:
*, ** Guidelines 12 and 13 each contains multiple semantic propositions. Since it is possible for only one of their points to be mentioned in a sentence, guidelines like #12 and #13 can potentially cause discrepancy among human raters when creating training examples and reviewing test results. So, it has been necessary to split them into multiple guidelines.

12-A. Antidepressants should not be stopped suddenly.
12-B. Abrupt cessation can cause discontinuation syndrome.

13-A. St John's Wort appears to be as effective as (tricyclic) antidepressants.
13-B. St John's Wort causes fewer side effects than (tricyclic) antidepressants.
13-C. Little is known about any long term adverse effects of St John's Wort.

Predicting Mortality of Sepsis Patients in a Multi-Site Healthcare System using Supervised Machine Learning

Bogle, Brittany[1]; Balduino, Ricardo[2]; Wolk, Donna M.[3]; Farag, Hosam A[4]; Kethireddy, Shravan[5]; Chatterjee, Avijit[6]; Abedi, Vida[7]

[1]Data Science Elite Team, IBM Corporation, 3039 E Cornwallis Road, Durham, North Carolina
[2]Data Science Elite Team, IBM Corporation, 555 Bailey Ave, San Jose, CA
[3]Geisinger Diagnostic Medicine Institute, 100 N Academy Avenue, Danville, PA
[4]Clinical and Molecular Microbiology, Geisinger Diagnostic Medicine Institute, Danville, PA
[5]Northeast Georgia Health System, 743 Spring St NE, Gainesville, GA
[6]Data Science Elite Team, IBM Corporation, 1 North Castle Drive, Armonk, New York
[7]Biomedical and Translational Informatics Institute, Geisinger Health System, 100 N Academy Ave, Danville, PA; Biocomplexity Institute, Virginia Tech, 1015 Life Sciences Circle, Blacksburg, VA

Abstract - ***Introduction***: *Sepsis patients suffer from high rates of mortality, but it is difficult to diagnose and accurately predict who experience death while in-hospital or post-discharge.* ***Methods***: *We trained and validated a supervised machine learning model to predict all-cause mortality between admission and 90-days after discharge using electronic healthcare record data from 10,593 patients with sepsis diagnosed during hospitalization at Geisinger Health System hospitals between 2006 and 2016.* ***Results***: *Our model had an AUC of 0.8561, with recall and precision of 0.7732 and 0.6931 respectively.* ***Conclusions***: *We have developed a predictive model for sepsis. This is a move towards providing personalized care for sepsis patients and help prevent death. Future work is needed to further refine this model.*

Keywords: Sepsis; Electronic Healthcare Records; EHR; Machine Learning; Mortality Prediction Model

1 Introduction

Sepsis is a life-threatening organ dysfunction caused by a dysregulated host response to infection [1]. Annually, more than 1.6 million people in the U.S. are diagnosed with sepsis and about 250,000 die from sepsis– one every 2 minutes [2]. As many as 80% of sepsis deaths could be prevented with rapid diagnosis and treatment[3], since every hour of delay in treatment increases the probability of death by 7.6%. [3] Sepsis survivors have a reduced life expectancy, are more likely to suffer from an impaired quality of life, and are 42% more likely to commit suicide [4], [5]. Finally, sepsis is the most expensive condition to treat in the US, costing the US healthcare system more than $24 billion annually. [6]

The proliferation of Electronic Health Record (EHR) data brings opportunities to use machine learning (ML) to build predictive models that may provide data-driven decision support to health care providers and improve care while reducing costs. In fact, there is increasing evidence that the use of EHR or administrative data can be used to enhance healthcare quality in integrated healthcare hospital systems[7][8][9]. However, using EHR data for research poses its own unique challenges [10] and requires customized pre-processing[11]–[14]. Furthermore, EHR data can contain thousands of features for a patient, which contributes to a complex modeling environment. Feature extraction techniques should be used to reduce the dimensionality and improve the predictive power of these models.

Utilization of administrative data in combination with genetic screening and mobile tracking could drive personalized health and preventive measures that are tailored to each individual. For instance, in a large multi-center study, Dr. Kethireddy and his team demonstrated that patients with culture-negative septic shock behave similarly to those with culture-positive septic shock in nearly all respects but early appropriate antimicrobial therapy appears to improve mortality [15]. In that study, the EHR data from 28 academic and community hospitals in three countries between 1997 and 2010 were analyzed. These large multi-center studies are needed to identify trends, highlight where more research is warrant and guide management and policy changes. For instance, in a systematic review [16] of sepsis in patients admitted to ICU, critical care interventions and surgery-related factors were modifiable factors associated with sepsis, suggesting that improving the care of surgical patients and effective management of critical care interventions may decrease the risk of sepsis in these patients. Early recognition and eradication of infection is the most obvious effective strategy to improve hospital survival [17] [18], but ML can further facilitate identification of other non-intuitive factors and improve our predictive capabilities, by transforming data into insight and knowledge.

While models exist to predict sepsis severity and inpatient outcomes,[19] no such model has been developed to predict all-cause inpatient and post-discharge mortality among sepsis patients using EHR from a large integrated health care system. In the present study, we sought to develop and validate a model for sepsis patients within Geisinger Health System. Geisinger provides valuable longitudinal clinical data for translational and clinical research studies. The EHR data associated with active patients spans multiple years, with a median of 116 laboratory results. We have reported phenotype data of our active patient population in two recent publications. [20][21]

2 Methods

2.1 Patient Population

Patients were eligible for inclusion in our study if they had an inpatient admission at one of Geisinger's hospitals between 2006 and 2016, had an admission or discharge diagnosis of sepsis (ICD 9: 995.9x; ICD 10: A41.xx, A40.xx, B37.7) or septic shock (ICD-9 785.52; ICD-10: R65.2). Patients under the age of 18 ~~or over the age of 100~~, or had invalid vasopressor durations (negative values) were excluded.

2.2 Outcomes

Our objective was to predict death that occurred either during the index hospitalization (in-hospital death) or within 90 days post-discharge. Patient deaths are recorded by Geisinger upon report by kin or upon receipt of a death reported by the Pennsylvania Department of Health Knowledge Center Health Incident Management System (KC-HIMS). In-hospital mortality was defined as death between admission to the emergency department/inpatient hospital admission and discharge. All in-hospital deaths were required to have a discharge disposition indicating death during the hospitalization. For patients with a date of death recorded, the number of days between the index hospitalization's discharge date and the date of death were calculated, and mortality within 90 days post-discharge was derived from this calculation.

2.3 Data Sources

We performed a retrospective study of de-identified inpatient patients with a primary or secondary discharge diagnosis of sepsis from Geisinger Health System (Geisinger). IRB Determination Notice approved that this research activity did not involve "Human Subjects" and therefore did not require submission of the proposed work to the IRB for further review/approval. Data extraction from the EHR and de-identification were conducted through data-brokers from Geisinger Phenomic Analysis Core. Patient data were queried from Geisinger's data warehouse on specific domains and are summarized in Table 1.

2.4 Modeling Approach

We used data available on hospitalized patients from both during and up to 90 days prior to the hospitalization to predict death. A schematic is displayed in Figure 1.

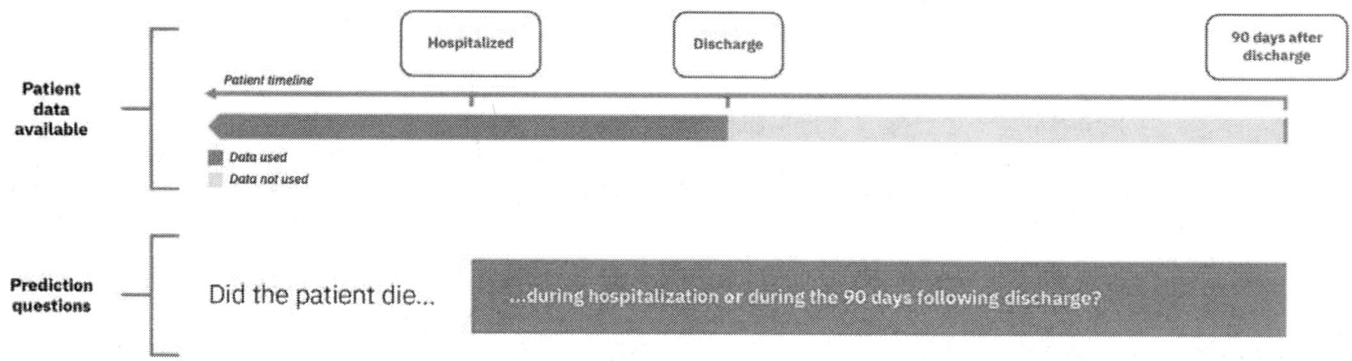

Figure 1: Modeling approach.

We used XGBoost, a widely used scalable system for tree boosting [22], to predict the binary outcome of in-hospital or 90-day post-discharge mortality. We used Python 3.5 to leverage XGBoost (version 0.7) as through *scikit-learn* package's wrapper interface[23]. XGBoost parameters were iteratively tuned on the training data to maximize the area under the curve (AUC). XGBoost selects the most important features and assigns corresponding weights to design a predictive model. All analysis was conducted in Python 3.5 using IBM's Data Science Experience Local platform (datascience.ibm.com), which supports single-click operationalization and end-to-end model lifecycle management.

Index hospitalizations were randomly split into training (60%) and testing (40%) datasets. In the training stages, 10-fold cross validation was employed, and 5-fold cross validation was used for tuning the parameters of the XGBoost model. These parameters are described in Table 3. During the tuning process, each parameter was tuned by iterating over a range of parameter values and the value that resulted in the highest AUC in the test dataset. The final model was used to estimate precision, recall, and the AU in both the training and testing datasets.

Table 1. Data description and example of elements. A total of 199 variables were used in this study.

Data Domain	Description	# features used
Admissions/ Discharge	Admission/discharge date; diagnosis; key treatments, demographics	43
Encounters	Basic information on a unique patient encounter	41
Surgeries	All surgeries during a patient encounter	2
Cultures	Specimen information and culture results	124
Social History	Self-reported history including tobacco and alcohol use	10
Comorbidity	Other diagnoses / conditions	19
Admission, discharge, and transfers	Movement/transfers within hospital system	1
Total		**199**

3 Results

3.1 Hospitalization Characteristics

Between 2006 and 2016, 10,593 hospitalizations at Geisinger met our study's inclusion criteria. All-cause mortality in this group was 2,670 (25.2%) during the hospitalization and 13.1% (1,389) within 90 days of discharge. Some patient and encounter characteristics, stratified by outcome, are displayed in Table 2.

Table 2: Patient and encounter characteristics.

	Overall (n=10,593)	Died (n=4059)	Survived (n=6534)	P-value (died vs. survived)
Age, mean (SD)	67 (16.4)	71 (14.1)	64 (17.1)	<0.001
Sex (% Female)	48%	47%	49%	0.0451
Race (%)				0.4887
White	97.6%	97.6%	98.0%	
Black/African American	2%	1%	2%	
American Indian/Alaska Native	0.1%	0.1%	0.1%	
Asian	0.2%	0.2%	0.3%	
Native Hawaiian/Pacific Islander	0.1%	0.1%	0.1%	
Hispanic/Latino (%)	1%	0.9%	1.6%	0.002
Current Smoker (%)	15%	11%	17%	< 0.0001
Admission Type (%)				0.0445
Emergency	78%	75%	79%	
Routine	3%	2.7%	3%	
Trauma	0.1%	0.3%	0.6%	
Urgent	19%	22%	17.2%	
Comorbidities prior to hospitalization (%)				
Cancer	24%	32%	19%	< 0.0001
Chronic pulmonary disease	31%	31%	31%	1.000
Chronic kidney disease, Stage 4	8%	9%	7%	0.0002
Diabetes Mellitus	33%	32%	34%	0.0336
End stage renal disease	6%	8%	5%	< 0.0001
Peripheral vascular disease	12%	14%	10%	< 0.0001
Transient ischemic attack/stroke	14%	16%	12%	< 0.0001
Hypertension	63%	65%	62%	0.0019
Surgeries within 30 days of hospitalization, mean (SD)	0.1 (0.7)	0.1 (0.6)	0.2 (0.8)	<0.001
Surgeries during hospitalization, mean (SD)	1.1 (2.4)	1.0 (2.4)	1.1 (2.4)	0.04
Cultures within 48 hours of hospitalization, mean (SD)	9.8 (10.37)	10.1 (11.1)	9.6 (9.7)	0.02

3.2 Model Characteristics

After tuning XGBoost parameters on the training dataset with a binary logistic objective, our final model was derived using the parameters seen in Table 3.

Table 3: Model parameters and the value used after tuning to train the final XGBoost model.

Parameter	Value	Description*
tree_method	hist	Tree construction algorithm. "Hist" uses a fast histogram optimized greedy algorithm.
learning_rate	0.15	Shrinkage step size
n_estimators	64	Number of boosted trees to fit
scale_pos_weight	1.6	Controls the balance of positive and negative weights
max_depth	4	Maximum depth of tree
min_child_weight	2	Minimum sum of instance weight for a child node
gamma	0	Minimum loss reduction required to make a further partition on a leaf node of the tree
colsample_bytree	0.9	Proportion of columns used to construct tree
subsample	0.9	Proportion of rows used to construct tree
reg_alpha	0	L1 regularization term
reg_lambda	1	L2 regularization term

*Description of parameters are summarized from http://xgboost.readthedocs.io/en/latest/parameter.html

Performance of the tuned XG Boost model was strong in the external test data (n=4238): AUC was 0.8561, precision was 0.6931, and recall was 0.7732. The model had a resulting F1 Score of 0.7124. Figure 2 displays the confusion matrix, and Figure 3 displays a summary of the model's performance.

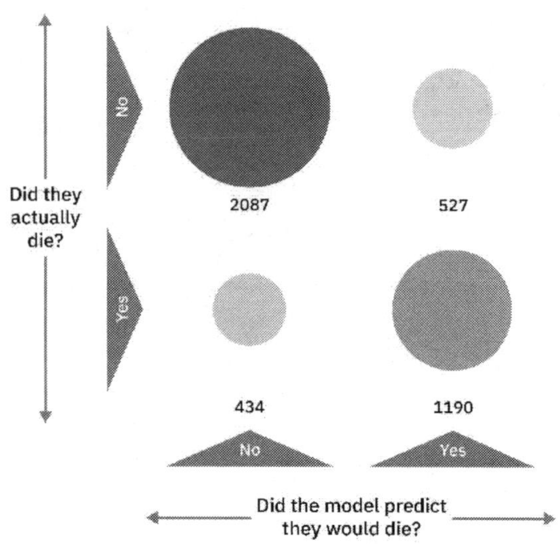

Figure 2: Confusion matrix on test data.

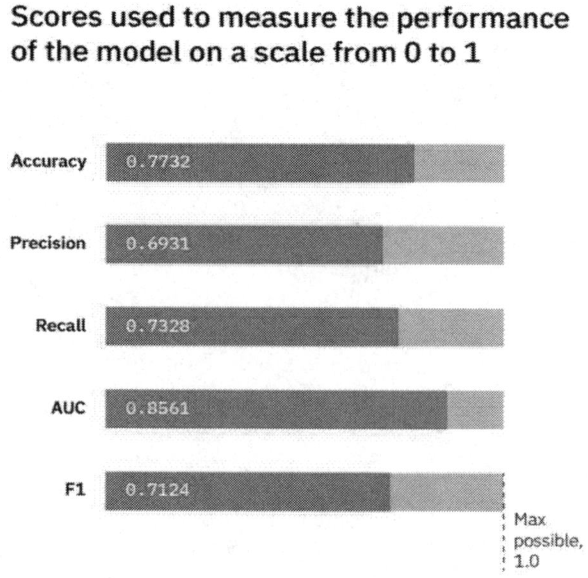

Figure 3: Performance of model on test data.

Our final model used 64 decision trees that were fitted and used to inform the boosted tree model. Of the 199 candidate features, 107 features were selected for inclusion in the final XGBoost model. The top 20 features are displayed in Figure 4. We defined feature importance as the expected percentage of patients for which that feature is used in predicting death. If a feature was the top branch of each of the 64 trees, the feature importance would be 100%, but in our model, no feature is the top branch in every tree. In fact, the top feature by this definition of importance is "age at admission", which is only used by 29.5% of patients to predict death. This implies that many of the important features may be associated with death in some subsets of patients, after conditioning upon other factors higher up in higher branches of the trees. *Note*: Feature importance does not inform whether that feature is positively or negatively associated with the outcome, so an important feature could be strongly predictive of death or strongly predictive of survival.

4 Discussion

We derived a predictive model for in-hospital or 90-day post-discharge mortality of patients who suffered from sepsis while admitted to a large healthcare system. The model produced from this study serves as a starting point for a more personalized care in acute care and infectious diseases, specifically sepsis. We envision refining this predictive model and training and validating it further in terms of its clinical utility and generalizability.

4.1 Strengths and Limitations

There are several important strengths and limitations to our study. While some of the predictive features occur prior to hospitalization, such as the 30-day history of surgeries preceding the hospitalization and comorbidities, many of the important features in our model were cross-sectional in nature.

Due to the combined retrospective and cross-sectional nature of our study, we cannot make causal inferences on mortality using the predictive features.

One strength of our study design is that it leverages real EHR data, with all its complexity and inherent noise. Many predictive models are derived using longitudinal cohort data, which are carefully measured and controlled but often differ from how such data are collected in a clinical setting, leading to bias and challenges in translating those models to a clinical setting. While we believe that ultimately deriving predictive models using clinical data has significant value, there are limitations to this approach. First, the accuracy of EHR data collection and recording processes may vary by clinician, hospital, and over time. Additionally, while our model had strong performance in both the derivation and testing/validation data, these datasets both came from within a single healthcare system. These data points may vary in how they are collected and stored outside of Geisinger Healthcare System. Thus, we cannot assume that our model is generalizable to all healthcare systems. Finally, as our patient population is a predominantly white population, additional work is needed to understand if these models are robust and generalizable, especially since race has been shown to be associated with developing sepsis [24]. Validating these findings in other populations will be important to understanding the generalizability of our model. We leave the evaluation of the model's robustness, including the need for re-calibration, to future work.

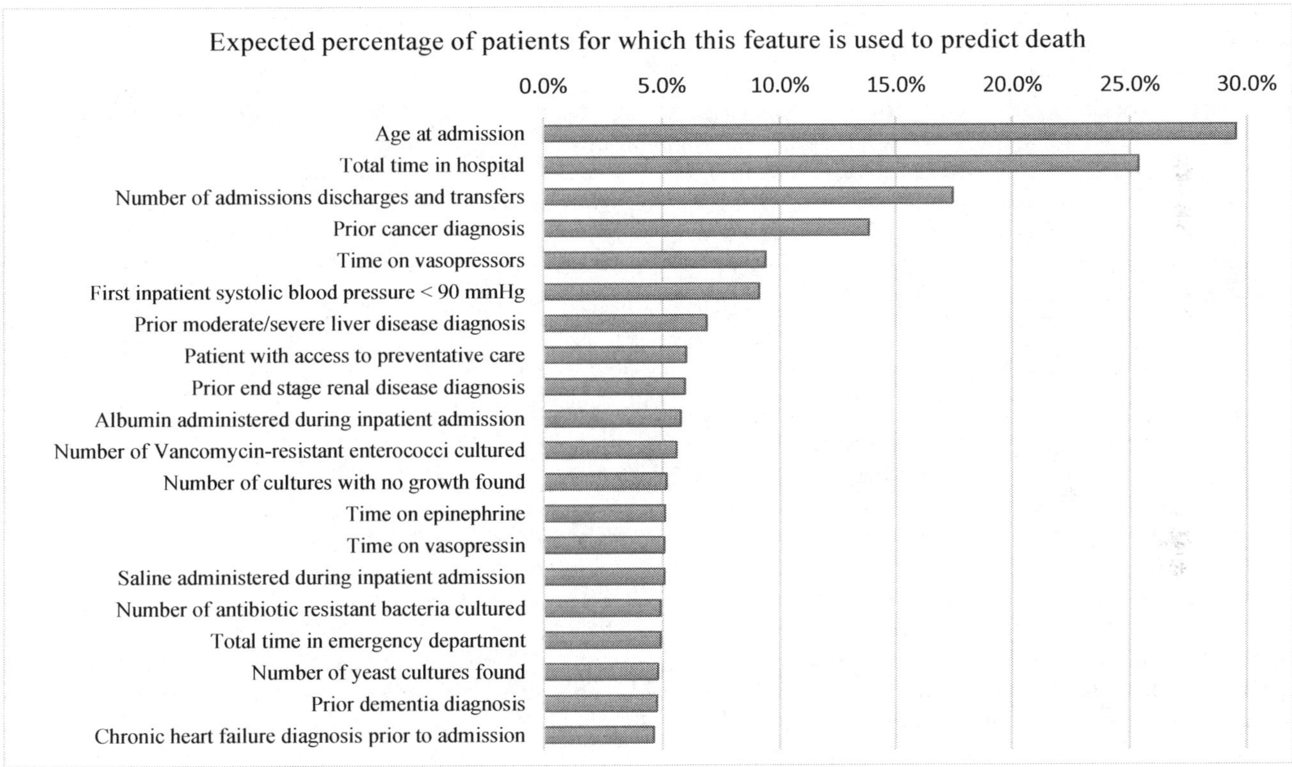

Figure 4: Feature importance of the 20 most important features in final model. Feature importance does not inform whether that feature is positively or negatively associated with the outcome.

Geisinger Healthcare System, like most modern healthcare systems in the United States, has a rapidly evolving clinical data warehouse infrastructure. Because of this, some hospitals within Geisinger may have a bias in data availability. For example, some hospitals did not begin storing vasopressor duration within the EHR until 2011. This missing data bias may have impacted the derivation of our model and would likely impact its validity in external populations. Limiting our analysis to more recent time period can alleviate some of these limitations, however, it will also significantly reduce our cohort size; expanding this work to 2017 and beyond will improve our model's predictive value. This study also provides some venues for further investigations. Due to data limitations, we defined sepsis according to discharge diagnosis codes and we plan to refine that definition using culture and antibiotic data in future studies.

In summary, we have identified clinical biomarkers that are associated with higher chances of death from sepsis infection. These include, age; time on vasopressors, saline and albumin; time in hospital; prior cancer diagnosis, resistant bacteria; decrease blood pressure. Many of features that were identified as important in our models are confirmed by published studies as associated with sepsis patient death. This provides reassurance that our machine learning model can identify well-known associations with sepsis death even among the noise of many unrelated variables.

As this study was the first phase of what we hope is the development of a comprehensive model for predicting sepsis patient outcomes, we anticipate several follow-up studies. First, since our study used complete case data only, we plan to incorporate chained or multiple imputation methods in future models. We have developed imputation method that is specifically designed for EHR data for complex diseases [14] that could be applied to this dataset as well. We are working to expand this study to include EHR data on sepsis patient hospitalizations from 2017; the latter can be used to further validate and refine our existing models. We are also including additional variables that may not directly have an association with sepsis, but taken together can provide a more granular view of the patient – these added variables include complete laboratory test results, problem lists, and complete vitals data among others. As an additional future direction, we will investigate the spatial distribution and socio-economic factors influencing the mortality rate of patients with sepsis in the catchment area of Geisinger in central Pennsylvania using patient's address information (available through patient Protected Health Information). Collectively, leveraging machine learning to predict sepsis mortality and identify biomarkers has the potential to improve efficiency and streamline resources to the most vulnerable sepsis patients and aids in creating personalized preventive care plans.

5 Acknowledgements

The authors would like to acknowledge Jason P. Brown, of Geisinger, who extracted and de-identified patient data and Debdipto Misra of Geisinger IT-Data Management, who provided an insightful perspective to this work. We would also like to thank Anna Hazard (IBM), who assisted with data visualization and figures and the preliminary analysis that Vinay Dandin (IBM) made to this work. We also received valuable insights from Bipin Karunakaran, Rameswara, Sashi Challa, and Satish Kalepalli (Geisinger), Aleksandr Petrov, Wanting Wang, Rajiv Joshi, Cheranellore Vasudevan, Alan Newman and Vidhya Shankar (IBM). This work was supported in part by funding from Geisinger Health System. Many thanks to the IBM Academy of Technology and IBM's executive sponsor Rob Thomas for approving this initiative.

6 References

[1] M. Singer *et al.*, "The Third International Consensus Definitions for Sepsis and Septic Shock (Sepsis-3)" *JAMA*, vol. 315, no. 8, pp. 801–10, Feb. 2016.

[2] CDC Data Reports, "Basic information on sepsis: Making Health Care Safer: Think Sepsis. Time Matters," *CDC*, 2016. [Online].https://www.cdc.gov/sepsis/datareports/index.html.

[3] A. Kumar *et al.*, "Duration of hypotension before initiation of effective antimicrobial therapy is the critical determinant of survival in human septic shock*," *Crit. Care Med.*, vol. 34, no. 6, pp. 1589–1596, Jun. 2006.

[4] B. D. Winters, M. Eberlein, J. Leung, D. M. Needham, P. J. Pronovost, and J. E. Sevransky, "Long-term mortality and quality of life in sepsis: A systematic review*," *Crit. Care Med.*, vol. 38, no. 5, pp. 1276–1283, May 2010.

[5] H. Lund-Sørensen *et al.*, "A Nationwide Cohort Study of the Association Between Hospitalization With Infection and Risk of Death by Suicide," *JAMA Psychiatry*, vol. 73, no. 9, p. 912, Sep. 2016.

[6] C. M. Torio and B. J. Moore, *National Inpatient Hospital Costs: The Most Expensive Conditions by Payer, 2013: Statistical Brief #204*. 2016.

[7] S. Chandra *et al.*, "The use of an electronic medical record based automatic calculation tool to quantify risk of unplanned readmission to the intensive care unit: a validation study.," *J. Crit. Care*, vol. 26, no. 6, p. 634.e9-634.e15, Dec. 2011.

[8] T. Lagu *et al.*, "Development and validation of a model that uses enhanced administrative data to predict mortality in patients with sepsis," *Crit. Care Med.*, vol. 39, no. 11, pp. 2425–2430, Nov. 2011.

[9] G. J. Escobar, J. C. LaGuardia, B. J. Turk, A. Ragins, P. Kipnis, and D. Draper, "Early detection of impending physiologic deterioration among patients who are not in intensive care: Development of predictive models using data from an automated electronic medical record," *J. Hosp. Med.*, vol. 7, no. 5, pp. 388–395, May 2012.

[10] V. Abedi *et al.*, "Novel Screening Tool for Stroke Using Artificial Neural Network," *Stroke*, vol. 48, no. 6, pp. 1678–1681, Jun. 2017.

[11] B. K. Beaulieu-Jones, D. R. Lavage, J. W. Snyder, J. H. Moore, S. A. Pendergrass, and C. R. Bauer, "Characterizing and Managing Missing Structured Data in Electronic Health Records," *bioRxiv*, p. 167858, Jul. 2017.

[12] B. K. BEAULIEU-JONES and J. H. MOORE, "Missing Data Imputation in the electronic health record using deeply learned autoencoders," in *Biocomputing 2017*, 2017, vol. 22, pp. 207–218.

[13] B. J. Wells, A. S. Nowacki, K. Chagin, and M. W. Kattan, "Strategies for Handling Missing Data in Electronic Health Record Derived Data," *eGEMs (Generating Evid. Methods to Improv. patient outcomes)*, vol. 1, no. 3, p. 7, Dec. 2013.

[14] V. Abedi *et al.*, "Latent-Based Imputation of Laboratory Measures from Electronic Health Records: Case for Complex Diseases," *bioRxiv*, p. 275743, Mar. 2018.

[15] S. Kethireddy *et al.*, "Culture-Negative Septic Shock Compared With Culture-Positive Septic Shock," *Crit. Care Med.*, vol. 46, no. 4, pp. 506–512, Apr. 2018.

[16] M. Fathi, N. Markazi-Moghaddam, and A. Ramezankhani, "A systematic review on risk factors associated with sepsis in patients admitted to intensive care units," *Aust. Crit. Care*, Mar. 2018.

[17] D. M. Wolk and A. B. Fiorello, "Code Sepsis: Rapid Methods To Diagnose Sepsis and Detect Hematopathogens," *Clin. Microbiol. Newsl.*, vol. 32, no. 6, pp. 41–49, Mar. 2010.

[18] S. S. Buehler *et al.*, "Effectiveness of Practices To Increase Timeliness of Providing Targeted Therapy for Inpatients with Bloodstream Infections: a Laboratory Medicine Best Practices Systematic Review and Meta-analysis," *Clin. Microbiol. Rev.*, vol. 29, no. 1, pp. 59–103, Jan. 2016.

[19] F. Sadaka, C. EthmaneAbouElMaali, M. A. Cytron, K. Fowler, V. M. Javaux, and J. O'Brien, "Predicting Mortality

of Patients With Sepsis: A Comparison of APACHE II and APACHE III Scoring Systems.," *J. Clin. Med. Res.*, vol. 9, no. 11, pp. 907–910, Nov. 2017.

[20] F. E. Dewey *et al.*, "Distribution and clinical impact of functional variants in 50,726 whole-exome sequences from the DiscovEHR study," *Science (80-.).*, vol. 354, no. 6319, p. aaf6814, Dec. 2016.

[21] N. S. Abul-Husn *et al.*, "Genetic identification of familial hypercholesterolemia within a single U.S. health care system," *Science (80-.).*, vol. 354, no. 6319, p.7000, Dec. 2016.

Shaping Future Patient-centered Healthcare Research through a Modified Delphi Process

Huanmei Wu[1], Hao Yu[1], Tammy Toscos[2], Amy Miller[1], Brad Doebbeling[3]
[1]Department of BioHealth Informatics, School of Informatics and Computing, IUPUI, Indianapolis, IN, USA,
[2]Indianapolis Parkview Mirro Center for Research & Innovation, Fort Wayne, IN, USA
[3]School of Science Health Care Delivery and Department of Biomedical Informatics,
College of Health Solutions, Arizona State University, Phoenix, AZ, USA

Abstract - *For our patient center project, which aims to improve patient care access, to further develop and refine future research and clinical-oriented projects, we held an interactive modified interactive Delphi panel of all stakeholders (patients, care providers, clinical staff, healthcare policymakers, and other professionals associated with healthcare). We shared our project and ideas for next steps with the participants in small groups, and then solicited their suggestions on meaningful next-step work. Voting results were analyzed and categorized to determine the top priorities for future actions. We found the broad stakeholder groups interested in training and other strategies to foster organizational culture change, as well as more significant applications to HIT and health data analytics for the improvement of care and operations. This interactive approach can be a useful method for engaging participants in considering, expanding and prioritizing a broad range of health system redesign and quality improvement options.*

Keywords: Patient-centered health care, Delphi panel, Health data analytics

1 Introduction

There is substantial evidence showing that the impact of limited access to be a significant burden on the U.S. population [1]. Moreover, access to health care is not improving in the U.S. [2, 3]. Translational research is needed to develop, implement and spread effective systems interventions to impact the experience of patients needs to access the health care system [3, 4].

Our project, titled "*Improving Healthcare Systems for Access to Care by Underserved Patients,*" funded by Patient-Centered Outcomes Research Institute (PCORI), focused on identifying effective practices to providing better healthcare access for under- and uninsured patients. The project investigators had interviewed and analyzed nearly 100 key stakeholders (including patients, staff, and providers) from community health clinics (CHCs) across Indiana to understand and collect successful approaches used to improve access [5-7]. These findings were used to create a list of potential interventions to improve access in CHCs.

Previous investigations have identified many innovative strategies. The highest ranked ones were expanding open-access scheduling, fostering a culture of customer service and accountability, and providing dashboards regarding access measures for feedback [5-9]. We also created a community data warehouse, composed of electronic health records (EHRs), clinic operational data, and financial data from all 7 CHC systems representing 40 individual clinics to support the project.

We partnered with three of the seven participating CHCs to coach their intervention implementation. This multi-component intervention included: 1) expanding and optimizing open-access scheduling, 2) creating a culture of customer service, focusing not only on interactions between CHC staff and patients but also among staff; and 3) developing and sharing role-specific dashboards to provide feedback on progress and foster continued engagement by stakeholders [10-12].

Our project is examining the impact of the intervention on access measures, patient satisfaction, and other essential metrics. Initial results based on feedback from stakeholders and CHC system leaders are promising. The outcomes demonstrate high engagement and satisfaction by the intervention clinics, an improvement in appointment no-show rates, and broad interest from all participating clinics in implementation and spread of the intervention. In the final stage of our current PCORI, we hosted a dissemination meeting to disseminate results and provide reflections of all stakeholders.

All the dissemination attendees were either under-served patient populations or critical stakeholders involved in providing healthcare through CHCs for the under-served communities. During the meeting, we organized a modified Delphi panel [13, 14] with these stakeholders. The primary panel goals are:

- Gather ideas of what practices and behaviors may be useful in improving access to primary care for under-served patients;

- Discover the pressing concerns and expectations for next-step actions in clinic-oriented projects;

- Expand and prioritize future ideas for patient-centered care research in this area.

2 Methods

We applied the modified Delphi panel for the panel discussions, led by two project investigators. The panel attendees randomly separated into four groups. Only one group of attendees participated in the panel discussions each time. The other three groups had concurrent professional training and demonstration activities at the same time.

Figure 1 illustrated the modified panel process. Initially, the panel leaders shared a concise list of future working directions or advocated project ideas (4 suggestions in this specific case). This initial list, denoted as L_0, written on Post-it® Self-Stick Wall Pad (size: 25" x 30") and placed on the wall of a conference room. It is the starting point for the panel discussion. Upon arriving each group of panelists, the leaders briefly introduced the goal of the panel and quickly went over the existing suggestions.

Thus, for Group 1 attendees, after explaining the initial list, L_0, the attendees were then arbitrarily separated into 2 or 3 sub-groups, each consisting of 4-6 panelists for active participation. Each sub-group had a short period of discussions and identified additional ideas. The leaders wrote the recommendations, attaching to the initial list of the sticky easel paper. Combining all the items from group 1 with the initial ones generated the updated list, noted L_1.

Then each attendee as given the opportunity to select the most important (top three) suggestions from L_1 and showed his/her choices by sticking the corresponding item with a small Post-it note (size: 1.375 x 1.875") on the wallpapers. There was no ranking order for the three selected preferences. This voting result generated the first ranking list, noted as R_1. After the group left, we recorded the voting results and removed the small Post-it notes from the wall.

When Group 2 attendees came, the discussions were based on the updated list L_1. The same procedure applied as what happened to Group 1: explaining the goals, describing the previous list, discussing among the sub-group, providing more suggestions, identifying their top three items from the updated list (L_2), and placing their votes on the wall summaries. The panel leaders recorded the results and cleaned the papers. The same procedures happened to the attendees of Groups 3 and 4.

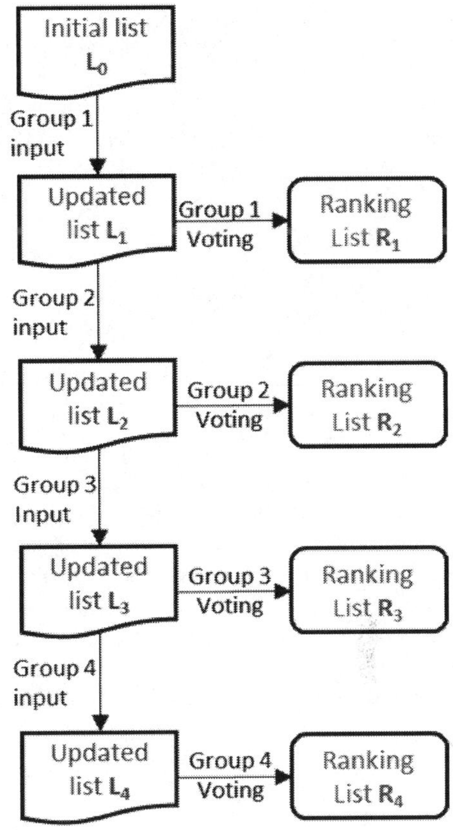

Figure 1– Flow diagram of the interactive panel process.

3 Results

3.1 Attendees information

There were total 65 participants. Among them, there are 21 Clinical professionals from nine geographical separated Community Health Centers (CHCs) across Indiana. They served different roles in CHCs, including clinical administrators (such as CEOs, CFOs, or CTOs), medical providers (such as medical doctors, nurse practitioners, physician assistants, or nurses), and CHC staff (such as the front desk or financial counseling staff).

There are 13 patients (6 males and 7 females), representing under-served populations in the Indianapolis areas. They came from a variety of race and ethnicity categories. Each had different health conditions and financial situations.

We invited 15 guests from various healthcare organizations around Indiana. The guests included representatives and medical/Medicaid related staff from the Indiana State Department of Health, the Indiana Congressional offices, and the Marion County Health Department. Some guests were healthcare researchers from different academic units, such as Indiana University (IU) Health, IU School of Nursing, IU School of Medicine, and IU School of Informatics and Computer Health Informatics.

Some researchers were from organizations in biomedical and healthcare research and services, such as the Regenstrief Institute, VA Medical Center, the Indiana Primary Health Care Association (IPHCA), Indiana CTSI (Clinical and Translational Sciences Institute), and Parkview Health Mirro Center for Research and Innovation. We also had participants from hospitals, including Eskenazi Health, and Parkview Health.

Total 16 of PCORI team members attended the activities, including five investigators, six graduate students, one consultant for clinical interventions, and four staff members.

3.2 Panel Suggestions

The overall strategic suggestions are listed in Table 1, shaded into four voting sub-lists. The initial suggestions by the panel leaders are the listed items 1 to 4. The specific suggestions proposed by attendees Group 1, Group 2, Group 3, and Group 4 are item lists [4, 13], [14, 17], [18, 26], and [27, 31], respectively. The suggestions of all the four groups were classified into six major topics, based on discussions among the investigators. Table 2 summarized the categorization results. The total votes for each suggestion and topics from all the four groups are also listed in Tables 1 and 2. Below is the summary of the six topics:

T1. *Create training modules:* Participants were interested in training sessions on how to best implement patient-centered culture change for both staff and patients to better use EHR systems and web portals, to understand health and wellbeing in the community, and to educate patients for timely preventative care.

T2. *Improve patient experiences:* Participants suggested approaches to improving the patient experience by paying more attention to patient history, accessing more information, focusing more on preventative care, and increasing face-time with providers.

T3. *Spread access interventions:* In addition to developing new technology guided access interventions, participants suggested adopting, implementing and spreading our access interventions to other clinics.

T4. *Shared decision making:* Attendees suggested all CHC stakeholders, including providers, patients, communities, and others work together regularly to make shared decisions for better patient care, such as establishing priorities, providing patient care options, and promoting team care.

T5. *Expand community data warehouses and analytics:* Participants favored improving the features and functionality of community data warehouses, such as developing more dashboards, data analytics and use to balance quality triage (Control-Improve-Plan), and anticipate changes to address emerging healthcare trends.

T6. *Optimize the use of EHR and other HIT Systems:* Participants favored expanded capabilities for HIT assistance for data collection, EHR system integration, new tool development, and improved user-centered design of the EHR to enhance patients' experience.

3.3 Voting Results

The voting results for each suggestion from each round are illustrated in Table 1 and Figure 2. There are several interesting observations. First, the voting of the attendees spread over all the suggestions, not only focusing on the new ones they just mentioned by the specific group. Second, some of the ideas were highly rated over several groups. Given the iterative design, the late suggestions proposed by

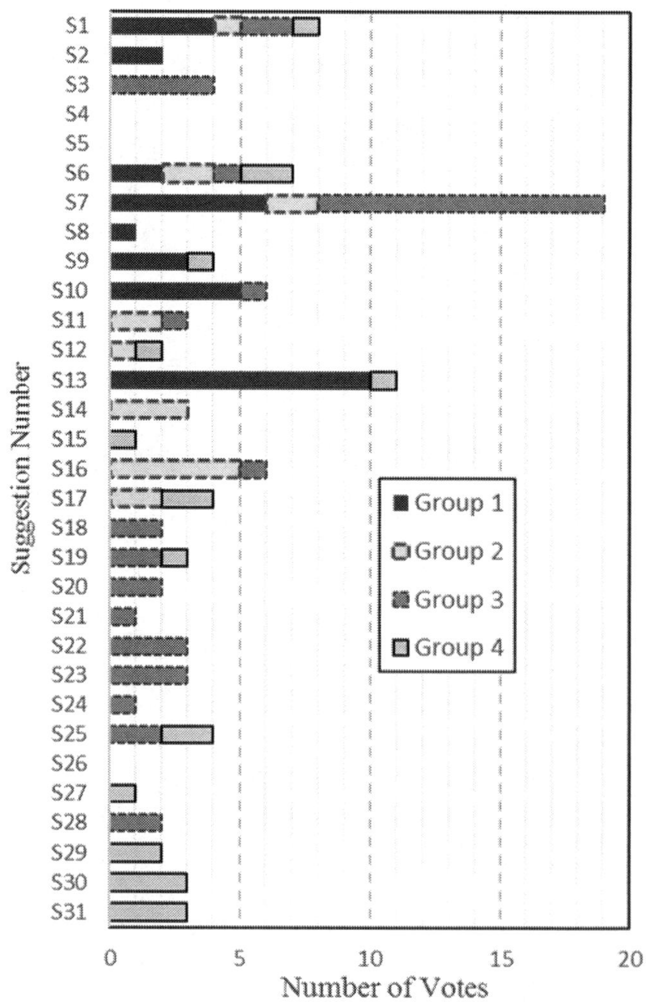

Figure 2– The voting results for each suggestion by the four groups of panel attendees.

Table 1– – Lists of suggestions and voting results for each panel round.

#	Suggestions	Voting				
		G1	G2	G3	G4	Sum
1	Spread intervention to other clinics	4	1	2	1	8
2	Develop new technology/interventions to increase accessibility	2				2
3	Adopt others' or new clinical interventions to tackle more problems			4		4
4	Improve clinical disease warehouse					0
5	More dashboards and analytics					0
6	Use data to educate/communicate/engage patients/provider in priorities for changes	2	2	1	2	7
7	Implement culture change for both staff and patients	6	2	10		19
8	Assist in ongoing data collection without interruption	1				1
9	Utilize scribes to up MD focus	3			1	4
10	Use EHR system to enhance patients' experience	5		1		6
11	Align multiple competing priorities yet still focus on Quality Culture		2	1		3
12	Use data to balance quality triage (Control-Improve-Plan)		1		1	2
13	Use data and quality improvement dashboards to balance workload for professionals	10			1	11
14	Better observing the patient experience and history		3			3
15	Improve patient access to more information in emergency/urgent care				1	1
16	More user friendly EHR systems		4	1		6
17	Change the understanding of health and wellbeing in community		2		2	4
18	Develop patient focused dashboards for visual learners			2		2
19	Continue to monitor intervention progress from other clinics			2	1	3
20	Have a clinical manager present during patient visits			2		2
21	Improve EHR Training			1		1
22	Clinical Integration: HIE and EHR system			3		3
23	Focus more on preventative Care			3		3
24	Facilitate decision choices between: family practitioner, emergency room, and specialist			1		1
25	Educate patient portal			2	2	4
26	Improve patients' experience by increasing face-time with Physicians			2		0
27	Have a back-up plan for patients not be able to get the same day appointment					1
28	Review data, evaluate trends				1	2
29	Form patient liaison/navigators to get care needed				2	2
30	Have a stakeholder panel to meet regularly with pts, doctors and healthcare workers				3	3
31	Education for patients who are reluctance to go to clinic				3	3
	Sub-total voting:	**33**	**18**	**39**	**21**	**111**

Table 2– Categorizing the panel suggestions and summarizing the voting results.

Major Topics	Suggestion #s	Group 1 Votes #	Group 2 Votes #	Group 3 Votes #	Group 4 Votes #	Total Votes
T1. Create training modules	7, 17, 21, 25, 31	6	4	24	7	**31**
T2. Improve patient experiences	10, 14, 15, 20, 23, 26	5	3	8	1	**17**
T3. Spread access interventions	1, 2, 3, 19	6	1	8	8	**17**
T4. Shared decision making	6, 11, 24, 27, 29, 30	2	4	3	3	**16**
T5. Expand community data warehouses and analytics	4, 5, 12, 13, 28, 18	10	1	2	2	**16**
T6. Optimize the use of EHR and other HIT Systems	8, 9, 16, 22	4	5	4	4	**14**

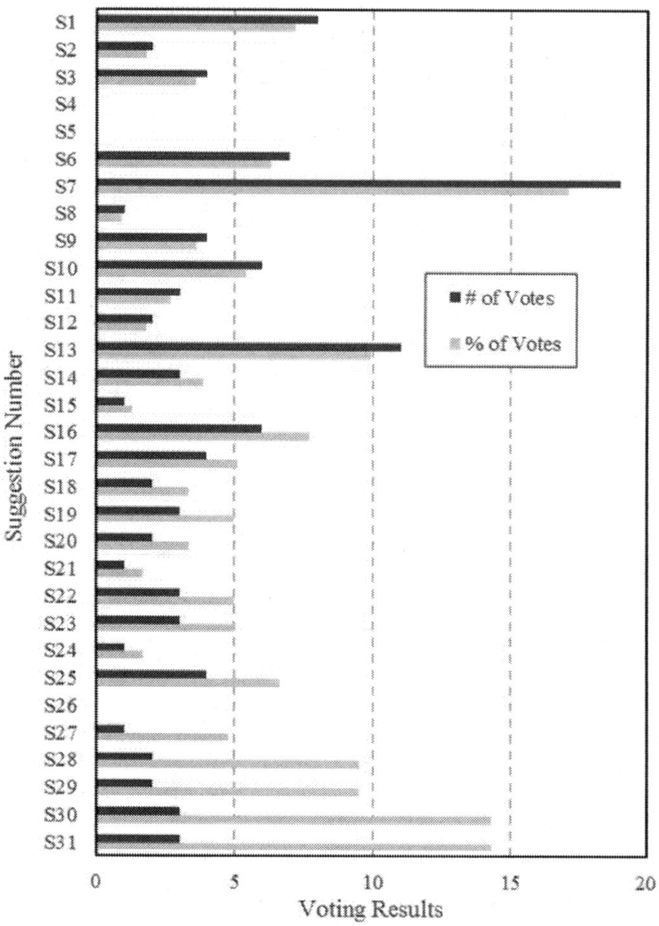

Figure 3 – The exact number of votes and the percentage of votes cast for each topic.

the subsequent groups were not visible to the previous attendees and thus were voted on by fewer attendees. Third, to interpret the importance of each suggestion, Figure 3 illustrated the calculated percentages of the votes. The percentage for each item involved dividing the number of votes for the specific item by the total potential maximum votes on it (*i.e.,* the number of attendees who voted on it). Notably, the # of votes and % of votes were similar, except for the last few suggestions, which were only voted on by the group 4 attendees.

The voting results also showed there were relatively few common concerns across all the attendees. The suggestion, which had the maximum vote, #7, was for implementing culture change for both staff and patients to work more towards patient-centered healthcare culture. It had 17 votes out of 111, which was about 17% of all voters. The next highest voting number went to Suggestion #13, which was to use clinical warehouse data and dashboards to identify essential priorities for QI and provide feedback for staff and providers on progress. It had 10% of all the votes.

When considering the scaled % of votes, the last few suggestions also stand out. These questions focused on education, training, and joint decision making among different stakeholders to improve patient care.

3.4 Importance of the Major Topic

Table 2 and Figure 4 summarized the voting results for the six major topics. These topics were of interest to all four groups, being voted by each group. On the other hand, the "creating training modules" stood out with the most popular votes (28% votes out of all votes). The other five had similar values (ranging from 13% to 15% of all the votes).

ANOVA-test [15] was performed to explore if it is significant for the voting results among different groups of attendees, or different major topics. The test results showed no significant difference in the voting of groups of attendees or across the major topics.

For example, the one way ANOVA test showed that voting results by the four groups on the six topics were not significant (with the f-ratio value of 1.40549 and the p-value of 0.27). Similar, the ANOCA test results showed that the distributions of the voting results on the six topics were not significant among the four groups. Thus, we found no evidence in these data of bias.

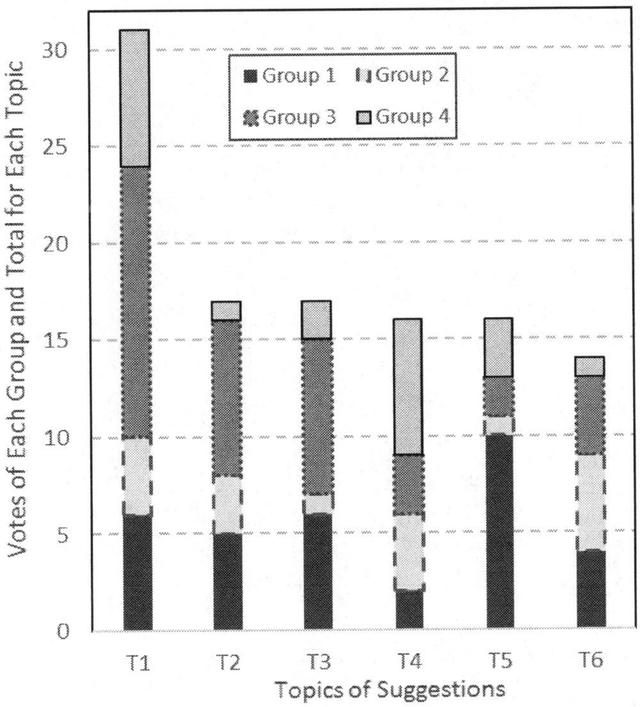

Figure 4– The voting results for each topic.

4 Discussions

We learned several lessons from the meeting and came with a few strategic ideas for future improvements.

4.1 Topics Priorities for Future Patient Care

The most pressing issues for community health centers using this approach was the creation of new training modules (Topic 1). Here, participants rated the most necessary training was to implement culture changes to focus more on patient-centered care for both staff and patients (suggestion 7, which has the most votes).

Culture changes in the CHCs are challenging, due to limited available resources, staff turnover, the burden of illness and the limited understanding of health and wellbeing in the community. We found a high interest in fostering the development of the culture to treat all patients the same with the limited resources, no matter the background, the religious status, the social standard, and the income conditions of the patients.

Participants also rated high for the education and engagement of patients in monitoring their health conditions, to get updated information from the patient portal, and to overcome challenges in keeping current in receiving preventative care.

The panelists were also looking for the development and deployment of an innovative HIT to improve patient experiences (Topic 2) and to adopt and spread interventions, which would enhance patient access to all the CHCs and other healthcare organizations (Topic 3). It was also highly required to have shared decision-making (Topic 4), and to enhance the usability and features of EHR systems (Topic 6). Many panelists mentioned that healthcare data analysis (Topic 5) were highly needed in CHCs. They did not have the resources to perform the analytical work. Collaboration with Academic partners would be an ideal solution for them.

There was considerable demand for a community data warehouse, such as that developed in the project, and applying data analytics in clinical operations and improving patient care. Notably, the high interest in our access to care dashboard, for CHC leadership, staff and for patients, demonstrated the value of applied data analytics for community healthcare stakeholders. They observed the great benefit of modifiable HIT resources for targeting improvements in patient care.

4.2 Expected Results

The suggestions and ranking results of the panelists are expected based on our previous work. The combined six topics also manifested our ongoing work with our clinical partners and primary care collaborators. The Delphi panel suggestions conformed to our past study on the healthcare needs of the underserved populations [11].

Our project team members had been working in all these topical areas. For example, to address the demand for data warehouse, we had developed a multidimensional data warehouse and coherent healthcare system [12, 17]. The group has also been actively working on data analytics over electronic health records [18].

4.3 Lessons Learned

Although the interactive panel helped to identify some critical future foci of CHC patient care, there were a few lessons learned to guide for future efforts:

First, each attendee provided their three top choices, although there was no specific order of the three options from the attendees. The ranking of these preferences may be of great interest to analyze.

Second, the grouping of the participants could be improved and more balanced. We chose to form random groups for this panel, based on initial seating arrangements for the previous didactic presentations. The numbers of panelists were not equally distributed.

Third, we did not allocate time to combine similar ideas, which might have resulted in a smaller or more parsimonious list. Elongated the panel session would help for future events.

Last, the voting did not record the role of the attendees. It would have been interesting to discover the top priorities for different attendees based on their work or stakeholder roles. For example, we anticipate that the concerns from the front desk scheduling staff will be different from the priorities of the medical providers.

5 Conclusions

An interactive modified Delphi panel was applied in the dissemination meeting of a patient-centered systems redesign project, whose goal was to improve patient access to health care for the underserved population. The panel process and the attendee voting results were analyzed to determine potential directions in advancing patient-centered access to health care. We found this broad stakeholder groups interested in training and other strategies to foster organizational culture change, as well as a prominent application of HIT and health data analytics to improve care and operations.

We will be exploring opportunities to carry out some of the suggested research projects. Additionally, this approach can be a useful method for engaging participants in considering, expanding and prioritizing a broad range of health system redesign and quality improvement options.

Acknowledgments

This research was funded through a Patient-Centered Outcomes Research Institute (PCORI) Award # IH-12-11-5488. The statements presented in this publication are solely the responsibility of the author(s).

6 References

[1] P. Gabow, G. Halvorson, G. Kaplan, Marshaling leadership for high-value health care: an Institute of Medicine discussion paper. JAMA: the journal of the American Medical Association. 308(3), 239-240, 2012.

[2] Agency for Healthcare Research and Quality (AHRQ). 2010 National Healthcare Disparities

[3] Report. U.S. Department of Health and Human Services; 2011.

[4] B. Bette and L. Martin. Culture in clinical care: Strategies for competence. Slack, 2013.

[5] A. Ghorob and T. Bodenheimer, Sharing the care to improve access to primary care. New England Journal of Medicine, 366(21), pp.1955-1957. 2012.

[6] U.S. Department of Health and Human Services, Health Resources and Services Administration. What is a Health Center? http://www.bphc.hrsa.gov/about/what-is-a-health-center/index.html; retrieved 10/08/15. 2015

[7] R.A. Rosenblatt, C.H.A. Andrilla, T. Curtin and L.G. Hart, Shortages of medical personnel at community health centers: implications for planned expansion. Jama, 295(9), pp.1042-1049. 2006.

[8] V.A. Lewis, C.H. Colla, K.E. Schoenherr, S.M. Shortell, and E.S. Fisher. Innovation in the safety net: integrating community health centers through accountable care. Journal of general internal medicine, 29(11),1484-1490. 2014.

[9] H. Song, et. al. Results of the Community Health Applied Research Network (CHARN) National Research Capacity Survey of Community Health Centers. Progress in community health partnerships: research, education, and action, 9(2), pp.229-242. 2012

[10] L. Ku, B.K. Frogner, E. Steinmetz, and P. Pittman, Community health centers employ diverse staffing patterns, which can provide productivity lessons for medical practices. Health Affairs, 34(1), pp.95-103, 2015

[11] I. Mohammadi, S. Hashemikhabir, T. Toscos, and H. Wu, Health Care Needs of Underserved Populations in the City of Indianapolis. In Proceedings of the 7th ACM International Conference on Bioinformatics, Computational Biology, and Health Informatics, 512-513, 2016.

[12] K. Kunjan, T. Toscos, A. Turkcan and B.N. Doebbeling, A Multidimensional Data Warehouse for Community Health Centers. In AMIA Annual Symposium Proceedings, p. 1976, 2015.

[13] A. Turkcan, T. Toscos, BN Doebbeling, Patient-Centered Appointment Scheduling Using Agent-Based Simulation. AMIA Annu Symp Proc. eCollection 2014.

[14] H.M. Oranga and E. Nordberg, The Delphi panel method for generating health information. Health policy and planning, 8(4), pp.405-412, 1993.

[15] C. Powell. The Delphi technique: myths and realities. Journal of advanced nursing, 41(4), pp.376-382, 2003.

[16] A. Cuevas, M. Febrero and R. Fraiman, An anova test for functional data. Computational statistics & data analysis, 47(1), pp.111-122, 2004.

[17] H Wu, A Ambavane, S Mukherjee, S Mao, A Coherent Healthcare System with RDBMS, NoSQL and GIS Databases, Proceedings of the 32nd International Conference on Computers and Their Applications, CATA p. 313-318, 2017.

[18] S Mukherjee, H Wu, J Jones, Healthcare Data Analytics for Parkinson's Disease Patients: A Study of Hospital Cost and Utilization in the United States, AMIA Annual Symposium Proceedings. 2017 Feb 10; 2016: 1950-1958.

Securing Electronic Health Records (EHRs) in OpenStack

Ashwini Devi Ventrapragada and Jigang Liu

Department of Computer Science and Cybersecurity
Metropolitan State University
St. Paul, Minnesota, USA

Abstract— **Electronic Health Records (EHRs) have been ever increasingly implemented and wildly used in the healthcare industry since Amazon introduced its Elastic Compute Cloud in 2006. Although the cloud computing has accelerated the adoption of EHRs due to its benefits in sharing information, the risk in alternating, losing, and exposing patient's private information rises significantly. In this paper, a critical issue in storing and accessing EHRs in OpenStack, one of the common cloud computing platforms, is addressed. To avoid revealing the entire information in a particular patient record regardless the credential of reviewers, an enhanced mechanism with a prototyped framework in dealing with the issue is proposed. Based the analysis and discussion, the new framework shows its promising potential in efficiently and effectively strengthening the protection of EHRs in the cloud.**

I. INTRODUCTION

The online access of Electronic Health Records (EHRs) via a cloud based storage has been adopted to help accessing and sharing the information among the various agencies in the management of EHRs in a centralized way for more than a decade. Although cloud based EHR systems provide an efficient and effective way in storing, sharing, and managing the EHR records, they expose the vulnerability in control and safety guard of the EHR records regarding security and privacy.

Under a cloud based EHR system, one can access the system from anywhere with an internet access. This not only reduces the expense on both software and hardware in hosting the system, it also saves the overhead in hiring for managing the system and handling daily operation. In addition, mobile EHR users can also be benefited in a way in which they can access the EHR system from anywhere and at anytime. Moreover, the potential issues in security and privacy exposed by the cloud based EHR systems can be effectively handled through a centralized manner.

Although the security issue is critical, the most concern in an EHR system is the privacy. HIPAA, Health Information Portability and Accountability Act, is a U.S. federal law that was designed to protect patient privacy. All EHR systems should be compliance with the HIPAA in terms of encrypted data transmissions, secure and redundant offsite data storage, and user authentication and access controls. The HIPAA security rule requires appropriate administrative, physical, and technical safeguards to ensure the confidentiality, integrity, and availability of EHRs. Under the technical safeguards guideline, the access control forms a major standard that needs to be fulfilled. According to the standard we need to implement technical policies and procedures for electronic information systems that maintain electronic protected health information to allow the access only to those persons or software programs that have been granted the access rights as specified in §164.308(a)(4) [10].

Even though cloud-based EHRs have received considerable attention since it would help achieve lower operational cost and better interoperability with other healthcare providers, the adoption of security-aware cloud systems has become an extremely important prerequisite for bringing interoperability and efficient management to the healthcare industry [1, 3]. The rest of the paper is organized as follows: an overview of cloud platforms is provided in the next section. In section III, the architecture and storage layout of OpenStack is discussed. The access control enhancement of OpenStack's Swift is proposed in section IV followed by discussion and assessment in section V. Finally, in section VI, the conclusion and future work is provided.

II. CLOUD COMPUTING PLATFORMS

Since Amazon introduced its Elastic Compute Cloud in 2006, cloud computing has been involved in many technology advancement, including EHR systems. Based on the definitions given by NIST, cloud computing provides three fundamental services, namely SaaS (Software as a Service), PaaS (Platform as a Service), and IaaS (Infrastructure as a Service), an EHR system is commonly supported by an IaaS cloud platform due to its nature of the application. Cloud services are fighting for market share and are developing the next generation of cloud management systems. Arguably the four biggest players in the market currently are OpenStack, CloudStack, Eucalyptus and OpenNebula. Each of them is creating new ways for organizations to connect various cloud services. There's no doubt that, right now, OpenStack is leading the way. However, cloud interconnectivity, API architectures, and the influences of the end-user will ultimately dictate the future of the cloud. Whatever the outcome, the business, and the of course the end-user, will certainly benefit.

As presented in [9], the four well known cloud computing platforms, especially for IaaS (Infrastructure as a Service), are compared and analyzed against their advantages and disadvantages as summarized in Table 1 below. "Checks" in the table means the advantages. The number of the checks means the level of the advantage, e.g. the more checks the better.

Table 1: Feature Comparison of IaaS Cloud Platforms [9]

	OpenStack	Eucalyptus 2.0	Nimbus	OpenNebula
Interfaces	EC2 and S3, Rest Interface. Working on OCCI ✓✓	EC2 and S3, Rest Interface. Working on OCCI ✓✓	EC2 and S3, Rest Interface ✓	Native XML/RPC, EC2 and S3, OCCI, Rest Interface ✓✓✓
Hypervisor	KVM, XEN, VMware Vsphere, LXC, UML and MS HyperV ✓✓✓	KVM and XEN. VMWare in the enterprise edition. ✓✓	KVM and XEN ✓	KVM, XEN and VMWare ✓✓
Networking	- Two modes: (a) Flat networking (b) VLAN networking -Creates Bridges automatically -Uses IP forwarding for public IP -VMs only have private IPs ✓✓✓	- Four modes: (a) managed; (b) managed-novLAN; (c) system; and (d) static - In (a) & (b) bridges are created automatically - IP forwarding for public IP -VMs only have private IPs ✓✓✓	- IP assigned using a DHCP server that can be configured in two ways. - Bridges must exists in the compute nodes ✓✓	- Networks can be defined to support Ebtable, Open vSwitch and 802.1Q tagging -Bridges must exists in the compute nodes -IP are setup inside VM ✓✓✓
Software deployment	- Software is composed by component that can be placed in different machines. - Compute nodes need to install OpenStack software ✓	- Software is composed by component that can be placed in different machines. - Compute nodes need to install OpenStack software ✓	Software is installed in frontend and compute nodes ✓✓	Software is installed in frontend ✓✓✓
DevOps deployment	Chef, Crowbar, Puppet ✓✓✓	Chef*, Puppet* ✓ (*according to vendor)	no	Chef, Puppet ✓✓
Storage (Image Transference)	- Swift (http/s) - Unix filesystem (ssh) ✓	Walrus (http/s) ✓	Cumulus (http/https) ✓	Unix Filesystem (ssh, shared filesystem or LVM with CoW) ✓
Authentication	X509 credentials, LDAP ✓✓✓	X509 credentials ✓	X509 credentials, Grids ✓✓	X509 credential, ssh rsa keypair, password, LDAP ✓✓✓
Avg. Release Frequency	<4month	>4 month ✓	<4 month	>6 month ✓
License	OpenSource - Apache ✓	OpenSource / Commercial	OpenSource Apache ✓	OpenSource Apache ✓

OpenNebula was started as a research venture project and was first publicly released in 2008. Since it looks more like a product than a working platform, OpenNebula provides a better interface designed than others as indicated in Table 1. Led by the researchers from Argonne National Laboratory and University of Chicago, Nimbus is based on an international collaboration for providing researchers with a powerful platform in building their own IaaS for their specific scientific computing needs. While Eucalyptus is the most developed one among the four IaaS platforms, many early cloud computing applications developed on it. Initiated and led by NASA, the first version of OpenStack, Austin, was released in 2010. Due to its openness and flexibility, the OpenStack project was quickly joined by some well-known companies, such as IBM, HP, and DELL. Although OpenNebula and OpenStack look like equally impressive based on the comparison shown in Table 1, the openness and flexibility in arranging computing power gives OpenStack the edge for being used in building an EHR system. Moreover, OpenStack's valuable potential is also indicated in a recently published paper on the journal of the future generation compute systems [12]. In next section, we will discuss the architecture as well as the design philosophy of OpenStack in detail to illustrate why OpenStack is an ideal choice for building an EHR system.

III. OPENSTACK AND SWIFT

Before initiating the OpenStack project, NASA was using Eucalyptus as its cloud computing platform. Due to the scalability limitation as well as the openness concern, NASA dropped Eucalyptus and collaborated with Rackspace for the OpenStack project. As the name of the platform suggests, OpenStack is built on multiple modules with a true open source environment. Although the learning curve for adopting OpenStack is relative high, the flexibility and the openness create a healthy environment for the users as well as its developers. In addition, if the vendor lock-in is one of the biggest concerns for adopting cloud computing, OpenStack is a better choice based on its lower level openness to the developers. To have an overall view of OpenStack, Figure 1 below shows its architecture.

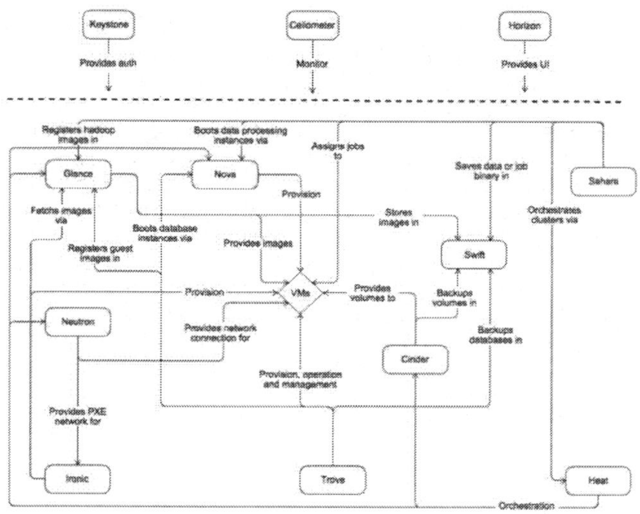

Figure 1 OpenStack Architecture [11]

There are three core components for an IaaS cloud computing platform: computing power, network configuration, and storage management. For OpenStack as shown in figure 1, Nova provides the computing power, networking is supported by Neutron, and Swift is the base for the storage. In Swift, the files are uploaded as objects and organized into containers, which makes it simpler to integrate, scale, manage, and unify storage at massive scale [11]. While accessing to those containers is critical in terms of security and privacy, Swift uses Access Control Lists (ACLs) to protect those containers.

The access control is commonly used for the prevention of unauthorized use of a resource. Access control begins with authentication, which provides the identity of the user or client systems attempting to gain entry. And then it is granting the permitted user to access to some specific data based on the previously defined rules and the user's clearance level. In other words, access control emphasizes on three areas: 1) subject, which is the entity that is given permission to the access the data; 2) object, which is the actual item being protected; and 3) access right, which is the means that the level of the control is established. As a result, access control mechanisms can be classified into four main classes in 1) discretionary where the data owner determines who can to what; 2) mandatory where users do not have much freedom to determine who can access their data but rely on the rules and trust in terms of security clearance level of the users as well as the classification of their data; 3) Role-based, where the access is determined by the jobs or roles users are granted; 4) Attribute-based, where the access right is granted through the user of the previously defined policies. Swift's access control is illustrated in Figure 2 below:

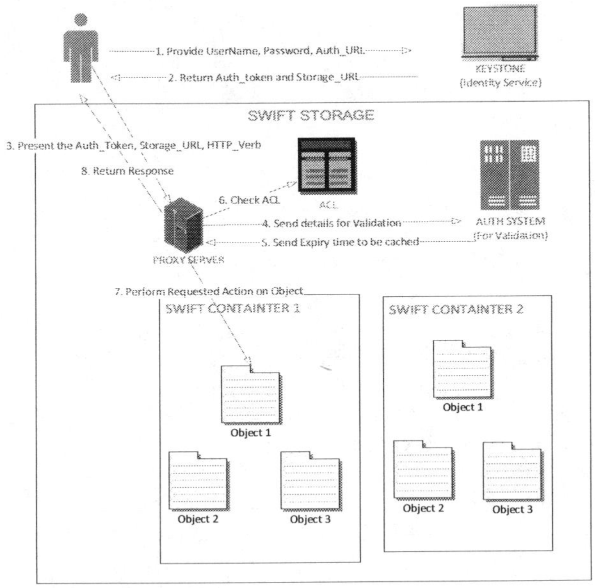

Figure 2: Access control flow in Swift

The eight steps involved in Swift's access control, shown in Figure 2 above, are explained as follows:

1)	KeyStone Identity Service: KeyStone is a key component of OpenStack, which is used to check the identity of the user;
2)	Keystone responds with Auth_token and Storage_URL;
3)	A user presents the Auth_token and Storage_URL and the HTTP_verb to the proxy server of the Swift Storage;
4)	The proxy server forwards the token details to the Auth System (external/ internal) for verification;
5)	If the token is valid, the Auth System responds with the expiry time limit of the token which is cached by Swift. The token does not change from request to request, but has a time limit;
6)	The Proxy server then retrieves the ACL for the user and validates the requested action;
7)	Performs the requested action. Note that the actions are the REST calls like GET, POST and PUT;
8)	Returns the response and response code. The response codes returned are also the regular HTTP response codes.

Based on the discussion above, it is obvious that once an object is accessible to someone, they could have the access to the entire content of the object, which means that the ACL in Swift only controls the access to the object's container, not beyond. As a result, the access control follows the principle of "all or nothing" approach, which is a vulnerable point for using Swift to store EHR records if a patient record is stored as an object in a Swift's container.

Since the access to these containers is restricted by the use of Access Control Lists (ACLs), it is important to provide restricted accesses to access the EHRs of patients depending on their privileges. As the current system of access control in Swift follows the rule that once a container is accessible to someone, they are granted the full right to access all the objects in the container as well as all the content in each of the objects in the container. As a result, the EHRs stored on Swift would violate the HIPPA principles in "need to know" and "minimum necessary" because any of the hospital staff would be granted the access to the entire patient record no matter for a medical appointment scheduler or the patient's doctor. This would have much serious impact on securing the sharing of EHRs between the various domains of healthcare systems like pharmacy, clinical lab and primary care, etc. In next section, an enhancement of Swift's ACL is proposed to mitigate the potential vulnerability existed in Swift.

IV. ACCESS CONTROL ENHANCEMENT IN SWIFT

To overcome the drawbacks of the existing system, the proposed system should be able to provide a partial access to an object. In other words, the system should provide the access control based on the content, not the object, depending on the role of a particular user. This would eliminate the "all or nothing" vulnerability resided in Swift's access control. The design goals of the proposed enhancement to Swift access control are listed as follows:

- To facilitate sharing of Electronic Health Records between the various domains of healthcare systems like pharmacy, clinical lab, primary care etc.;
- To provide restricted access to the user access the EHR of the patient depending on his privilege to access it;
- To increase the performance and efficiency of the system by minimizing the overhead caused by the storage of additional information;
- To create a systematic and standardized format for storing the EHR in OpenStack;
- To store the records in both XML and JSON format in the OpenStack Swift Storage.

Managing access control with explicit ACL's is time consuming even on a single machine, and scales poorly in the cloud due to the presence of data migration [8]. Although the Label Based Access Control model (LaBAC) proposed in [6] is an attribute based access control model used to specify authorization policies, its framework can be borrowed to construct an LaBAC for dealing with the content level access control for Swift as demonstrated in Figure 3 below. The Label based access control model we propose here is a content level access control model used to enforce the access to the authorized portion of the content of the object, e.g. EHR records. In order to protect a JSON document stored as a Swift object, the model assigns each JSON item (i.e. value of a JSON key) an object-label and each user a user-label. Then we specify policies in the form of (user-label values, action, object-label values) which means that objects labeled with any of 'object_label' values are allowed to be accessed by the users labeled with any of 'user-label' values for the specific 'action'.

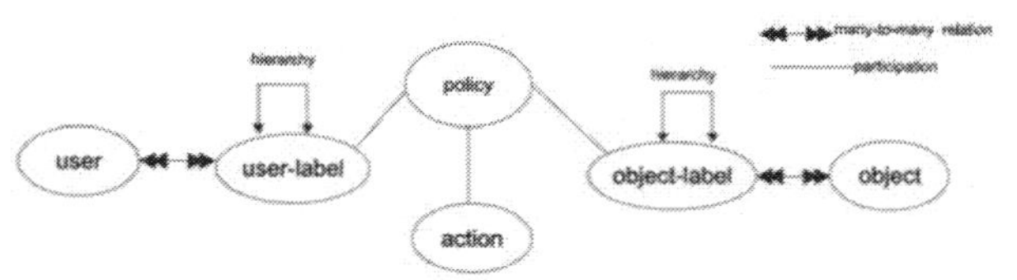

Figure 3: LaBAC Model Demonstration

Therefore, as shown in Figure 3 above, the Content-Level access mechanism can be implemented as follows:

- Using proposed system, the hospital management system can use objects of content-type 'Application/JSON' or XML to store patient's records;
- Each record / object is viewed as a collection of sections/ arrays. Each section is supposed to be accessed by the staff of a specific role defined in the hierarchy;
- The principle of hierarchy states that users can view a particular object content only at or below their own user security level. They would not have the access to the object content at above their own security level;
- At the container level, the label-policy is stored, which contains the users who are permitted to access the corresponding sections of the objects. The path of a particular section that is allowed to be accessed is defined in JSONPath or XPath;
- When a request for the operation on the object is made to the proxy server, the ACL is checked to determine if the user is authorized to access the object;
- Once the ACL authorizes the user, the label-policy in the metadata of the container is checked to determine what content of the object is the part that the user is authorized to access;
- Then the requested operation is made on the content authorized for the user and the partial content of the resultant object is returned;
- This would enforce the health care providers to access the patient information based on "need to know" and "minimum necessary" principles under the HIPAA guidelines.

The proposed enhancement for Swift's ACL can also be illustrated in Figure 4. Comparing with Figure 2, where a standard Swift's operation, a new action in step 7, "Check the label policy," is added to ensure a content level access control is implemented. By giving access to only partial content of the file, the content of the file can be protected. Hence, the content level security is enforced.

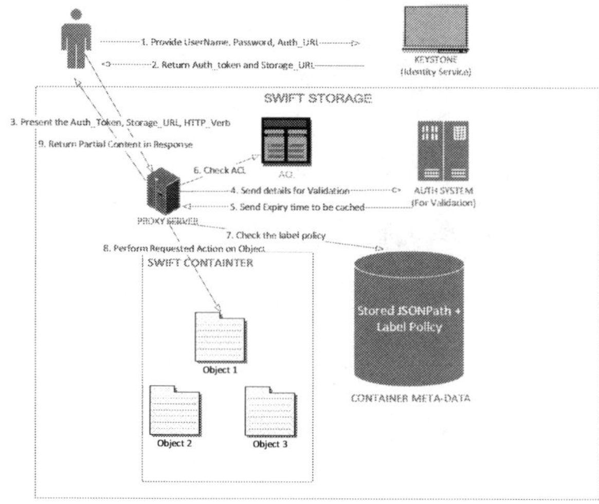

Figure 4: Proposed Enhancement for Swift's ACL

In the case of EHR records, when accessing the patient's information, each user can access only a part of the overall information. The user authorization on the content of the object is defined in the user hierarchy. Each EHR object is stored as JSON/XML and is grouped internally into sections according to the staff usage. Each JSON item or XML item can be labelled with their respective JSONPath and XPath. Each user is assigned to a role in which the user_label is stored. The user_label, json_path and the action are together specified in the Label_Policy. The label policy is validated before granting access to the user. Hence, the content level security is enforced. In next section, an example is used to illustrate how the proposed enhancement can be implemented within Swift.

V. Discussion and Assessment

By following the implementation steps detailed in section IV, the proposed enhancement could be well used to provide a restricted access at a content level. The user authorization on the content of the object is defined in the user hierarchy. However, as an extension to the LABAC model, the proposed system eliminates the need of Object-label in the implementation, thus decreasing the overhead of the metadata. The labels are stored in the container metadata as each container would be a homogeneous collection of objects for EHR. In the proposed system, EHRs can be stored as 'application/JSON' or XML objects. Each EHR object is grouped internally into sections according to the staff usage. Each json item or xml item can be labelled with their respective JSONPath and XPath. Each user is assigned a role in which the user-label is stored. The user-label, json-path and the action are together specified in the Label-Policy {'user-label','action','json-path'}. Hence, when the request is made, the Label Policy is validated additionally in the container meta-data and the access to the partial content authorized by the user is returned.

Even though the content level access control is achieved by the model and partial content is delivered to the user, it still faces the challenges. First, there are two different policies stored in the meta data of the Swift object: 1) The label policy defined for the content level access uses the additional user_label and object_label to specify the action between them. For instances, (user-label, action, object-label) and ('Manager', 'read', 'sensitive'); 2) The object_label is the JSON path and it gives the path of each element in the document starting from the root. The second challenge is that the storage of additional labels would be a limitation as anything extra added to the metadata would decrease the performance of the LaBAC implementation which was stated in [6]. In addition, for a homogeneous collection of objects, in case of EHR records of patients, the format in which the records are stored is similar. It would be redundant to store the same labels for each and every object. This would decrease the performance in many ways. Last but not least, the implementation of the model is limited to 'application/json' format. Most of the objects are also stored in the xml format in the cloud.

VI. Conclusion & Future Work

Cloud computing is growing fast in the IT industry. However, many businesses and individuals continue to view cloud computing as a technology that risks exposing their data to unauthorized users [7]. The system would enable the content level partial access to the object depending on the role of the user. This would eliminate the "all or nothing" drawback of the swift storage. When a check is made with the ACL and ACL denies the request, nothing is checked further. But if the ACL accepts the request and declares the user as a valid user, then the content that the user is authorized of is returned. This would enforce the health care providers to access the patient information based on "need to know" and "minimum necessary" principles under the HIPAA guidelines. Although the proposed enhancement to Swift's ACL implementation is promising, the next step of the project is to run an experiment to evaluate the performance of the enhancement of Swift's ACL as a proof of the concept.

References

[1] Wu, R., "*Secure sharing of electronic medical records in cloud computing*," the proceedings of the 8th International Conference on Collaborative Computing: Networking, Applications and Worksharing, Pittsburgh, PA, Oct. 14 -17, 2012

[2] Eichelberg, M., Aden, T., Riesmeier, J., Dogac, A., & Laleci, G. B., "*A survey and analysis of electronic healthcare record standards*," ACM Computing Surveys, 2005, *37*(4), pp. 277-315.

[3] Wu, R., *et.al.*, "*ACaaS: Access Control as a Service for IaaS Cloud,*" the proceedings of the 5th ASE/IEEE International Conference on Information Privacy, Security, Risk and Trust, Washington D.C., Sept. 8 -14, 2013.

[4] Ahn, G. J., Hu, H., Lee, J., & Meng, Y., "*Representing and reasoning about web access control policies*," the proceedings of the 34th IEEE Annual Conference on Computer Software and Applications, Seoul, South Korea, July 19 - 23, 2010 .

[5] Sefraoui, O., Aissaoui, M., & Eleuldj, M., "*OpenStack: toward an open-source solution for cloud computing*," International Journal of Computer Applications, 2012,*55*(3), pp. 38-42.

[6] Biswas, P., Patwa, F., & Sandhu, R., "*Content Level Access Control for OpenStack Swift Storage*," the proceedings of the 5th ACM Conference on Data and Application Security and Privacy, San Antonio, Texas, March 2 - 4, 2015

[7] Paladi, N., Michalas, A., & Gehrmann, C., "*Domain based storage protection with secure access control for the cloud,*" *the proceedings of the 2nd International Workshop on Security in Cloud Computing, Kyoto, Japan, June 3, 2014*

[8] Bates, A., Mood, B., Valafar, M., & Butler, K., "*Towards secure provenance-based access control in cloud environments,*" *the proceedings of the third ACM Conference on Data and Application Security and Privacy, San Antonio, Texas, Feb. 18 - 20, 2013*

[9] Laszewski, G. v., Diaz, J., Wang, F., Fox, G. C., "*Comparison of Multiple Cloud Frameworks*," the proceedings of the 5th IEEE International Conference on Cloud Computing, Honolulu, HI, June 24 - 29, 2012

[10] Department of Health & Human Services (USA), "*HIPAA Administrative Simplification Regulation Text*," March, 2013, pp. 64, last accessed on May 10, 2018, at https://www.hhs.gov/sites/default/files/hipaa-simplification-201303.pdf

[11] OpenStack, *OpenStack Conceptual Architecture*, accessed on May 10, 2018, at https://docs.openstack.org/

[12] Brinckman, A., et.al., "*Computing environments for reproducibility: Capturing the "Whole Tale"*," the Journal of Future Generation Computer Systems, 2018

ISBN: 1-60132-479-0, CSREA Press ©

Using IoT in Emergency Mobile Health Care

Daniela America da Silva, Gildarcio Goncalves Sousa, Samara Cardoso dos Santos, Marcelo Paiva Ramos, Alexandre Nascimento, Johnny Marques, Luiz Alberto Vieira Dias, Adilson Marques da Cunha, Paulo Marcelo Tasinaffo,

Brazilian Aeronautics Institute of Technology, São José dos Campos, São Paulo, Brazil

Abstract - *During the 2nd Semester of 2017, at the Brazilian Aeronautics Institute of Technology (Instituto Tecnológico de Aeronáutica - ITA), a successful Interdisciplinary Problem-Based Learning (IPBL) experience took place. At that time, almost 50 undergrad and graduate students from 4 different courses within just 16 academic weeks had the opportunity of conceptualizing, modeling, and developing a Computer System (software and hardware) involving Patients, Doctors, Hospitals and Suppliers for real-time decision making. The academic research project was named in Portuguese as "Projeto Interdisciplinar de Soluções Tecnológicas Aplicáveis às Mídias e Produtos de Saúde em Tempo Real (STAMPS-TR)", meaning in English "Technological Solutions Applicable for Health Care in Real Time - TSA4HCRT". Unlike other products from Universities, Research Institutes, Government Agencies, or Public and/or Private Enterprises, this product was developed and verified for quality, reliability, safety, and testability in just 16 academic weeks.*

Keywords: health care system; big data; Internet of Things; Agile method and testing; real time; interdisciplinarity.

1 Introduction

This paper tackles the development of an academic project using the Interdisciplinary Problem-Based Learning (IPBL). It has provided the integration of four different courses taught, during the 2nd Semester of 2017, at the Brazilian Aeronautics Institute of Technology (Instituto Tecnológico de Aeronáutica - ITA): CE-230 Software Quality, Reliability, and Safety; CES-65 Embedded Software Systems; CE-235 Real-Time Embedded Systems Project; and CE-237 Advanced Topics in Software Testing.

It describes a practical application of interdisciplinary concepts, by using the agile method [1][2]. This academic project was driven by the ITA to generate expertise on developing, integrating, and managing a real time embedded system applied to the Emergency Mobile Health Care environment [4]. This project was named in Portuguese "Projeto Interdisciplinar de Soluções Tecnológicas Aplicáveis às Mídias e Produtos de Saúde em Tempo Real (STAMPS-TR)", meaning in English "Technological Solutions Applicable for Health Care in Real Time - TSA4HCRT". It considered the development of a Computer System (software and hardware) involving Patients, Doctors, Hospitals, and Suppliers, for real-time decision making, by using agile methods; and software quality, reliability, safety, and testability.

The Scrum agile method and its best practices were used, in order to develop a computer system to satisfy project requirements in a time frame of just 16 academic weeks.The TSA4HCRT project was divided into the following four groups of application: Patients, Physicians, Hospitals, and Suppliers, by sharing its development among the four student teams, which were responsible for the ownership and verification of different functional requirements' definition and application of quality, reliability, safety, and testability.

The TSA4HCRT project was developed by using: the SCADE Suite® (Safety Critical Application Development Environment, from ANSYS Inc. / Esterel Technologies), an Integrated Computer Aided Software Engineering Environment (I-CASE-E); Docker and Python OpenFace from Phyton; Apache Kafka from Apache Software; Lego MindStorms Robot, from Lego; NoSQL databases, from MongoDB, among other technologies. During this collaborative project development, almost 50 students have practiced the roles of Product Owners (POs), Scrum Masters (SMs), and Team Developers (TDs).

At the end of the project, a total of 97 User Stories (USs) had been planned to compose the Product Backlog. However, only 46 of them were developed within 3 monthly sprints, and at the end of each sprint, reviews and retrospective meetings took place. Moreover, the Acceptance Test Driven Development (ATDD) [7] technique was applied generating a minimum, necessary, and sufficient set of artifacts stored within the Internet portal https://sites.google.com/site/stampsacademicorealtime/ [4]. For each User Story (US), more than one test case and acceptance test were developed. The integration strategy between groups of subsystem components was applied using GrayLog, a tool allowing data to be available and accessed from a central location. By using GrayLog, it was possible to display data by segments in dashboards, as shown in Figure 1.

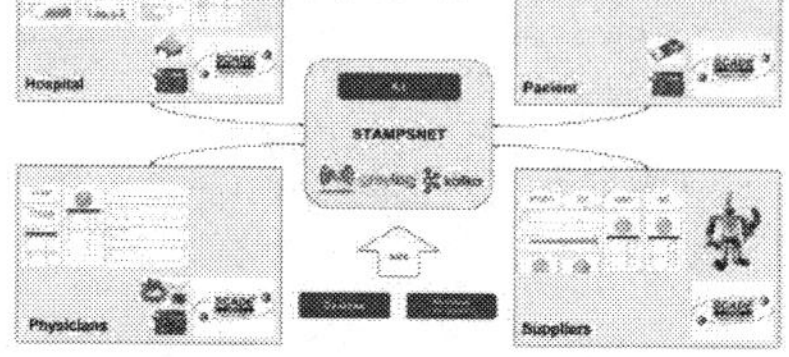

Figure 1. The TSA4HCRT Central Architecture

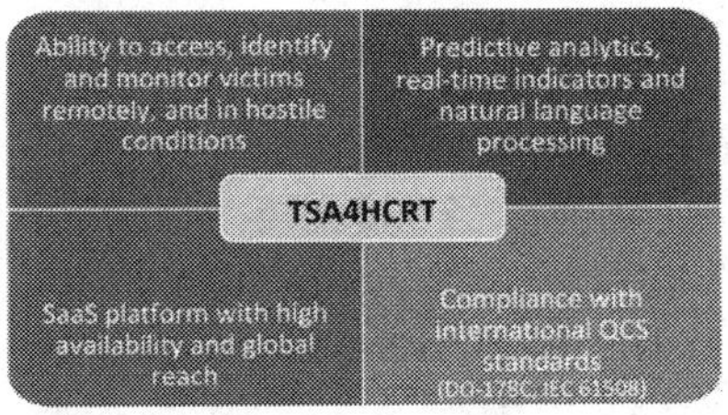

Figure 2. The TSA4HCRT Benefits

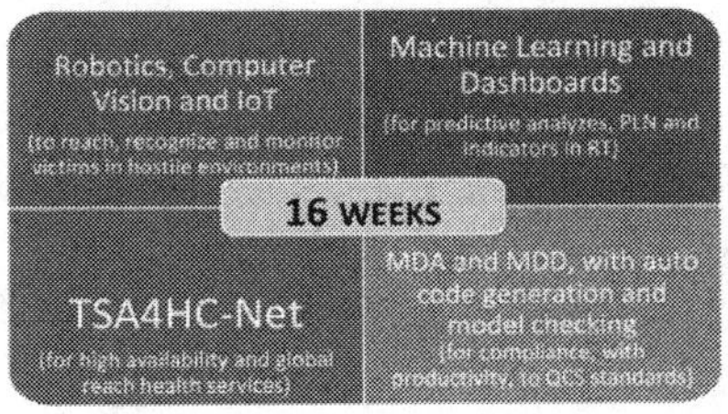

Figure 3. The TSA4HCRT Deliverables Overview

Thus, at the end of this TSA4HCRT academic project, a case study simulated mission was assigned, as a Proof of Concept (PoC), demonstrating it should be able to provide appropriate crises management and control, as described in section IV. The Figure 2 presents the benefits propitiated by the TSA4HCRT project and the Figure 3 presents an overview of the deliverables provided by TSA4HCRT project.

2 Interdisciplinarity

2.1 The Scrum Agile Method and its best practices

The STAMPS Academic Project has involved the following four undergrad and graduate courses:

- CE-230 Software Quality, Reliability, and Safety, involving the understanding of the development of software as process, product, and/or service with quality, reliability, and safety;

- CES-65 Embedded Software Systems and CE-235 Real-Time Embedded Systems Project, involving the understanding of agile development of embedded and real-time software systems, and also the understanding of software as process, product, and/or service; and

- CE-237 Advanced Topics in Software Testing, tackling the main advanced techniques used for software testing.

During this TSA4HCRT academic project development, all students participated as members of Team Developers (TDs). Both CES-65 and CE-235 course students were responsible: for modeling and programming, by using SCADE; and also for evaluating the compliance with other software tools such as Lego for Scrum, Docker, and Python OpenFace libraries. While the CE-237 course students were responsible for the definition and execution of the acceptance testings and its oracles, the CE-230 course students were responsible for validating and delivering intermediate product values with quality, reliability, safety, and testability.

Product Owners (POs) and Scrum Masters (SMs) have offered guidance to teams, trying to correct: the development progress in the event of any delay; the prioritization of the Backlog Product; and also the creation of some Scrum quick guides and videos to facilitate the understanding of the process. Scrum Masters helped teams to define and adhere to the process and to make sure the work was done to the best of students' ability, as shown in Figure 4.

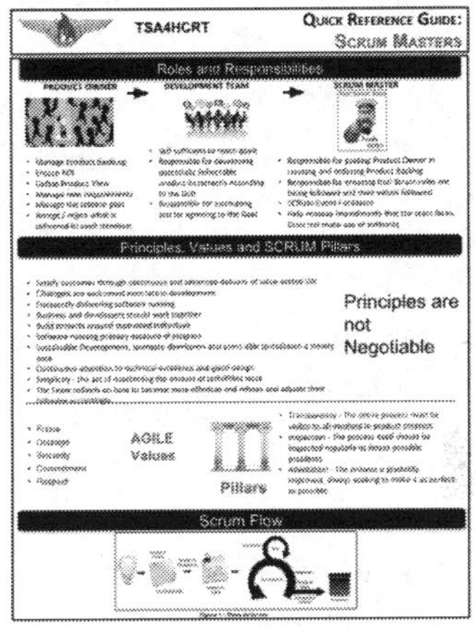

Figure 4. Some Produced TSA4HCRT Scrum Guides and Videos

2.2 The Importance of Internet of Things in Health Care

The Nacional Bank for Social and Economic Development (Banco Nacional de Desenvolvimento Econômico e Social - BNDES) has performed a study about an Action Plan for the Internet of Things in Brazil. This study was conducted by the Mckinsey, the CPqD Foundation, and Pereira Neto Macedo, aiming to conduct a diagnosis and propose some public policies involving Internet of Things in Brazil. This study was organized in 4 phases:

- General diagnosis and aspiration for Brazil;
- Selection of vertical and horizontal;
- Instruction and elaboration of action plan from 2018 up to 2022); and
- Detailing the main initiatives of the action plan.

According to this study, Health Care was considered as the main area with high demand, high development capacity and great supply in Brazil.

Its objective was to accelerate the implementation of the Internet of Things as an instrument for the sustainable development of the Brazilian society, becoming it to be capable of increasing the competitiveness of the economy, strengthening national productive chains, and promoting the improvement of life quality. Specifically in Health Care, the goal is to contribute to the expansion of access to quality health in Brazil through the creation of an integrated vision of patients, decentralization of health care, and improvement of the efficiency of health care units.

On this study, the main strategic objectives in Health Care were focused in 4 areas:

- Chronic Diseases - to improve the effectiveness of people treatment with chronic diseases through continuous monitoring of patients;
- Promotion and Prevention - to prevent risk situations and control the emergence of epidemics and infectious diseases through IoT solutions;
- Management Efficiency - to increase the efficiency of the Brazilian Health Care Unified System (Sistema Unificado de Saúde - SUS), hospitals, and primary health care units, through the adoption of IoT solutions; and
- Innovation - to promote the adoption of locally developed solutions to environmental challenges.

2.3 The Testing Methods

The TSA4HCRT project was developed, by using the TDD (Test Development Driven) technique, with requirements transformed into test cases and the development performed by taking into account specifications of test cases.

On this TSA4HCRT project, intermediate deliverable values of the end product have been validated against these test cases, on each week of each Sprint, through an iterative development process, where requirements evolve through collaboration between development team members, product owners, and stakeholders. Teams were self-organized and have defined problems in advance, differently from conventional methods, when tests usually performed only after implementation, in this new and innovative scenario, tests were performed even before and during the project implementation.

Team developers from the CE-237 Topics in Software Testing discipline have built and tested spreadsheets, performed some tests, and verified results through videos for checking and validating deliveries for each Sprint. Evidences from tests were published together with some test cases.

3 The Proof of Concept (PoC) Demo as an Assigned Mission

3.1 The Assigned Mission

The TSA4HCRT academic project was inspired from the needs of public and/or private organizations involved in crisis management with health events (e.g. huge car accidents), which need to manage data and information for decision making. With that in mind, it was chosen to analyze how to automate the emergency care of the following real accident that happened in Brazil, São Paulo State, in August 2017.

On a regular work day, a major accident involving 36 vehicles and causing fire and death has occurred at the Carvalho Pinto Highway in Jacareí county, SP, around 07:40 pm on August 30, 2017, at KM 75, from São Paulo towards Rio de Laneiro.

The State Highway Police has reported that 36 vehicles were involved in the accident, with 12 cars and two trucks being hit by the flames. At 09:10 am, the fire was extinguished, according to the fire department.

The events that caused the accident occurred in sequence as demonstrated in Table 1.

TABLE 1. THE ACCIDENT SEQUENCE OF EVENTS

Event	Impact
Visibility	Smoke under the bridge, off the road, caused a loss of visibility on the highway;
Visibility	There was a clouding because of the poor visibility;
Collision	A truck that carried paints could not stop and collided with cars already involved in the pile;
Collision	One car collided with another, pressing a car between two trucks;
Collision	Other vehicles also got involved in the piling;
Explosion	An explosion in the paint truck started a major fire; and
Road Blocked	The flames spread among other vehicles, involving a total of 2 trucks and 14 cars burned.

The highway was interdicted in the direction of SP inland and only partially available around 11:45 am of that day. In the afternoon, an on-site survey found that there was no damage to the structure of the viaduct.

Teams from the Highway Concessionary, the Fire Department, and an Eagle Military Police helicopter have participated in the rescue of the victims and the occurrence and aftermath at the scene of the accident.

Among the people (PATIENTS) involved there were helped as per Emergency Care numbers described in Table 2.

TABLE 2. EMERGENCY CARE NUMBERS

Accident Numbers	Details
Death	02 (two) confirmed deaths;
<1 Day in the Hospital	12 (twelve) victims in a light state, rescued in the Holy House of Jacareí, who were discharged on the same day;
1 Day in the Hospital	02 (two) victims, who remained hospitalized in the Municipal Hospital of São José and were discharged the following day;
>1 Day in the Hospital	03 (three) victims, who were hospitalized for more than one day at Vivalle Hospital in São José dos Campos; and
Attended in the local of the Accident	The other victims would have been attended and released at the scene of the accident.

Based upon the previously reported accident, the development of the TSA4HCRT (Technological Solutions Applicable to Means and Health Products in Real Time) project should be able to provide adequate management and control of accidents and/or crises of this type, providing an appropriate management of data and/or information coming from sensors, acting in real time as presented in Table 3.

TABLE 3. EMERGENCY CARE SYSTEM REQUIREMENTS

Segment	Requirements
PATIENT	The first victim(s) (PATIENT) may be appropriately diagnosed or the subsequent patient(s) is(are) readily identified and/or treated(s);
PHYSICIAN	The PHYSICIAN(s) and/or Rescuer(s) have computer tool(s) of the kind involved in the TSA4HCRT Project, which are able to provide preventive and appropriate care such as heart rate measurements, arterial pressure monitoring using a defibrillator, and a cardiopulmonary resuscitation procedure for resuscitation of the victim, among others;
SUPPLIERS	The PHYSICIAN(s) and/or Rescuer(s) have computer tool(s) of the type involved in the TSA4HCTR Project, which are capable of using appropriate technologies to provide efficient screening methods, prioritization of care and HOSPITAL locations for victims' emergency services, according to their criticalities and needs for specialized treatment;
HOSPITAL	HOSPITALS in the region have adequate computational means to collaborate in the process of managing large flows of efficient PATIENTS, using appropriate technologies and efficient emergency screening methods;
SUPPLIERS and HOSPITAL	The Health Units or HOSPITALS involved and their SUPPLIERS of medicines, devices and/or technologies also have appropriate tools to participate in a logistics process and/or supplies used to attend emergencies to victims of accidents or PATIENTS, regardless of where they have occurred;
PATIENT, HOSPITAL and SUPPLIER	Each confirmed case of PATIENT can generate, within the inventory control of a HOSPITAL, the release of care kits containing materials and medications, according to the size of the occurrence. In these cases, in addition to medicines, other supplies can also be considered important, such as blood bags for transfusion, as victims of accidents need quick rescue and accidents kill for blood loss;
HOSPITAL	The population/society has a computer tool of the type System Project involving TSA4HCTR capable of providing appropriate records, management, and controls of restricted and improper access roads; and
HOSPITAL and SUPPLIER	Public administration has reliable data and comprehensive situational awareness for decision making for accidents and/or crises.

3.2 The Proposed IoT and Big Data Solution

The proposed steps for automated system using IoT and Big Data to speed up emergency care is described in table 5.

TABLE 5. THE TSA4HCRT RESPONSE

Segment	Requirements
PATIENT and PHYSICIANS (Predictive Model)	Rescue team receives information about the proportion of the accident (e.g. number of cars involved and patients at the accident site);
PATIENT and PHYSICIANS (Predictive Model)	A predictive model will generate a prediction of the type of trauma and medications, and the size of the rescue team needed to attend to the occurrence. (eg given an accident will have three patients who will need neurosurgery, 3 orthopedists and estimation of blood bag use, estimate number of patients who will need a certain type of examination - radiography, resonance.
PHYSICIAN and SUPPLIERS (Predictive Model)	Based on this prediction the predictive model already activates the hospitals, the suppliers and warns the authorities according to the capacity of attention of the surrounding cities. And also sends a suitable number of first responders to camp.
PATIENT (Voice Command)	In the field, first responders began first aid, checking pulse, and using electrocardiogram when needed, and may also request additional instructions from voice command, based on the state of the victims.
SUPPLIER (Rescue Robot and Face Recognition)	The life-saving robot provides the live stream from the accident site to a remote first aid team to assist the team in the field. And it also initiates the identification of the victim via facial recognition. Once the victim is identified, it is also possible to access the medical history and identify if there is any preexisting disease (for example if the patient is cardiac).
SUPPLIER (Rescue Robot and Face Recognition)	The victim is moved to the ambulance, and transported to the hospital with the capacity to attend to the patient according to the trauma suffered and already with the data of the patient identified by the robot can inform the family and the authorities.
SUPPLIER and HOSPITAL (Drug Cart Robot)	The robot drug cart will be preventively supplied by providers according to the predictive model of the size of the occurrence, and will automatically circulate in the hospital to attend the floors where the patients were received. The supply of the cart will continue according to the queue and the average waiting time and the permanence of the victims in the hospital.
HOSPITAL (Gray Log Dashboard)	During the patient care period, the dashboard will be updated, informing how many victims remain hospitalized and for how long, and how many victims were discharged from the hospital in the course of the day. (important to inform the hospitals X beds in the authorities dashboard)
HOSPITAL (Gray Log Dashboard)	The queue and waiting time inside the hospital are also indicators for another hospital to be activated for care and receiving of the victims - in addition to those that were triggered by a predictive model.
HOSPITAL (Gray Log Dashboard)	The queue and waiting time inside the hospital are also indicators for another hospital to be activated for care and receiving of the victims - in addition to those that were triggered by a predictive model.
PATIENT, PHYSICIANS, HOSPITAL and SUPPLIER (Next Emergency Occurrence)	The team of first responders, the life-saving robot and the remote relief team will be available to attend to a next occurrence after all patients have been admitted to the hospitals taking care of the occurrence.

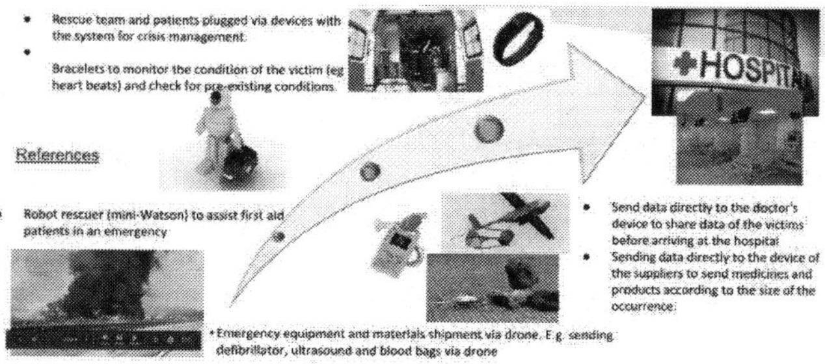

Figure 5. The Product Vision

4 The TSA4HCRT Project Subsystems Structure

The TSA4HCRT Academic project prototype was divided into 4 development teams composed by students from those 4 different courses. Each team with an average of 5 plus or minus 2 students was responsible for choosing and developing specific subsystem components.

In order to satisfy the requirements of the technology applied to mobile midia and health care solutions, in a time frame of just 16 academic weeks, the TSA4HCRT Academic project prototype was also divided into 4 groups of application subsystem components classified according to their high cohesion and low coupling characteristics as PATIENTS, PHYSICIANS, HOSPITALS, and SUPPLIERS.

4.1 The PATIENTS Application Subsystem

Within the PATIENTS Application Subsystem, for the development of the TSA4HCRT Academic Project, and its segments, which needed to integrate data for emergency response, the team Patients was responsible for developing solutions that interact with patients to map trends and potential critical patients. Unlike the other teams, the Patient team aimed to create connectivity technologies and real-time embedded systems to obtain and process patient information, streamlining the initial diagnosis setting, enabling physicians and paramedics to make decisions on the occurrence of disastrous events.

The main deliverable value of the Patient team was to develop a Voice Recognition system that could capture symptoms from Patients and automatically provide to the rescue team a potential list of diagnosis, as shown in Figure 6.

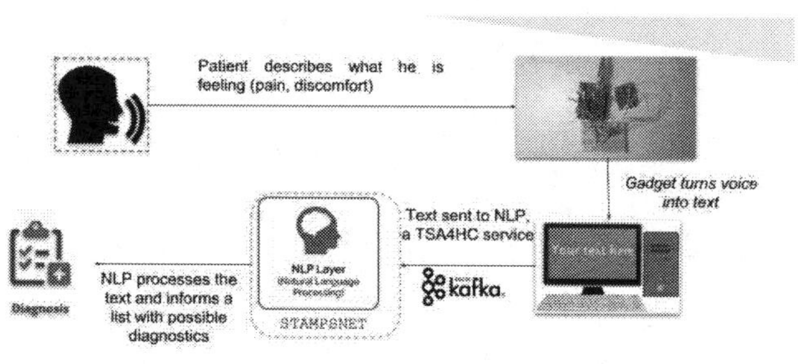

Figure 6. The Voice Recognition Subsystem

4.2 The PHYSICIANS Application Subsystem

Within the PHYSICIANS subsystem, for the development of this TSA4HCRT Academic Project and its segments, which will need to integrate data for emergency response, the Physicians team was responsible for the development of solutions for both life-saving and on-duty physicians.

Unlike other teams, the Physicians team aims to create connectivity technologies, real-time embedded systems, and machine learning, with the guarantee of quality, reliability, safety, and testability, to provide information to physicians and public health managers, so that resources are optimized in the event of disastrous events.

The main deliverable of the Physicians team was to develop a predictive system that could identify required resources based upon initial diagnosis of Patients and required resources in Health Care.

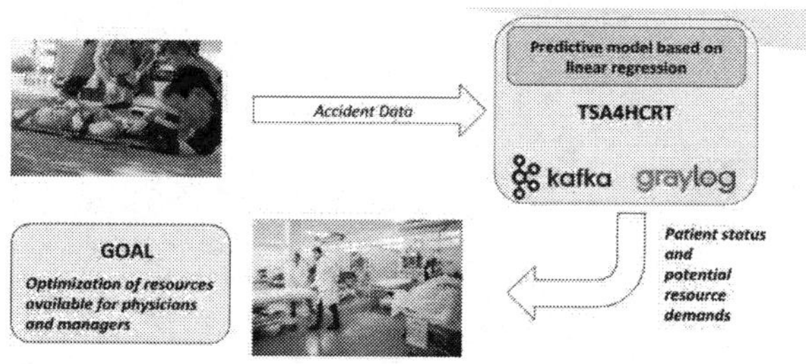

Figure 7. The Physicians Predictive Subsystem

4.3 The HOSPITALS Application Subsystem

For the development of this TSA4HCRT Academic Project and its segments, which will need to integrate data for emergency response, the follow-up of Hospitals was responsible for the study of technologies and the development of solutions, involving the segment of Hospitals and Ambulances.

Unlike other teams, the Hospitals segment was mainly concerned with the management of people, resources, hospital infrastructure, and emergency care (ambulances) in the region, in order to respond to victims in a fast and efficient way, offering advanced monitoring and availability facilities in real time, aiming the attendance in the shortest possible time, providing greater life expectancy and patient safety.

The main deliverable of the Hospitals team was to monitor were the occurrence has happened, get the incident report straight from the local of the emergency, monitor hospital bed occupancy, and patient satisfaction.

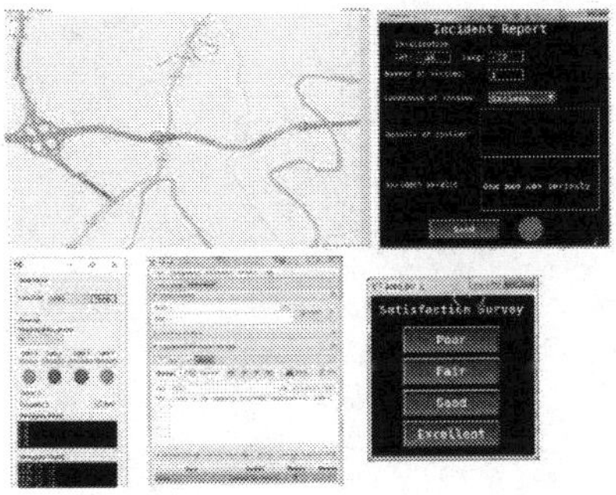

Figure 8. The Hospital Subsystem

4.4 The SUPPLIERS Application Subsystem

For the development of the TSA4HCRT Project and its segments, which will need to integrate data for emergency response, the Supplier Segment was responsible for the study of technologies and the development of its solutions.

Unlike other teams, the Team Scrum 04 was concerned to promptly identify victims served at the scene, through technologies involving robotics, central control of the robot, recognition and facial identification, by using the best practices and cutting-edge technologies, with quality, reliability, safety, and testability, in order to mitigate the incorrect and/or incomplete identification of patients and reduce the occurrence of incidents.

The main deliverable value of the Supplier team was to perform a face recognition, by using a rescue robot in the scene of the accident, and also to propose a framework to connect IoTs in the scene of the accident.

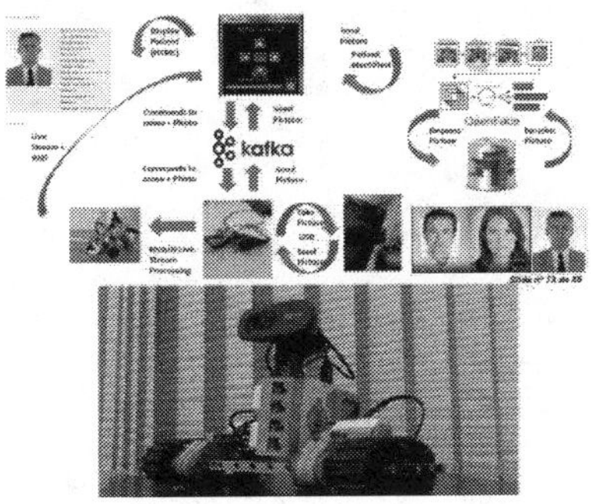

Figure 9. The Supplier Subsystem - Face Recognition using Rescue Robot

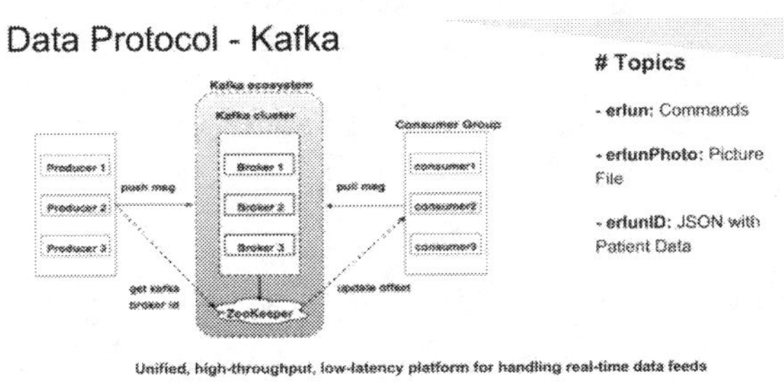

Figure 10. The IoT Framework

5 Conclusions

This paper aimed to describe the development of an academic interdisciplinary project using Scrum agile method and its best practices, in order to develop a prototype for a Proof of Concept (PoC), by using IoT resources.

It has described an Integrated Problem-Based Learning (IPBL) project, named TSA4HCRT Academic Project Prototype, a Computer System based on Big Data, Internet of Things (IoT), and other emerging Information Technologies (ITs) for governmental organization and private sector. The purpose of this system was to aggregate data and integrate sectors such as PATIENTS, HOSPITALS, PHYSICIANS, and HEALTH SUPPLIERS for the decision making process related to crisis management of events in the health system, involving big accidents.

The TSA4HCRT project was developed by students from four different Computer Science courses taught at the Brazilian Aeronautics Institute of Technology (Instituto Tecnológico de Aeronáutica – ITA), on the 2nd semester of 2017.

5.1 Specific Conclusions

The use of interdisciplinarity in 4 courses of Computer Science has worked as expected, since students were able to know how to work in teams to successfully develop a complex computer system. The cloud computing environment has been widely used by students to enable collaborative work from distance, using remote meetings, personal websites, and an official project website.

The Scrum framework has been adapted to the reality of the interdisciplinary academic environment of ITA, helping the entire team of almost 50 students to offer value to stakeholders at the end of each sprint and also at the end of this project.

The application of Test Driven Development (TDD) and Acceptance Testing Driven Development (ATDD) techniques in the project was closely related to the interdisciplinary approach adopted, since acceptance tests were created by CE-237 course students, while the embedded software was implemented by CE-230, CES-65, and CE-235 course students. Kafka, Graylog, and Mosquitto software applications were hosted on the AWS cloud services and represented rhe main tools applied in integrating the services of each subsystem.

The main results obtained from the use of the TSA4HCRT project prototype were successful. Its operating logic was established and all teams were able to perform development integration, by defining and accomplishing the phases of the Assigned Mission, mapping User Stories to functionalities for each segment needing integration with other segments, which variables and detailed characteristics would be changed as inputs and/or outputs.

At the end of this project, in just 16 weeks, it was possible to demonstrate the building of the Interdisciplinary Project TSA4HCRT, without completeness, but following a model with quality, reliability, safety, and testability, following norms and standards applicable to a product of this nature.

Finally, students have presented the TSA4HCRT Academic Project Prototype, as the final project for their courses, as a Proof of Concept (PoC) to professors, entrepreneurs, and some invited guests from industry and academia.

5.2 General Conclusions

The academic development of a critical intelligent system is a rewarding experience that can be used in different undergrad and graduate courses. The use of interdisciplinarity, cloud computing, SCADE programming for an embedded system, and agile methods seems to be an interesting novel and exciting way to achieve academic goals, in just one semester of 16 weeks and can also be extended to other knowledge domains.

It is possible to integrate products generated with SCADE, from different teams, with different technologies, from a minimal organization between teams, defining intervening variables to be exchanged between each of them, from collective planning among all involved.

This integration can be extended to other devices, running on different machines or even on their own control devices shown from its Project Technical Architecture.

5.3 Recommendations

It is strongly recommended the use of automated testing tools and procedures to speed up the development process, increasing product quality. Automation testing tools that use Python can be also used, as they provide some automation of testing, but there was no time for students to fully utilize this in the Scrum Team 4.

It is recommended to continue this Project, starting from what has already been possible to obtain and execute, with the next classes, new Sprints, generating the possibility of increasing completeness. It is also recommended to take a closer approach to hardware in conjunction with SCADE, and use more sensors to prevent and or to attend accidents and crises patients.

For the next year, it is also recommended to hold SCADE detailed Courses and/or Lectures with some representatives from ANSYS/Esterel Technologies in Brazil involving some SCADE Environment Specialists.

5.4 Future Work

It is suggested that the process used in this TSA4HCRT academic project prototype can be extended to other embedded systems projects and predictive systems, in order to improve estimation of efforts and resources to attend an emergency. It is also suggested the use of some simulation processes to measure emergency care with and without the use of technology supports of health management.

Finally, for future work, it is suggested to expand some cooperation among the ITA, hospitals, innovation foundations, medical suppliers, industries and public and private enterprises, in order to get a selection of academic projects aligned to updated needs from the market.

6 Acknowledgement

The authors would like to thank the Esterel Technologies, a subsidiary of ANSYS Inc., the Brazilian Aeronautics Institute of Technology, and The Casimiro Montenegro Filho Foundation (FCMF) for their support, during the development of this TSA4HCRT Project.

7 References

[1] Sutherland J., 2010, SCRUM Handbook, Scrum Training Institute Press.
[2] Cohen D., et al., 2004, An Introduction to Agile Methods, Fraunhofer Center for Experimental Software Engineering, ADVANCES IN COMPUTERS, VOL. 62.
[3] STAMPS, 2017, Technological Solutions Applicable to Medias and Products in Health, https://sites.google.com/site/stampsacademicorealtime/
[4] RTCA. Software Considerations in Airbone Systems and Equipment Certification: DO-178C. Washington D.C. 2011.
[5] JORGENSEN, P. C. "Software Testing - A Craftsman's Approach". 4th Edition. Boca Ratin, FL: CRC Press, 2014.
[6] SCADE SUITE. Technical Data Sheet. SCADE Suite R18. Available in http://goo.gl/ED54Ua, acessado em 01/agosto/2017
[7] BNDES,2017, IoT Um plano de ação para o Brasil, acessed in Maio 2018, available in https://www.bndes.gov.br/wps/portal/site/home/conhecimento/estudos/chamada-publica-internet-coisas/estudo-internet-das-coisas-um-plano-de-acao-para-o-brasil
[8]LEGO Mindstorms. Available: http://mindstorms.lego.com, access in August, 16th 2013.
[9] Shaw A., 2001, Real-Time Systems and Software, New York.
[10] Andrea J., 2010, Acceptance Test-Driven Development: Not as Optional as You Think, Available: http://www.agileconnection.com/article/acceptancetest-driven-development-not-optional-you-think, access in June, 06th 2014.
[11] Crispin L, Gregory J., 2009, Agile Testing: A Practical Guide for Testers and Agile Teams, Addison-Wesley, Pearson Education, Inc.
[12] Copeland L., 2004, A Practioner's Guide to Software Testing Design, Arctech House.
[13] Cohn M., 2010, Succeeding with agile: Software development using Scrum, 1st Edition, Pearson Education, Inc.
[14] Leandog, 2012, Agile Discussion Guide, Version 3.1, Cleaveland, Ohio.
[15] Schwaber K., Sutherland J., 2013, The Scrum Guide. Available: https://www.scrum.org/scrumguide, access in March, 07th, 2014.
[16] Jell, T., 2018, BigIOT Overview and NG Use Case, Available in http://big-iot.eu/f

A Study of Evidence-Based Practice Level, Knowledge and Implementation amongst Health Care Practitioners in Riyadh City Hospitals

Deena M. Barakah; DDS, M.Sc.; Registrar HI and
Dental Clinic Department, King Saud Medical City, Ministry of Health, Riyadh, Saudi Arabia
Email: drbarakah@ksmc.med.sa

Haifa M. A. Barakah;
BDS, M.Sc.; Registrar RDS
College Of Dentistry, King Saud University,
Riyadh , Saudi Arabia
Email: hbarakah@ksu.edu.sa

Reem S Alwakeel
Senior dental student ,College of Dentistry ,
King Saud Bin Abdulaziz University ,
Riyadh, Saudi Arabia
Email: alwakeel519@ksau-hs.edu.sa

Abstract— **Evidence-based practice (EBP) requires physicians, dentists and health care practitioners to investigate , value and incorporate research literature with clinical experience and patient' perspectives. EBP is expected to creates a new decision-making approach and policies that positively impact all fields of healthcare and clinical domain.**

Currently, few studies were carried out about EBP at Saudi hospitals and medical and dental staff attitudes to EBP. Little is known about their awareness and implementation levels of EBP , existing and available resources to them for implementing EBP in their daily practice at their hospitals.

In this research, we present early results of our study for levels of awareness , knowledge of EBP, and Level of practice and implementation of EBP at two dental Saudi hospitals namely: King Saud Medical City dental hospital and college of dentistry hospital at King Saud university in Riyadh, Saudi Arabia

A questionnaire was developed and distributed for seeking information about EBP issues among medical staff of this research study. The findings of this study show that using EBP approach in Clinical tasks context has an overall average equals to 61.1% of all participants. Awareness about "evidence-based dentistry and medicine is relatively reasonable, as about (56.8%) agreed that they have good understanding of it.

Index Terms— ***Evidence based practice in clinical practice, Evidence based practice in Saudi health System.***

I. INTRODUCTION

In today modern hospitals, the concept of evidence-based practice (EBP) is becoming more and more important in dental and medical clinical practice. EBP strengths the coordination between the current research outcomes, information and communication technologies along with clinical practice , patients needs to quality improve health-care decisions[1-4]. EBP gives higher weight for new and better treatments or results and new IT based tools in deciding the rejection of ineffective treatments. The EBP aim is to develop advanced dental and medical profession, to achieve better patient care, to produce new health policies and a reduced health care cost [4,5].

Historically, the "evidence-based" term was first mentioned in Canada in 1992 , by a clinical group at McMaster University[6] . Later on , this expression were widely used in dental and medical resources , journals, curriculums , books , and practice and research centers located in different universities and countries [7-11]. In dental practice in particular , the American Dental Association (ADA) and other academic and research organization stressed and supported heavily the incorporation of EBP into dentistry clinical practice in the United States, and the development of evidence-based dentistry [10-13]. Other similar studies of EBP were carried in many other countries for EBP enhancements [14-17].

Few research studies have been carried out in Saudi Arabia for EBP awareness and perception. A study that aims to assess nurses' knowledge/skills and attitude about evidence based practice in King Khalid Eye Specialist Hospital (KKESH) and King Faisal Specialist Hospital Research Centre (KFSCRC) was carried in 2009 [18]. Another study was performed to investigate the knowledge, attitude, and barriers using evidence based practice (EBP) by dental and medical final year students and new graduates at King Abdulaziz University, Jeddah, Saudi Arabia during the 2012 to 2013 academic year [19].

Reference [20] present an early research study conducted to assess the perception and attitude of dental students at King Saud University, Riyadh, Saudi Arabia.

The research of this paper is therefore one study of a collection of a larger research project studies accomplished to explore the awareness and implementation levels of EBP by Saudi dentists , physicians and healthcare practitioners at major Saudi Hospitals.

II. RESEARCH STUDY SETTING

King Saud Medical City is ranked as tertiary-care hospitals for and surgery and medicine and is located in Riyadh, Saudi Arabia. It consists of several medical centers and three major hospitals namely: Dental hospital and center ; General Hospital, Obstetrics and Gynecology hospital and a Pediatrics hospital. KSMC other centers include: Spinal and Neurosurgery and Dialysis Centers. Work force size of KSMC is 1412 health care practitioners and bed capacity is 140 intensive-care unit beds and 1473 ward beds[21].

College of Dentistry at King Saud university is the first university-based dental training institution in Saudi Arabia. The College mission is to develop competent dental professionals and contribute to research and community service; through an environment that stimulates acquisition, dissemination and production of oral health knowledge, adopting technology, and building local and international partnerships. Most recently a new dental hospital was added to the college facilities for tremendously training of male and female dentists and providing dental care for Riyadh city residents [22].

III. Participants, Research Data Management and Mythology

A questionnaire was developed and distributed for seeking information about EBP issues among medical and dental staff of this research study. The questionnaire was distributed to physicians , dentists , pharmacists , interim medical students and health care employees to get their feedback. Each participant is asked to fill out the questionnaire indicating his or her agreement of disagreement with each statement, mostly on a Likert-type scale.

Our study was carried out in Riyadh, Saudi Arabia at two dental hospitals namely: King Saud Medical City (KSMC) dental hospital and college of dentistry hospital at King Saud University (KSU). The survey questionnaire instrument consisted of four parts, with questions about (1) Personal , Socio-Demographic & Educational Information, (2) Levels of Awareness and Knowledge of Evidence Based Dentistry & Medicine (EBP) (3) Level of practice and Implementation of Evidence Based Dentistry& Medicine (EBP) for Clinical Tasks and Practice (4) Barriers to Evidence Based Dentistry & Medicine (EBP). The questionnaire was organized in a multitude format with two to five choices including yes/no questions or 2-to 5-point Likert scales.

Two hundred participants of the study were selected in 2017. A total of 95 participants completed the questionnaire. The demographic distribution of the study sample participants was 63 (66.3 %) male , 32 (33.7%) female. Majority of participants were Saudi nationals (81.1%). Age group ranges were from below 25 (27.4%) years old up to above 50 years (5.3%). Two third of participants were from KSMC ,while about one third from KSU. The respondents' experience varied from less than 2 years (43.2%) to more than 10 years (29.5%) , and has various rank positions (e.g. internship and post graduate trainees, dental assistant, general practitioner, dental and medical consultants) reflecting the population from which the sample was drawn. The majority of participations were General practitioners (9.5%) , Prosthodontist (9.5%) , Endodontic (8.5%) ; Restorative Dentist (7.4%) ; Dermatologist (6.3%), Medical surgeon (5.3%) ,and undergraduate students at college of dentistry (5.3 %). Regarding job title : 31.6 % were specialists , 27.4% consultants , 16.8% residents , 9.5 % internship and 7.2 % dental students.

The collected questionnaire data was processed and went through various analysis using Google Forms. Future work will include subsequent analysis using the Statistical Package for Social Sciences software(SPSS).

IV. Major Statistical Results

In what follows we present major research results (as obtained from the statistical analysis of questionnaire responses):

- **Awareness about the term "evidence-based dentistry& Medicine"**
  - Good understanding 56.8%
  - Have a vague idea 36.8%
  - No idea 6.3 %
- **Period length of knowing about EBP**
  - < 2 years (72.6%)
  - 2-5 years (12.6%)
  - 5-10 years (8.4%)
  - > 10 years (6.3%)
- **Ways of knowing about EBP**

  Ways of knowing about EBP include: Reading a book about EBP (14.7%) , Reading Journal article about EBP (24.2%) , Attending a lecture about EBP (48.4%) , Attending a workshop about EBP(6.3%) , From friends (2.1%) , Part of our practice and training in the hospital (1.15%) .

- **Level Rank of understanding of the concept of EBP**
  - Poor 18.9 %
  - Fair 34.2 %
  - Good 43.2% %

- **Level of knowledge of a selection of EBDM tools**

  Fig. 1. shows the knowledge level for selection of various EBP tools. These include : EBDM tool , P-value , Relative risk , Sensitivity , Meta-analysis , Odds ratio . Publication bias , Confidence interval , Systematic Review , Randomization Heterogeneity, Blinding , Likelihood Ratio Specificity , and Absolute Risk.

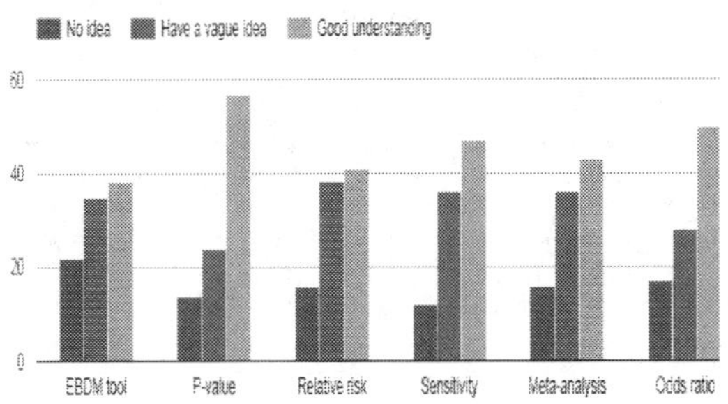

Fig. 1.a knowledge level of a selection of various EBP tools

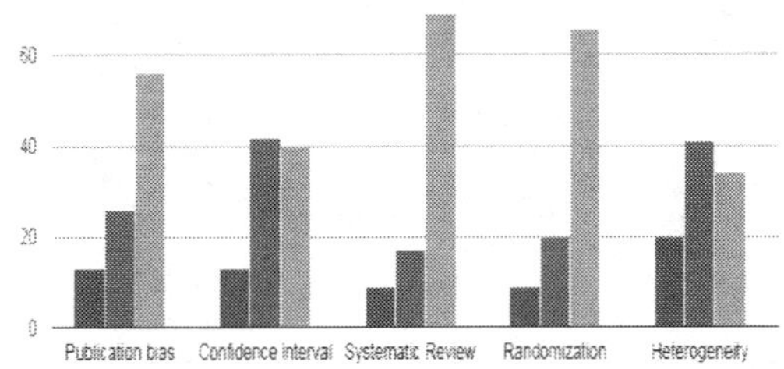

Fig. 1.b knowledge level of a selection of various EBP tools

.

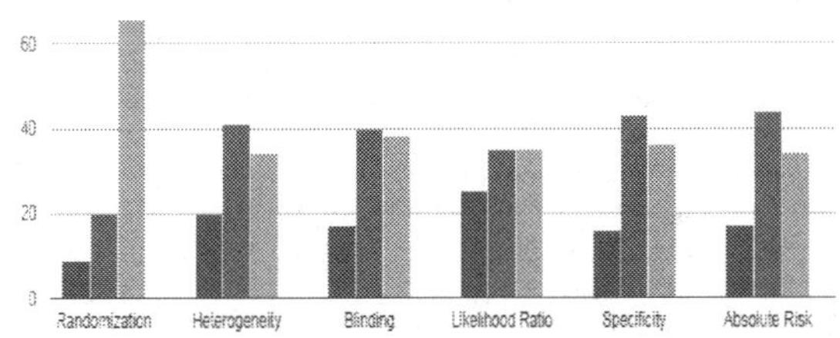

Fig. 1.c knowledge level of a selection of EBP tools .

- **Level of applying the EBP approach in daily practice**
  - +ve answer (Yes) 61.1 %
  - –ve answer (No) (38.9%)
- **Extent of practice of EBP**
  - Almost always (5.3%)
  - Most of the time (18.9 %)
  - Sometimes (35.8%)
  - Rarely (40 %)
- **Attitude towards EBP**
  - potential to improve health care outcome. (Agree 94.7 %)
  - willing to attend workshops/courses on EBDM (Agree 93.7 %)
  - support implementing EBDM in my working place (Agree 95.8%)
- **Main Barriers to Evidence Based Dentistry & Medicine (EBP) Agreement Level**
  - Lack of training (89.3 %)
  - Lack of access to EPB resources (90%)
  - Difficulty of EBP concepts (72%)
  - Resistance to change (68.4 %)
  - Lack of EBP skills (53.6%)
  - Availability of the evidence (73.6%)
  - Access to Internet in work environment (78.9%)
  - Lack of wireless Net connectivity during patient treatment (81.1%)
  - Lack of personal computing in work place (74.7%)

V. Discussion of Findings

The findings of this study show that using EBP approach in Clinical tasks context has an overall average equals to 61.1% of all participants. When comparing the extent of practice of EBP, the highest average rate for EBP usage was for rarely (40%). A relatively low percentage of participants (5.3%) reported that they use EBP almost always. Awareness about "evidence-based dentistry& Medicine" is relatively reasonable as about (56.8%) agreed that they have good understanding of it. Also , there was reasonable Level of understanding of the concept of EBP with 77.4 % of participants has good or fair understanding of EBP

Other statistics about IT tools availability at work place for access to EBP resources shows that lack of such tools is main barrier to applying EBP , as lack of Access to Internet (78.9%) , lack of wireless Net connectivity during patient treatment (81.1%) and lack of personal computing in work place (74.7%) were among major barriers.

Based on the above, it can be deduced that providing more EBP resources , training and IT tools at work places (e.g. wireless Internet) are however needed to increase the practice and awareness about EBP for enhancing medical knowledge and patients treatment.

VI. Conclusions And Future Work

This research study at King Saud Medical City and college of dentistry hospital at King Saud university in Riyadh, Saudi Arabia, addressed the assessment of the awareness , perceptions and practice of EBP amongst medical and healthcare providers at these hospitals. Results of this research is early results obtained and will be followed by extensive study through subsequent analysis using the SPSS software. Such study is very important and essential in an age of rapid IT technological development and new advances in medicine. It produces a clear understanding of medical staff and health care practitioners perceptions of EBP, related resources and needs necessary to develop a successful implementation of EBP in King Saud medical city (KSMC) and other Saudi hospitals. This research results will generate various recommendations for using EBP for improving the quality of medical education, research , patient treatment and health care services at KSMC and other Riyadh City hospitals.

ACKNOWLEDGMENT

This work was supported by King Saud Medical City Research Center, Ministry of health , Riyadh , Saudi Arabia. The authors would like to thank the KSMC and research center officials for their support. Also, the authors would also like to thanks Prof. Sami Alwakeel at King Saud University for his valuable comments and suggestions throughout the work of this research.

REFERENCES

[1] Kitto S, Grant R. Revisiting evidence-based checklists: interprofessionalism, safety culture and collective competence. J Interprof Care 2014; 14: 1-3.

[2] Sackett DL, Rosenberg WM, Gray JA, Haynes RB, Richardson WS. Evidence based medicine: what it is and what it isn't. BMJ 1996; 312: 71-72.

[3] Coleman P, Nicholl J. Influence of evidence-based guidance on health policy and clinical practice in England. Qual Health Care 2001; 10: 229-237.

[4] Ubbink DT, Guyatt GH, Vermeulen H. Framework of policy recommendations for implementation of evidence-based practice: a systematic scooping review. BMJ Open 2013; 24: 3.

[5] Clarkson J, Harrison JE, Ismail AI, Needleman I, Worthington H. Evidence based dentistry for effective practice. London (UK): Martin Dunitz Publishers; 2003.

[6] Evidence-Based Medicine Working Group. Evidence based medicine. JAMA 1992; 268: 2420-2425.

[7] Institute of Medicine. Crossing the quality chasm: A new health system for the 21st century: Washington (DC): National Academy Press; 2001.

[8] White B. Making evidence-based medicine doable in everyday practice. Fam Pract Manag 2004; 11: 51-58.

[9] Rabb-Waytowich D. You ask, we answer: Evidence-based dentistry: Part 1. an over-view. J Can Dent Assoc 2009; 75: 27-28.

[10] ADA Center for Evidence-Based Dentistry. Data Base of Systematic Reviews from: http://ebd.ada.org.

[11] Lang LA, Teich ST. A critical appraisal of evidence-based dentistry: The best available evidence. J Prosthet Dent 2014; 111: 485-492.

[12] Winning T, Needleman I, Rohlin M, et al. Evidence-based care and the curriculum. Eur J Dent Educ 2008; 12(Suppl. 1): 48-63.

[13] Cheryl L. Straub-Morarend; Teresa A. Marshall; David C. Holmes; Michael W. Finkelstein. Toward Defining Dentists' Evidence-Based Practice: Influence of Decade of Dental School Graduation and Scope of Practice on Implementation and Perceived Obstacles, Journal of Dental Education 2013; 77(2): 137-45.

[14] Aitken LM, Hackwood B, Crouch S, Clayton S, West N, Carney D, et al. Creating an environment to implement and sustain evidence based practice: A developmental process. Aust Crit Care 2011; 24: 244-254.

[15] Syed Muzzami , Ali Salah , Khawaja Muhammad Saquib, Syed Ahmed Omar , Daud Mirza , Ameer Ali ; Awareness , knoweldge , & Practice of Evidence Based Dentistry Amongest Dentist in Karachi ; Pakistan Oral & Dental Journal Vol 35, No. 2 ;June 2015.

[16] Nermin Yamalik, Secil Karakoca Nemli, Eunice Carrilho, Simona Dianiskova, Paulo Melo, Anna Lella, Joel Trouillet and Vladimer Margvelashvili. Implementation of evidence-based dentistry into practice: analysis of awareness, perceptions and attitudes of dentists in the World Dental Federation–European Regional Organization zone through a multicentre questionnaire, International Dental Journal 2015; 10: 121-26.

[17] Rabe P1, Holmén A, Sjögren P. ; Attitudes, awareness and perceptions on evidence based dentistry and scientific publications among dental professionals in the county of Halland, Sweden: a questionnaire survey.; Swedeen Dent J. 2007;31(3):113-20.

[18] Olfat A . Salem; Aishah Alamrani and Monirah M Alblouchi Knowledge, Practice and Attitude of Evidence Based Practice Among Nurses in Kingdom of Saudi Arabia; Med. J. Cairo Univ., Vol. 77, No. 2, September: 121-128, 2009

[19] Maha A. Bahammam, , Amal I. Linjawi, Knowledge, attitude, and barriers towards the use of evidence based practice among senior dental and medical students in western Saudi Arabia; Saudi Med J; Vol. 35 (10); 2014

[20] Fedorowicz Z, Almas K, Keenan J. Perceptions and attitudes towards the use of evidence based dentistry (EBD) among final year students and interns at King Saud University, College of Dentistry in Riyadh Saudi Arabia. Brazilian Journal Of Oral Sciences 2004; 3: 470-474.

[21] King Saud Medical City Web site: URL : https://www.ksmc.med.sa/en/pages/default.aspx Accessed April 15, 2018.

[22] King Saud University,College of Dentistry Web site: URL http://dent.ksu.edu.sa/en Accessed April 15, 2018.

Deena M. Barakah has a Master's of Science degree in Health informatics, from King Saud bin Abdulaziz University for Health Sciences , Riyadh , Saudi Arabia and a Bachelor's of Science degree in Dental Medicine & Surgery, from Dentistry College, at Damascus University.

She is currently working as a Dentist and Dental Informatics Specialist at King Saud Medical City (KSMC) , Riyadh , Saudi Arabia. Previously she was the head of Dental Department at Children Hospital in King Fahd Medical City and at Sulimina Children Hospital , Riyadh, Saudi Arabia.

Dr. Deena is an author for several journal and conferences articles on health Informatics and a co-author for a chapter in a book titled" Handbook of Medical and Healthcare Technologies "published by Springer.

Dr. Deena Barakah is a Licensed Dentist, Health Informatics Register , by the Saudi Commission for Health Specialties and a member of the Saudi Health informatics society.

Haifa M. A. Barakah; has a Bachelor's of Science degree in Dental Medicine & Surgery from Dentistry College, a Master's of Science degree in dentistry , and holds the Saudi board in Restorative Dentistry (RDS). She is currently working as a lecturer in college of dentistry at King Saud University (KSU) , Riyadh , Saudi Arabia.

Reem Sami Alwakeel, a senior dental student at King Saud bin Abdulaziz University for Health Sciences, College of Dentistry, Riyadh, Saudi Arabia. She has previously published a paper in an international journal and several poster presentations at National Saudi conferences. She is currently working in applying an orthodontic postgraduate program. The author has attended multiple medical education programs. In addition, the author has participated in multiple extra-curricular activities.

Using Twitter Stream Data for Real-time Influenza-Like Illness Detection and Prediction

Dan Li
Department of Computer Science
Eastern Washington University
Cheney, WA, U.S.A.

Abstract - *Flu represents a significant public health problem that affects millions of Americans and is associated with hospitalizations and deaths in people of all ages every year in the United States. Early insights into the timing and intensity of the flu season could be very useful to public health agencies for vaccination campaigns, communicating to the public, allocating resources, and implementing strategies to combat the spread of flu disease. Since Twitter data have accurate time and location information, real-time information from tweets has become a popular source of public health information. In addition to tracking the outbreaks of disease, the spatio-temporal Twitter data can also be used to get ahead of the curve and predict where and when illnesses will spread. This research targets at this goal to build a real-time health informatics system to provide invaluable information for public health agencies. The proposed system has two major components. The first one is to identify influenza-like illness (ILI) related tweets efficiently and accurately using a combination of lexicon-based approaches and machine learning approaches; the second component uses visualization techniques to provide a real-time map of disease outbreaks. In addition, it predicts the occurrences and the spread of the illnesses in both geographical and temporal dimensions.*

Keywords: Influenza-Like Illness; Twitter Stream; Real-time; Spatial and Temporal Prediction; Health Informatics.

1 Introduction

With the advent of social media, social data have become an important source of insight into the activities and events around the world. Websites like Facebook, Twitter, LinkedIn, and many others hold vast quantities of information about the people using them. Such data can be used to track and predict social trends, map relationships between users, analyze public opinions, and make product recommendations. Recently, there have been increasing interests in monitoring and predicting disease outbreaks using searches and social media data. One of the earliest examples was Google Flu Trends, which began offering real-time data to the public in 2008 [5]. Based on people's Internet searches for flu-related terms, this tool monitored flu outbreaks and provided data nearly as precise as the data from Centers for Disease Control and Prevention (CDC) while having the advantage of being one to two weeks faster. However, Google discontinued this tool in 2015 due to its lack of accuracy in estimation. Since Twitter can provide more contextual information than search queries, it has become a favorite social media source for monitoring the spreads of infectious disease.

2 Related Work

Initial work in this direction has been presented in [3, 8, 13, 14, 15]. Traditional supervised learning algorithms are commonly used to identify disease-related tweets from Twitter. For instance, a Support Vector Machine (SVM) based regression approach is adopted to determine the relative contribution of each tweet [15]. It produces a non-linear model that minimizes a pre-defined cost function. Each input tweet is described as a collection of values on a known set of variables or features where the feature set is defined from a collection of terms in the dictionary generated from all tweets. Similarly, a binary predictive model using SVM is created to identify flu-like tweets in [14]. It further predicts the health state of any individual by leveraging the interplay of location and friendship information obtained from Twitter. Another regression-based model is built in [8]. It uses a keyword-based approach to compute a weighed flu-score from Twitter corpus, and the selected features are then used in a linear regression model to determine the relevance in tweets. Since keyword-based approach is prone to overfitting when too many keywords are added, it is necessary to use a greater number of high quality training data to obtain more reliable result from keyword selection [3]. A semi-supervised cascade learning approach is introduced to improve the quality of such learning models [18]. In addition to machine learning approaches, there exist other works using lexicon-based approaches to enhance the tracking of ILI messages from Twitter [2, 4].

While there has been quite a bit of work on tweet analysis to detect or predict prevalence of infectious disease, there has been limited work on methods for real-time analysis integrating both geographical and temporal information from tweets [18]. Real-time analytics challenges the traditional architecture and methods and is complicated in its design and delivery because traditional data analytics collection and analysis usually requires long periods of time to complete. To build effective real-time big data applications, several challenges need to be addressed including real-time data transfer, real-time analytics, and real-time representation of knowledge. This project aims to develop a health informatics system that (1) uses efficient steaming techniques for Twitter data collection and storage, (2) accurately detects tweets related to influenza-like illnesses (ILI), (3) constructs a high-performance architecture for real-time spatio-temporal data analysis, and (4) provides data visualization interface to help interpret the results.

3 Methodologies

Figure 1 shows the basic architecture of the proposed system. It consists of two modules: (1) batch data preprocessing and learning, and (2) real-time data visualization and prediction. The first module aims at collecting an expanded set of tweets using Twitter's new streaming Application Programming Interface (API) with the intent of accurately identifying ILI tweets. The second module targets at efficient processing of data and providing real-time visualization and prediction of disease outbreaks.

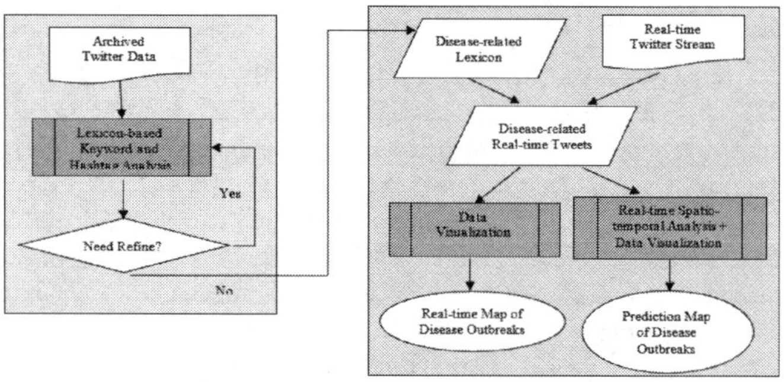

Figure 1. System Architecture

3.1 Identifying ILI Tweets

There exist two categories of approaches for detecting influenza-like illness (ILI) messages from Twitter data, lexicon-based approaches and machine learning approaches. In lexicon-based approaches, a Twitter message is represented as a bag of keywords. Following this representation of message, we need to decide if a given tweet is a disease-related message [7].

In original lexicon-based approaches, a small set of disease-related keywords is collected manually as an initial seed. Well-known dictionaries are then used to expand the set of keywords by adding their synonyms and antonyms [12]. Such dictionary-based approaches are not able to find words that are domain specific. Corpus-based lexicon approaches overcome this limitation by finding syntactic or co-occurrence phrases and patterns from a large domain-specific corpus. Both dictionary and corpus based approaches need to count on domain experts to identify a set of words to begin with. We plan to use a set of ILI related keywords and phrases developed in [4] as initial seed and further refine it by incorporating rich semantic information contained in Twitter messages such as negation, intensification, hashtags, and emoji. As discussed in Section 2, keyword-based approaches are prone to overfitting when too many keywords are added. To overcome this, we combine lexicon-based approaches with machine learning approaches to refine the result.

Machine learning approaches use supervised learning methods such as Naïve Bayes, Neural Networks, and Support Vector Machines to build a predictive model from a large training corpus of annotated data. Such predictive model is later used on unannotated data to determine if a given tweet is an ILI message. Two main challenges need to be addressed in machine learning approaches. The first one is to construct a large collection of high quality annotated training corpus. To obtain such a dataset, we have already started collecting Twitter messages by using Twitter's publically available streaming API. Since our ultimate goal is to provide real-time visualization of disease outbreaks, we apply various filtering strategies to target at the tweets that have geo-location information. In addition, we use a subset of data published in [11] which included the messages gathered between 2009 and 2010 through a combination of queries to Twitter's public search API as well as messages obtained from the *Gardenhose* stream, a sample of all public Twitter messages.

The second challenge in identifying ILI messages using machine learning approaches lies in the intrinsic imbalanced characteristic of datasets, as the majority of Twitter massages are not relevant to influenza-like illnesses. Standard machine learning algorithms tend to produce unsatisfactory results when dealing with imbalanced datasets [10]. To overcome this, we plan to build multiple learning models from existing Twitter data and a weighted ensemble model will be constructed to ensure high quality of learning model.

3.2 Real-time Visualization and Prediction of ILI

The second module in the proposed health informatics system targets at efficient processing of Twitter steam data to provide real-time visualization and prediction of disease outbreaks.

3.2.1 Real-time Visualization

Stream data are arriving continuously in high speed and large volume; therefore, unlike traditional data analysis solutions, it is infeasible to re-scan or even perform a multi-scan of the entire database. A single scan of data is essential and necessary for data stream analysis. In addition, the unbounded feature of data streams makes it challenging to utilize limited memory storage to discovery dynamic patterns efficiently and effectively. To ensure real-time stream data processing, we build the system on a Hadoop Distributed File System (HDFS) for high-performance parallel processing.

Since Twitter messages potentially include geo-location information, this provides us the capability to visualize the outbreaks of ILI in real-time. Tableau has gained popularity recently due to its simple, drag and drop based user interface. It allows easy transfer of data to or from popular file formats and the user can draw up charts and histograms of varying complexities as and when needed [17]. Figure 2 is a sample map generated by Tableau which depicts a County View Health Index from the healthiest to the least healthy counties. The proposed health informatics system uses Tableau as an interactive data visualization tool.

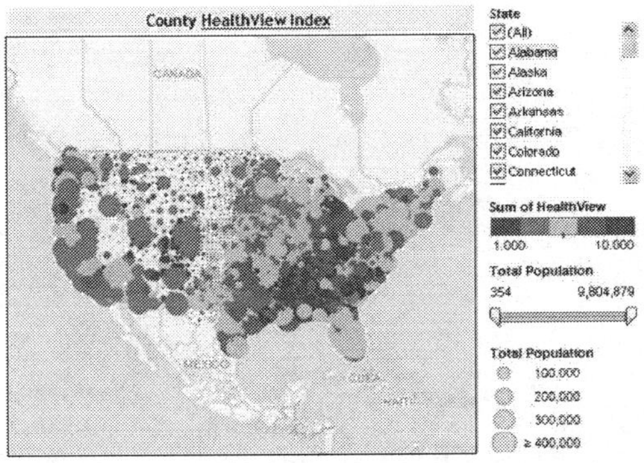

Figure 2. A sample map generated by Tableau [Image Credit: https://public.tableau.com/s/]

3.2.2 ILI Prediction

Besides tracking the current status of disease outbreaks, it is essential to predict the occurrences and the spread of the illnesses in a timely manner. This task is challenging because it involves both geographical analysis and temporal analysis.

Density-based cluster analysis techniques will be used for geographical analysis. Density-based clustering refers to unsupervised learning methods that identify distinctive clusters in the data, based on the idea that a cluster in a data space is a contiguous region of high point density, separated from other such clusters by contiguous regions of low point density. Environmental and climatic data including temperature, humidity, vegetation, meteorology, and related demographical information can be collected for spatial cluster analysis. To be more flexible in analysis, we will employ soft computing techniques to investigate boundary overlap situations. Boundary overlap has been used to assess relationships between edaphic factors and vegetation boundaries [6]. The similar idea can be used in this project to identify the relationship between disease outbreaks and other environmental factors.

The temporal analysis focuses on finding particular patterns of temporal variation, whether it is periodic or whether is a long-term trend. This involves the study of historical ILI data collected from CDC to identify useful temporal patterns. Sequential pattern discovery techniques incorporate the temporal ordering information into the pattern discovery process, thus can be used to identify temporal disease patterns from historical data. To make the prediction more accurate, the model-based prediction will be individually adjusted for each object based on the basic statistics of the distribution of the original values. To effectively deal with real-time stream data, the statistics will be computed and updated constantly in the model description file together with other information about the clustering groups.

However, another challenge that needs to be addressed in Twitter stream data is that, other than the huge data volume, data streams are also characterized by their drifting concepts. The underlying data generating mechanism or the concept that we try to learn from the data is constantly evolving. The fundamental problem we need to solve is that given an infinite amount of continuous measurements, how do we model them in order to capture time-evolving trends and patterns in the stream? In other words, the mining method of data streams needs to adapt to the evolving data distribution [16].

A compact data structure, the closed enumeration tree (CET), is introduced in [1] to maintain a dynamically selected set of patterns over a sliding window. We have previously developed another efficient tree structure, the ordered suffix tree (OST), to discover subsequent patterns in large text databases [9]. Combining the features from CET and OST, we propose a new compact suffix tree structure to ensure single-scan of Twitter data while utilizing limited memory storage. The proposed tree structure will be used to maintain a dynamically selected set of temporal patterns over a sliding window. Concept drifts in the data streams will be reflected by the boundary movements in the windows, and thus can be easily and efficiently captured. Once evolving changes have been identified and confirmed, the system will adjust the input parameters automatically or interactively to adapt to the evolving changes.

4 Conclusions

Early insights into the timing and intensity of the flu season could be very useful to public health agencies. This study proposes a high-performance health informatics system to detect and predict the spread of influenza-like illnesses in real-time by analyzing Twitter stream data and historical health data. To build a successful system, we need to ensure the efficient and accurate detection of influenza-like illness messages from Twitter. While traditional lexicon-based text analysis methods help identify related messages quickly, simply applying them could potentially result in an over-fitted system. To address this issue, we propose to combine lexicon-based approaches with machine learning approaches to ensure the accuracy of the system. Once the real-time disease related messages have been identified, we propose to use Tableau as an underlying data visualization tool to provide a real-time map of disease outbreaks. In addition, spatial and temporal data analysis techniques will be used to study the historical and current health and geographical data. This would provide health agencies a useful tool for the prediction of the future outbreaks of influenza-like illnesses.

5 References

[1] Y. Chi, H. Wang, P. Yu, and R. Muntz, "Catch the Moment: Maintaining Closed Frequent Itemsets in a Data Stream Sliding Window", Knowledge and Information Systems, 10(3): 265-294.

[2] N. Collier, S. Nguyen, and M. Nguyen, "Omg u got flu? Analysis of shared health messages for bio-surveillance", Proceedings of the 4th Symposium on Semantic Mining in BioMedicine, Cambridge, UK, 2010.

[3] A. Culotta, "Towards detecting influenza epidemics by analyzing Twitter messages", Proceedings of the 1st

Workshop on Social Media Analytics, Washington, DC, July 2010.

[4] S. Doan, L. Ohno-Machado, and N. Collier, "Enhancing Twitter data analysis with simple semantic filtering: example in tracking influenza-like illnesses", Proceedings of 2012 IEEE 2nd International Conference on Healthcare Informatics, Imaging and Systems Biology, San Diego, CA, 2012.

[5] J. Ginsberg, M. Mohebbi, R. Patel, L. Brammer, M. Smolinski, and L. Brilliant, "Detecting influenza epidemics using search engine query data", Nature 457, 1012-1014, February 2009.

[6] G. Jacquez, "The map comparison problem: tests for the overlop of geographic boundaries", Statistics in Medicine 14:2343-61, 1995.

[7] A. Jurek, M. Mulvenna, and Y. Bi, "Improved lexicon-based sentiment analysis for social media analytics", Security Informatics (2015) 4: 9, 2015.

[8] V. Lampos, T. De Bie, and N. Cristianini, "Flu Detector - Tracking Epidemics on Twitter", Machine Learning and Knowledge Discovery in Databases, Lecture Notes in Computer Science, vol 6323. Springer, Berlin, Heidelberg, 2010.

[9] D. Li, K. Wang and J. Deogun, "An Efficient Algorithm for Pattern Discovery in Large Text Databases", Proceedings of the 2003 International Conference on Information and Knowledge Engineering, pp. 96-102, Las Vegas, NV, June 2003.

[10] V. López, A. Fernández, S. García, V. Palade, and F. Herrera, "An insight into classification with imbalanced data: Empirical results and current trends on using data intrinsic characteristics", Information Sciences, Vol. 250, pp. 113-141, November 2013.

[11] B. O'Connor, R. Balasubramanyan, B. Routledge, and N. Smith. "From Tweets to polls: Linking text sentiment to public opinion time series", Proceedings of International AAAI Conference on Weblogs and Social Media, Washington, D.C., 2010.

[12] Q. Rajput, S. Haider, and S. Ghani, "Lexicon-Based Sentiment Analysis of Teachers' Evaluation," Applied Computational Intelligence and Soft Computing, vol. 2016, Article ID 2385429, 12 pages, 2016.

[13] J. Ritterman, M. Osborne, and E. Klein. "Using prediction markets and Twitter to predict a swine flu pandemic", proceedings of the 1st International Workshop on Mining Social Media, 2009.

[14] A. Sadilek, H. Kautz, and V. Silenzio, "Predicting Disease Transmission from Geo-Tagged Micro-Blog Data", Proceedings of the 26th AAAI Conference on Artificial Intelligence, 2012.

[15] A. Signorini, A. Segre, and P. Polgreen, "The Use of Twitter to Track Levels of Disease Activity and Public Concern in the U.S. during the Influenza A H1N1 Pandemic", PLOS ONE 6(5): e19467, 2011.

[16] H. Wang, W. Fan, P. Yu and J. Han, "Finding Concept-Drifting Data Streams using Ensemble Classifiers", Proceedings of the 9th ACM International Conference on Knowledge Discovery and Data Mining (SIGKDD'03), Washington DC, USA, August 2003.

[17] R. Wesley, M. Eldridge, and P. Terlecki, "An Analytic Data Engine for Visualization in Tableau", Proceedings of the 2011 ACM SIGMOD International Conference on Management of data, 1185-1194, New York, NY, USA, 2011.

[18] K. Zhang, R. Arablouei, and R. Jurdak, "Predicting Prevalence of Influenza-Like Illness From Geo-Tagged Tweets", Proceedings of the 26th International Conference on World Wide Web Companion, 2017.

On Development of Health Care Digital Libraries and Health Care Data Analytics: An Adaptive Algorithmic Approach

Anastasia-Dimitra Lipitakis[1] **and Evangelia A.E.C. Lipitakis**[2]

(1) Department of Informatics and Telematics, Harokopio University, Athens, Hellas
adlipita@hua.gr
(2) Kent Business School, University of Kent, Canterbury, England
leacynthialipitakis@yahoo.com

Abstract

Some basic issues on the development of digital library environment supporting research at health care organizations and medical schools and research centres are presented. Digital libraries facilitate access to medical material produced by laboratories for both research and educational purposes. Adaptive algorithmic procedures for digital library supported workflows, medical and histological descriptions, and medical object data and metadata using special content manager constructs with digital libraries component are described. Several health care data analytics basic elements are also given.

Keywords and Phrases: *digital libraries, adaptive algorithms, health care libraries, health care data analytics, medical objects interaction, networks of human genes*

1. Introduction

Health care digital libraries facilitate greatly access to basic and advanced medical knowledge existing in health organization archives and produced by related scientific laboratories, research centres, university hospital and medical schools for research, educational and social services purposes. All the information and material collected can be diversified different in structures, types, forms, purposes, and should be created, classified and managed in appropriate ways allowing easy and simplified manner by the end-user groups according to their personal and collective requirements. The information collection management within integrated digital library environments should include automated collection definition, unified collection management, efficient functionality and interaction, fast and accurate collection search for a satisfactory overall system performance.

Several medical laboratories and health care centers operating in the framework of university hospitals, medical schools and research centers produce very large amounts of material, in the form of medical images, results, videos in digital formats, which can be exploited for research, educational and experimental purposes. Digital library systems can use advanced accessing capabilities for organizing and maintaining very large amounts of images, videos and related results of all medical material types (Borgman, 2002; Suh et al., 2002).

Various information collections can be considered including such related material described by core metadata sets without maintaining specific research and/or educational characteristics.

Note that the functionality of these schemes can be extended as follows:

(i) The gathered material can be used by the teaching and research personnel for presentation in lectures and added in the libraries characterizing educational and specialized research properties particularly useful for specific medical areas, and complicated metadata management schemes, such as IEEE Learning Object Metadata (IEEE, 2002) can be used for describing larger collections.

(ii) Digital libraries usually support multiple collections that follow specific orientations of individual research centres and organizations providing for each set of collections specific features and characteristics, determining predetermined types and structures of available digital materials. Metadata can be used for describing different collections and both the number and nature of supported collections are various crosswalks between metadata schemes should be supported (Yu et al., 2003).

(iii) The design of digital library architectures requires dynamical creation and administration of collections, since both number and nature of supported collections are not predefined. The creation and management of independent collections can

ISBN: 1-60132-479-0, CSREA Press ©

be achieved by using various nonprogrammable graphical interfaces.

(iv) In several medical archiving systems the required material is gathered and processed by specialized support units adding directly complex workflows by researchers participating in metadata creation and can be stored in digital libraries (Bristol University, 2000)

(v) Existing services in digital libraries should be functional for all collections without special programming effort.

(vi) The existing features should be multilingual supporting material characterization and user interfaces.

In the case of extended requirements in very large scale digital libraries special collection management techniques and implementation of respective features can be used with automated collection definition and unified collection management within integrated digital library environments. These operations facilitate implementation of provided digital library service under common guidelines in open environments, integration of heterogeneous collections in terms of material structure and metadata support and simplification of collection management (Lagoze and Van de Sompel, 2001).

Digital libraries are based on modular architectures and digital material is stored in special repositories for storing and accessing data and additional functionalities are implemented as independent software modules (services). The implementation of supported workflow applications resulting from active research participation in cataloguing workflow requires special attention in particular when multilingual support is used for digital library service implementation and efficient performance of the overall system especially during the collection searches. The services of digital libraries focusing on collection management, workflow services, operational functionality and implementation requirements, as well as issues concerning collection definition processes, metadata representation, dynamic collection management and implementation of supported services are of particular interest (Nikolaidou et al., 2005).

2. Digital Libraries Supported Services

Different collections can be used for each laboratory and most of metadata including descriptions, producers and formats need to be supported, while collection administration is performed by librarians of central libraries through the collection management services. Most collections are partially described by the same metadata sets allowing the librarians to define collections based on existing collection descriptions (Darmoni et al. 2001). The selection process of appropriate material is performed by laboratory staff according predetermined criteria related to specific medical file fields characterized by content based properties meaningful in medical research, such as images, videos etc. accompanied by descriptions indicating their significance written by researchers/specialist medical doctors in appropriate forms.

New medical material can be added in digital libraries by researchers and processing of such material and filling metadata fields can be done by both cataloguers and researchers, while the corresponding workflow is facilitated by medical object processing and cataloguing services, and create presentations and tutorial services. Different users groups may search collections using certain criteria based on metadata fields or digital material content written in multilingual languages, with the required access granted through web based applications.

Various heterogeneous collections in integrated digital library environment concerning structure, purpose, related metadata of collection directories, need to be supported. These collections include the following services:

(i) collection management services: with special capabilities such as
defining collections, extending and modifying collection definitions, defining collection relationships, accessing collections by a common access points, integrating collections supported by different implementation environments, independent of searching mechaisms and digital object storing (Witten et al., 2001; Arms et al., 2002; Van de Sompel and Lagoze, 2001; Bainbridge et al., 2003).
Collection properties involve structural information, access information and relationship s between different collections, while collection descriptions can be derived from existing ones by extending object structures and metadata models (Lightle and Ridgway, 2003).

(ii) Supported workflow services, including medical object processing, cataloguing and presentation/tutorial services, facilitating cooperation of researchers and cataloguers for developing collections.
Note that digital objects, i.e. digital material (compound objects, documents consisting of texts, images, sounds indexed by different tools) can be parts of other objects, and all objects

ISBN: 1-60132-479-0, CSREA Press ©

belonging in specific collections have the same structure.
Several digital objects in specific collections have common general metadata sets including the following metadata categories: descriptive, technical, educational and access control rights (Besser, 2002).
Collection properties involving structural information, access information and relationships between different collections search options and limitations can be defined (Light and Ridgway, 2003), while collection descriptions can be appropriately derived from existing descriptions by extending object structures and metadata models.
The digital library supported workflows can be described by the following pseudo-algorithmic scheme:

Algorithm DLW-1 (ε_{SP} SPMO, ε_{PI} PIVS, ε_{RM} RMO, ε_{CM} CMO, ε_{PM} PMO, ε_{UF} DLSW)
Purpose: This algorithm describes the digital library supported workflows

Input: store presentations and medical objects (SPMO), set primal images-videos-sounds (PIVS), review medical objects (RMO), catalogue medical objects (CMO), publication of medical objects (PMO), singular perturbation (sp) parameters ε_{SP}, ε_{PI}, ε_{RM}, ε_{CM}, ε_{PM} and uncertainty factor parameter ε_{UF}
Output: digital library supported workflows (DLSW)
Computational Procedure:
Step 0: read sp parameters ε_{SP}, ε_{PI}, ε_{RM}, ε_{CM}, ε_{PM}
Step 1: /part 1//researchers create presentation and tutorials/
/store presentations and tutorials, and add medical objects in presentations ε_{SP} (SPMO)/
Step 2:/part 2/
/researchers and cataloguers add, process and publish medical objects/
/set primal images-videos-sounds ε_{PI} (PIVS)/
Step 2.1: add images-video-sounds
/consider images-videos-sounds/
Step 2.2: review medical objects ε_{RM} (RMO)
/use primal images-videos-sounds/
Step 2.3: process images/videos/sounds
/consider medical objects/
Step 2.4: create medical objects
/use stored medical objects/
Step 2.5: catalogue medical objects ε_{CM} (CMO)
/use published medical objects/
Step 2.6: publish medical objects ε_{PM} (PMO)
Step 3: determine uncertainty factor parameter ε_{UF} and form the digital library supported workflows ε_{UF} (DLSW)

Completed medical objects can be published and metadata fields are filled by researchers and cataloguers for research and educational purposes.
(iii) collection search services: supporting the following:
simple searches on specific metadata fields;
combined search processes on same on multiple meta data fields;
combined search processes on multiple metadata and data fields facilitating several searching sub-collections of specific collections accompanied with certain limitations and special characteristics.
Note that the multilingual facility supporting metadata and digital objects can affect the performance rate of the overall process.

3. Digital library collection definitions

The creation of laboratories specific collections includes several definitions of generic medical collections with specific material type and common metadata sets. These definitions with various advantages includes the following:

(i) Medical collection definitions: consisting of three sub-collections, namely medical image collections, medical video collections, presentation collections. The first two objects contain original and derivative images-videos, thumbnail images and multilingual descriptions. Medical images archives and various health care applications can be used for descriptive and technical metadata of medical images-video objects (Sakai, 2001; Davenport-Robertson et al. 2001).
(ii) Histological collection definitions: satisfying needs of histology laboratories containing certain properties and restrictions of medical collection descriptions. Some medical and histological descriptions are indicated in the following pseudo-algorithmic form (algorithm Med-Histo-Descriptions-1):

Algorithm MHD-1 (ε_{MP} MPC, MVC, MIC, ε_{HC} HCO, PRC, HVC, HIC, ε_{UF} MHDMDL)
Purpose: This algorithm provides several medical and histological descriptions in the development of medical digital libraries

ISBN: 1-60132-479-0, CSREA Press ©

Input: medical collection MPC, medical video collections MVC, medical images collections MIC, histological collections HIC, sp parameters ε_{MP}, ε_{HC} and uncertainty factor parameter ε_{UF}
Output: medical and histological descriptions in the development of medical digital libraries MHDMDL
Computational procedure:
/part 1/
Step 1: consider medical and presentation collection ε_{MP} MPC
Step 1.1: consider presentation collections
Step 1.1:1: check object structure
Step 1.1.1.1: check object parts
Step 1.1.1.2: check technical metadata
Step 1.1.2: check metadata
Step 1.1.2.1: check educational part
Step 1.1.2.2: check technical part
Step 1.1.2.3: check administrative part
Step 1.1.2.4: check descriptive part
Step 1.2: consider medical video collections MVC
Step 1.2.1: check object structure
Step 1.2.1.1: consider original videos
Step 1.2.1.2: consider derived videos
Step 1.2.1.3: consider descriptions
Step 1.2.1.4: consider thumbnails
Step 1.2.2: consider metadata sets
Step 1.3: consider medical images collections MIC
Step 1.3.1: check object structure
Step 1.3.1.1: consider image
Step 1.3.1.2: consider derived images
Step 1.3.1.3: consider thumbnail
Step 1.3.1.4: consider description
Step 1.3.2: consider metadata
Step 1.3.2.1: consider educational part
Step 1.3.2.2: consider administrative part
Step 1.3.2.3: consider technical part
Step 1.3.2.4: consider descriptive part
Step 2: consider histological collections ε_{HC} HCO
Step 2.1: consider presentation collection PRC
Step 2.2: consider histological video collection HVC
Step 2.3: consider histological image collection HIC
Step 2.3.1: object structures
Step 2.3.1.1: check original image
Step 2.3.1.2: check derived image
Step 2.3.1.3: check thumbnail
Step 2.3.1.4: check description
Step 2.3.1.5: check watermarked images
Step 2.3.1.6: check screen size images
Step 2.3.2: consider metadata
Step 2.3.2.1: consider educational material
Step 2.3.2.2: consider administrative material
Step 2.3.2.3: consider technical material
Step 2.3.2.4: consider descriptive material
Step 3: determine uncertainty factor parameter ε_{UF} and form medical and histological descriptions in the development of medical digital libraries ε_{UF} MHDMDL

The algorithm MHD-1 provides medical and histological descriptions in the development of medical digital libraries.

(iii) Medical object implementation issues

Several collection repositories can be developed by using special content manager platforms. Note that most metadata fields supporting multilingualism and large numbers of restricted metadata value lists can increase significantly the system complexity. Various metadata information can be stored within the underlying databases and as tag structured text parts in corresponding medical digital objects for improving search performance. Medical object data and metadata internal representations using special content manager constructs, as well as digital libraries components can be described in the following pseudo-algorithmic form (Algorithm Med-Objects-1):

Algorithm MO-1 (ε_{DM} DMO, ISS, TSS, ε_{DL} DLC, CMP, CSS, MOPCW, PTW, ε_{UF} MODMIR)
Purpose: This algorithm describes medical object data and metadata internal representations using special content manager constructs, as well as digital libraries components
Input: documents of medical objects (DMO), image search server (ISS), text search server (TSS), digital library components (DLC), content manager platform) (CMP), collection search service (CSS), medical object processing and cataloguing workflow (MOPCW), presentations and tutorials workflow (PTW), sp parameters ε_{DM}, ε_{DL} and uncertainty factor parameter ε_{UF}
Output: medical object data and metadata internal representations using special content manager constructs, as well as digital libraries components (MODMIR)
Computational procedure:
Step 0: determine the sp parameters DMO and DLC
/part 1/
Step 1: consider documents of medical objects ε_{DM} (DMO)
Step 1.1: consider image search server (ISS)
Step 1.1.1: consider original images
Step 1.1.2: consider thumbnail images
Step 1.1.3: consider derivate images
Step 1.2: consider text search server (TSS)
Step 1.2.1: using multilingual description
Step 1.2.2: consider metadata (structured texts)
/part 2/
Step 2: use digital library components ε_{DL} (DLC)
Step 2.1: /use web browser/

ISBN: 1-60132-479-0, CSREA Press ©

use collection repository (content manager platform) (CMP)

Step 2.1.1: consider collection search service (CSS)

Step 2.1.2: consider medical object processing and cataloguing workflow (MOPCW)

Step 2.1.3: consider creating presentations and tutorials workflow (PTW)

Step 2.1.3.1: consider collection management service

Step 2.1.3.2: consider collection dictionary

Step 2.1.3.3: consider collection management clients

Step 3: Determine the uncertainty factor parameter ε_{UF} and form medical object data and metadata internal representations using special content manager constructs, as well as digital libraries components ε_{UF} (MODMIR)

Collection dictionaries can be used for maintaining collection related information and access control information. The collection repositories facilitate storing and searching various digital objects, while the collection management service is managing the collection dictionaries enabling unified access to all collections and transparent implementation of proposed services.

Other related digital library components include the following:

>Collection repository: consisting of content manager components, i.e. a middleware platform providing storing, searching and managing digital content tools.

>Collection management: providing elementary services for adding, deleting digital material by initiating collection search and forwarding several search results. This service is implemented by using component programming.

>End user services: contains graphical environment facilitating users and collection management. All related applications are modular easily implemented as Java applets.

Digital libraries require for the system development:

(i) efficient organization and administration of dynamically created collections

(ii) appropriate support of advanced workflow capabilities. The medical material of all forms can be added in the libraries directly by researchers and can be used for creating presentations, online tutorials stored in the libraries.

Dynamic collection management can provide automated collection definition and unified collection management within digital library integrated environments (Nikolaidou et al., 2005).

4. Health Care Data Analytics

4.1 Introductory Remarks

The Health Care data continuum includes a plethora of measurements, images, diagnostic tests, medical prescriptions and long lists of patients, specialists and doctors. In this huge mega-data sets several other related significant factors, such as the several networks of human genes linked to various diseases and disorders, human disease networks, health care ecosystems, bio-informatics, info-medical biology with complex structures of protein interaction networks, should be included (Lipitakis and Lipitakis, 2009).

The issue of the efficient very big data sets management is a significant research topic. In particular in the fields of bioinformatics, digital health care data, such as a great number of measurements, images, diagnostic tests, genetic profiles, liquid biopsies, electrocardiograms etc.. The so-called 'big data revolution' is considered to be a great transformation of medicine and bio-informatics. All these transforming technologies it is reported that have 'the consumers in the drivers' seat'.

In an artificial intelligence data healthcare command center information from several data streams in real time including patient health records, lab tests, emergency dispatch service updates, availability of hospital beds at any given time, can be performed by appropriate algorithms transferring proper messages to surgical teams. It has been reported that digital health is not exactly computer science or engineering sciences, but its social science and behavioral science (Fry and Mukherjee, 2018).

4.2 A Digital Health Care Ecosystem

A characteristic constellation of Health Care ecosystem basic components including measurements, images, diagnostic tests genetic profiles, liquid biopsies, electrocardiograms etc. can be described in the following pseudoalgorithmic form:

Algorithm HCDA-1 (ε_{PA} PAS, ε_{DA} DAC, ε_{PH} PHA, ε_{GO} GOV, ε_{IP} IPA, ε_{UF} HDHE)

Purpose: This algorithm describes a health care ecosystem basic components including measurements, images, diagnostic tests, genetic profiles, liquid biopsies, electrocardiograms and other related components

Input: Patient status PAS, doctor activities DAC, pharmaceutics PHA, government GOV, insurer/payer

ISBN: 1-60132-479-0, CSREA Press ©

IPA, sp parameters ε_{PA} , ε_{DA} , ε_{PH} , ε_{GO} , ε_{IP} , ε_{DM} and uncertainty factor parameter ε_{UF}
Output: Human Digital Health Ecosystem components (HDHE)
Computational Procedure:
Step 1: consider Patient status ε_{PA} (PAS)
Step 1.1: lab tests
Step 1.2: personal health records
Step 1.3: clinical history
Step 1.4: diseases
Step 1.4.1: cancer
Step 1.4.1.1: quality measures
Step 1.4.2: lung diseases
Step 1.4.3: diabetes
Step 1.4.4: stroke risk
Step 1.4.5: heart disease
Step 1.4.6: Alzheimer's neurological disease
Step 1.4.7: hypertension
Step 1.4.8: irregular heart rhythm
Step 1.4.9: kidney disease
Step 1.4.10: breath sensors
Step 1.4.11: various molecular biomarkers
Step 1.4.11.1: waste analysis
Step 1.4.12: imaging/scans
Step 1.4.12.1: social media
Step 1.4.12.2: smart phones
Step 1.4.12.3: Gps
Step 1.4.12.4: health applications
Step 1.4.12.5: cameras
Step 1.5: liquid biopsy
Step 1.5.1: biomarker
Step 1.5.2: health/fitness tracker
Step 1.5.2.1: DNA
Step 1.5.2.2: radio waves
Step 1.5.2.3: altimeter
Step 1.5.2.4: thermometer
Step 1.5.2.5: infrared optical sensor
Step 1.5.2.6: accelerometer
Step 1.5.2.7: gyroscope
Step 2: doctor activities ε_{DA} (DAC)
Step 2.1: doctors' notes and prescriptions
Step 2.2: telemedicine
Step 2.3: genetic data
Step 2.4: electronic health records
Step 2.5: prescription data
Step 3: pharmaceutics ε_{PH} (PHA)
Step 3.1: clinical trial data
Step 3.2: electronic health records
Step 3.3: economic data
Step 3.4: pharmacogenomics
Step 3.5: pharmacokinetics
Step 3.6: consumer spending
Step 3.7: id outbreaks
Step 4: government ε_{GO} (GOV)
Step 4.1: environmental data
Step 4.2: caretaker data
Step 4.3: electronic health data
Step 5: insurer/payer ε_{IP} (IPA)
Step 5.1: claims data
Step 5.2: microrna
Step 5.3: id breaks
Step 6: Form the Human Digital Health Ecosystem components ε_{UF} (HDHE)

The algorithm HCDA-1 describes a health care ecosystem basic components including measurements, images, diagnostic tests, genetic profiles, liquid biopsies, electrocardiograms and other related components. Several networks of human genes are linked to various diseases and disorders, and these genes associated with similar disorders are more likely to interact with other networks of genes.

5. Conclusion

Several important issues of the development of digital library environment supporting research at health care organizations and medical schools and research centers have been presented. The Digital health care libraries facilitate access to medical material produced by laboratories for both research and educational purposes. A set of adaptive algorithmic procedures for digital library supported workflows, medical and histological descriptions, and medical object data and metadata using special content manager constructs with digital libraries component are given. Several health care data analytics basic elements are also presented.

REFERENCES

Arms W. (2002): A spectrum in interoperability, D-Lib Magazine 8 (1), www.dlib.org.dlib/january02/01arms.html

Bainbridge D., Thomson J. and Witten I. (2003): Assembling and enriching digital library collections, Procs. Third Joint ACM/IEEE Conference, ACM Computer Press, NW, 323-334

Besser H. (2002): The next stage: moving from isolated collections to interoperable digital libraries, First Monday On line Journal 7 (6),

Borgman C. L. (2002): Challenges in building digital libraries for the 21st century, Procs of IACDL 2002, LNCS 2555, Springer Verlag, NY, 1-13

Bristol University (2000): TR: Bristol Biomedical Image Archive case study, http://ltsc.ieee.org/doc/wg12/LOM_WD6_4.pdf

Darmoni S., Leroy J., Baudic F., Douyere M., Piot M. and Thirion B. (2001): CISMeF: A structured health resource guide, Methods Information Medicine 39

ISBN: 1-60132-479-0, CSREA Press ©

(1), 30-35, http://firstmoday.org/issues/issue7_6/besser/index.html

Fry E. and Mukherjee S. (2018): Big Data meets biology, Fortune 4, 24-35

IEEE (2002): IEEE P1484.12.1/D6.4 draft standard for learning object metadata,

Lagoze C. and Van de Sompel H. (2001): The Open Archive Initiative: building a low barrier interoperability framework, Procs. First Joint ACM/IEEE Conference on Digital Library (JCDL 2001), ACM Computer Press, NY, 54-62

Lightle K. and Ridgway J. (2003): Generation of XML records across multiple metadata standards, D-Lib Magazine 9 (9), www.dlib.org.dlib/september03/lightle/09lightle.html

Lipitakis A. and Lipitakis E.A.E.C. (2009): Adaptive Algorithmic Modelling in e-Business and Strategy Management: The Case of e-Health Services. In Proceedings of the 14th International Symposium for Health Information Management Research (ISHIMR 2009 Conference), October 2009, Kalmar, Sweden.

Nikolaidou M., Anagnostopoulos D. and Hatzopoulos M. (2005): Development of a medical digital library managing multiple collections, The Electronic Library 23 (2), 221-236.

Suh E.B., Wang S.A.,Cheung H., Tangiral P. and Martino R.L. (2002): A we-based medical image archive system, Procs Medical Imaging 2002, Intern. Soc. For Optical Engng., www.brisbio.ac.uk

Van de Sompel H. and Lagoze C. (2001): The Open Archive Initiative Protocol for Metadata Harvesting, Open Archive Initiative, www.openarchives.org/OAI_protocol/openarchiveprotocol.html

Witten I., Banbridge D. and Boddie S. (2001): Greenstone: open source digital library software with end user collection building, On line Information Review 25 (5), 288-298

Yu S.C., Lu K.Y. and Chen R.S. (2003): Metadata management system: design and implementation, The Electronic Library 21 (2), 154-164.

ISBN: 1-60132-479-0, CSREA Press ©

SESSION

MEDICAL SYSTEMS, DEVICES AND SERVICES + MONITORING SYSTEMS + TOOLS FOR REHABILITATION

Chair(s)

TBA

ISBN: 1-60132-479-0, CSREA Press ©

Infrastructure and Procedure for Simulation of Cardiac Remote Monitoring: Experiences from the Telemedicine Agder Project

B.F. Smaradottir[1,2], C.E. Moe[3] and R.W. Fensli[1],
[1]Department of Information and Communication Technology, University of Agder, Grimstad, Norway
[2]Clinical Research Department, Sørlandet Hospital HF, Kristiansand, Norway
[3]Department of Information Systems, University of Agder, Kristiansand, Norway

Abstract - *Telemedicine are remote electronic clinical consultations using technology for delivery of health care services. Telemedicine can be offered as a service to citizens living at home with an aim of reducing the number of hospital visits or visits to the General Practitioner and improving long-term cost-effectiveness. In Norway, a recent health reform has caused municipalities to re-organize their design of health services, with an increased use of telemedicine. In this context, the "Telemedicine Agder" project focuses on the organization, implementation and operation of large scale telemedicine services. In the project, a simulation of a telemedicine service for monitoring of heart failure was made in a clinical laboratory together with a patient, nurses and physicians. In addition, there were technical professionals and a research team present. This paper presents the laboratory infrastructure for the simulation and experiences are shared from the research project.*

Keywords: Laboratory Infrastructure, Telemedicine, Simulation, Heart Failure

1 Introduction

Telemedicine can be defined as remote electronic clinical consultations using technology for the delivery of health care and the exchange of information across distance [1]. Telemedicine technology covers a diverse spectrum of applications, aiming to improve the equity of access to and the quality of health care services [2][3][4]. Telemedicine also aims to reduce the number of hospital visits and improve long-term cost-effectiveness of the health care budget [1]. In Norway, a health reform was adopted in 2012 targeting the care delivery and focusing on collaboration and the continuity of care [5]. The reform lead to municipalities starting to re-organize their service design of the health services, with an increased use of telemedicine to carry out care by distance. When modelling a new service design, there is a need to test and evaluate the technical solutions and service models. User-based simulation in a clinical laboratory provides a controlled environment for evaluation of technology and workflow interactions [6].

In this context, the research project *Telemedicine Agder* aims to evaluate service models and large-scale implementation of telemedicine technology [7]. The project is 3-year long (2016-2019) and includes three Norwegian municipalities, one hospital, two industry partners and one research institution. In an earlier project phase, simulation of diabetes remote monitoring was made [8]. In a following phase, the service design and the technical solution for telemedicine monitoring of heart failure patients was run as a simulation in a clinical laboratory together with the project participants. Based on the cardiac simulation experiences, this paper presents the technical and physical infrastructure of the clinical laboratory and lessons learned by the research team. The following two research questions (RQs) were addressed:

RQ1: What technical and physical infrastructure is suitable for simulation of cardiac telemedicine monitoring?

RQ2: What are the lessons learned from simulation of cardiac telemedicine monitoring that are transferable to other contexts?

After this introduction, the telemedicine technology is presented. In the next section, the simulation procedure and the technical and physical infrastructure for the clinical laboratory is described. The discussion reflects on lessons learned from carrying out the simulation. Finally, conclusions are drawn on the project contributions.

2 The technology

The telemedicine technology for remote monitoring was developed by the Danish vendor Open TeleHealth [9] and delivered by Siemens Healthineers [10] for implementation in Norway. The telemedicine technology consisted of a patient tablet with a remote monitoring application and an information and management system for remote follow-up by telemedicine nurses.

When a patient with heart failure is included to telemedicine monitoring at the municipal telemedicine center, (s)he receives a case containing the technical equipment and instructions. The patient has to log in to the tablet at home, see Figure 1.

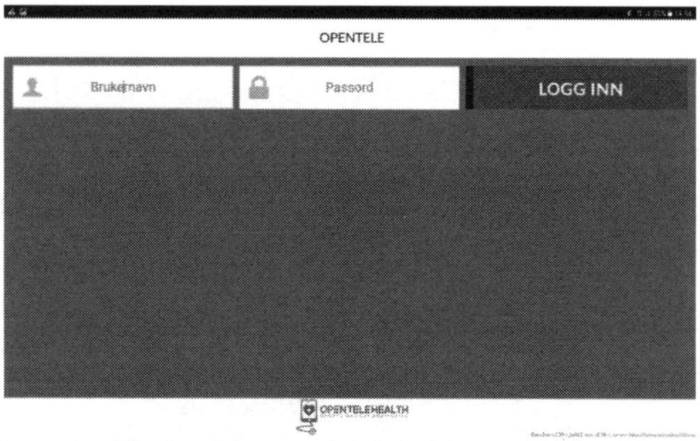

Figure 1. The log in screen for the tablet application.

The tablet is used for answering a symptom-specific questionnaire for heart failure and for sending physiological measurements to a server. The home screen also has a few administrative functions and overview of earlier measurements, see Figure 2.

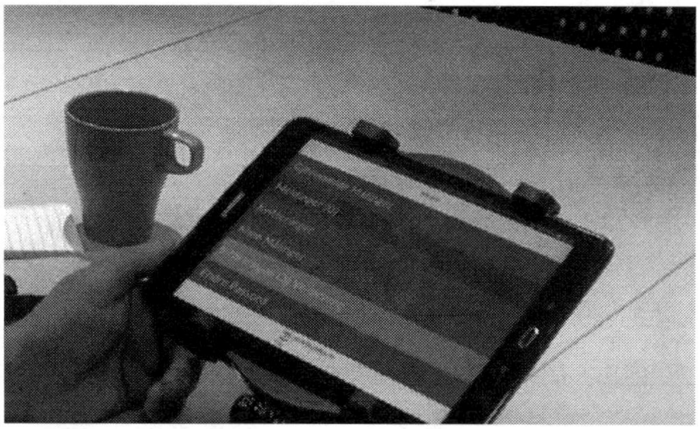

Figure 2. The tablet on a stand, showing the home screen.

The nurses at the telemedicine center accessed the measurements and questionnaire details through a specific information and management system for telemedicine, see Figure 3. The system had a video-consultation function.

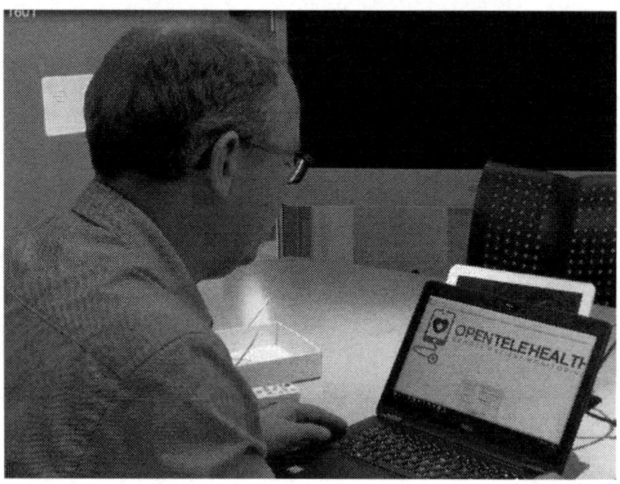

Figure 3. A nurse logging into the information and management system.

The system has an automated health assessment function with color-coded icons to show the severity of the patient's measurements and questionnaire answers. With a red alert, an immediate follow-up has to be made. There is a feedback function where the nurse can send an individual message to the patient's tablet.

3 The simulation infrastructure

A simulation with a task-based scenario for telemedicine monitoring of heart failure was made in the Clinical Laboratory at the University of Agder in Norway during April 2018. The simulation was organized and led by a research team consisting of three people with a health informatics background. Ten people from the *Telemedicine Agder* project's partners participated in the simulation.

3.1 Simulation scenarios

The test scenario targeted telemedicine monitoring situations for a heart failure patient. Before start, a 15 minutes long introduction was made of tasks and roles. Two different scenarios were carried out as a role-play in the clinical laboratory facilities. In the first scenario, a patient was included to telemedicine monitoring after a recent heart attack. He received the technical equipment and was instructed on the log in procedure by a technical instructor. The telemedicine center made a "first time" video-consultation for registrations of the cardiac status, for setting personal goals and for individual user training on the tablet. As a next step the patient made measurements of blood pressure, weight and pulse oximetry with Bluetooth transmission to the tablet and filled in a self-evaluation questionnaire on heart symptoms that was sent to the telemedicine center. The nurse at the telemedicine center evaluated the measurements and questionnaire answers and made an ordinary daily follow-up video-consultation. In the second scenario, the patient was elderly with hypertension, diabetes, obesity and heart failure. The remote measurements and questionnaire answers showed a worsening condition. The telemedicine nurse made a follow-up video-consultation based on a clinical worsening condition, also conferring with the patient's General Practitioner (GP) by phone for medical advices in the scenario.

3.2 The physical infrastructure

The simulations were performed in a clinical laboratory environment that had two separate test rooms and one control- and observation room. The physical infrastructure for the simulations is illustrated in Figure 4. Test room 1 represented the patient's home and Test room 2 the telemedicine center. In each test room, there was a separate recording camera source. In the observation room, the simulation was followed simultaneously on 4 monitors, one for each camera source and one monitor for merging and showing all sources simultaneously.

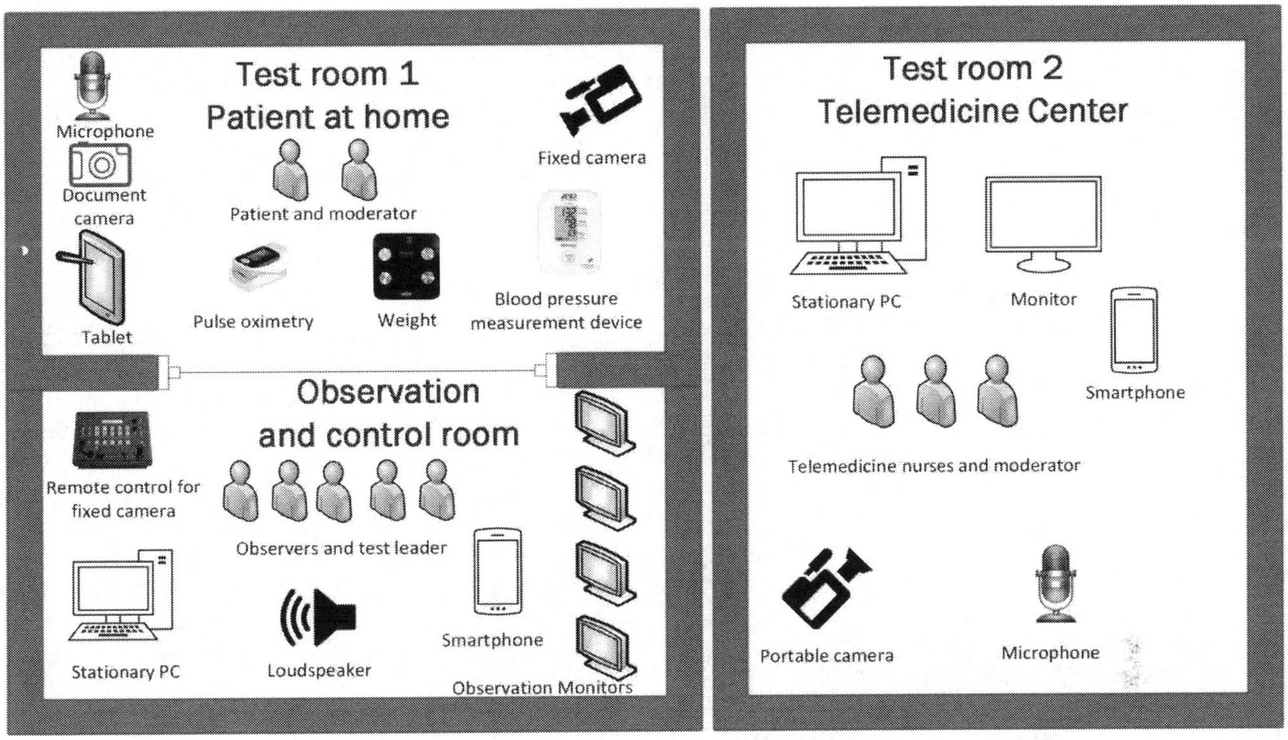

Figure 4. The technical and physical infrastructure for the simulation of cardiac telemedicine monitoring.

Between the Test room 1 and the control- and observation room there was a one-way mirror that allowed the observers to closely follow the simulation. In the Test room 1, the patient (played by a heart patient) used a device for blood pressure, a weight and a pulse oximetry device that sent the measurements to a tablet with Bluetooth transmission. The tablet had an application for remote monitoring and videoconference between the patient and the telemedicine nurse. In the Test room 2, a test application for the information and management system for remote monitoring was accessed and used in a desktop PC. There was also a smartphone available for communication with the patient and GP. The observation room had a desktop PC connected to four large monitors, allowing the observers to remotely follow the simulation and the interactions between the test rooms. Another monitor showed the camera sources simultaneously in one screen, using the software application Tricaster [11]. The operation of the fixed and portable cameras for recording purposes was made in the control- and observation room.

3.3 The technical infrastructure

The test rooms and the control and observation room were connected through a dedicated segment of the secured LAN infrastructure of the Centre for eHealth at University of Agder using VLAN technology. The same connection was also used for the IP-based streaming of video and audio signals from the test rooms. The recordings from the audio-visual sources were merged into one file including multiple video perspectives. For replication purposes the equipment used is listed.

Test room 1:

- Android Samsung A tablet device with Open TeleHealth application installed.
- A&D device model UA-651BLE for blood pressure and pulse measurement.
- A&D weight model UC-352BLE.
- Nonin device model 9560BT for pulse oximetry.
- Tobii eye-tracking equipment, camera and stand.
- Fixed Camera: SONY BRCZ330 HD 1/3 1CMOS P/T/Z 18x Optical Zoom (72x with Digital Zoom) Colour Video Camera.
- Sennheiser e912 Condenser Boundary Microphone.

Test room 2:

- Desktop for the Open TeleHealth information and management system (test version).
- 2x 27" monitors.
- Portable Camera: SONY HXR-NX30 Series.
- Logitech 886-000012 Boundary Microphone.
- Smartphone.

Control-and Observation room:

- Stationary PC: Mac Pro.
- Monitor: 4x 55".
- 27" Mac Monitor.
- Streaming: 2x Teradek RX Cube-455 TCP/IP 1080p H.264.
- Software Tricaster.
- Smartphone

3.4 The simulation procedure

The scenarios were performed as a telemedicine monitoring procedure where the interactions between the test rooms were made with use of technology. Both scenarios had a detailed description of the context, role and tasks for both the patient and the telemedicine nurse. In the patient role, there was a heart failure patient performing the defined tasks and measurements. In the telemedicine nurse role, there were two nurses from a telemedicine center carrying out the scenario together. The GP's role was acted in the observation room by a GP involved in the project team. In both the test rooms, there was a moderator from the project group to assist during the scenarios. In the observation room there were 7 people from the project participants observing the simulation and making annotations, (see Figure 5), and there was also one research team member controlling the recordings and simulation procedure. After both scenarios there was a group debrief with all participants to go through the task solving and actions made.

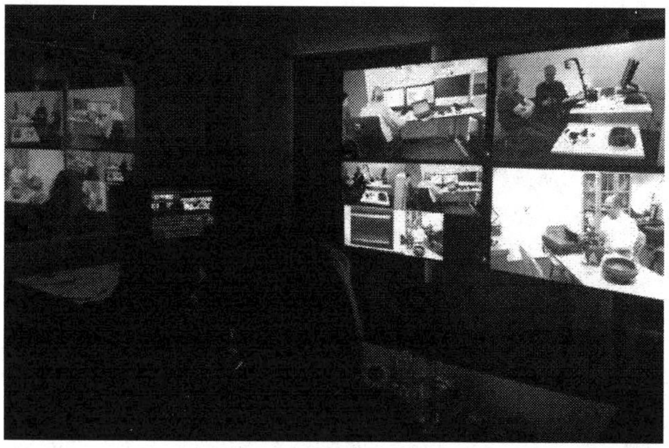

Figure 5. Observers in the control and observation room following the simulation in the test rooms and making annotations.

3.5 Ethical considerations

This research study was approved by the Norwegian Centre for Research Data with project number 53693 [12]. The participants received oral and written information about the project and they all signed an individual consent form.

4 Discussion

This paper has presented a technical and physical infrastructure for simulation of telemedicine monitoring, based on the research project *Telemedicine Agder*. The experiences shared by the research team performing the simulation could be useful for other projects within telemedicine and health informatics.

The two research questions (RQs) are answered based on the study. RQ1 asked about a suitable technical and physical infrastructure for simulation of cardiac telemedicine monitoring. When simulating a clinical scenario, it is of importance to create a realistic environment for performance of tasks and roles. The infrastructure needs to have the flexibility to adapt to changes in the scenarios, roles and technical equipment, both during a simulation but also between different contexts. We recommend using different test rooms simultaneously to add a dynamic dimension and to study interactions and work processes in addition to the technical solution, in line with [6]. The use of different test rooms requires technical equipment to record multiple sources simultaneously. We recommend recording both in separate files for detailed analysis, and in one synchronized file to ease the analysis retrospectively.

RQ2 asked about lessons learned from the cardiac telemedicine simulation that can be transferable to other contexts. Test and evaluation of technology under development is important to identify errors that need refinements, but simulating clinical models and workflow is also of importance. Simulations are complex when involving different user groups that interact with each other between the test rooms. It is of importance to involve multiple user groups as observers in the control and observation room to follow and annotate the scenarios, users who are experts of the user context and work processes. A group debrief that combines the practical experiences of the test participants and the observations of the observers is highly recommended, to discuss errors and need for refinements in the technology and clinical logistics. The group debrief allows the participants to speak more freely, compared to the simulation scenarios where there are defined tasks solve, so we recommend recording the debrief for retrospective analysis. For safety reasons, a participant should never be left alone in a test room, but always be accompanied by a moderator as being observed in laboratory can be a stressful experience and for avoiding claustrophobia. The test leader should have a detailed knowledge of the scenarios and the tested technology, to be able to make the correct decisions and lead the participants through a simulation.

We experienced some technical issues regarding the infrastructure and recording equipment and needed immediate technical assistance. We recommend having technical support available on short notice to avoid interference and distortion of the results. In addition, two external technicians with expertise on the telemedicine technology participated during the simulation to assist in case of technical failure. We needed the expertise during the simulation to be able to use the technology as intended.

The patient in the simulation had chronic heart failure for real. For ethical reasons, it is important to instruct the patient very clearly that (s)he is playing a role in the simulation and the main contribution is sharing experiences on using technology and procedures, and not sharing sensitive medical information. To illustrate this, our patient played both the role of a male and a female during the simulation, and one of them in a severe condition. It is important to consider that simulation can be exhausting for a patient, and we recommend multiple breaks and facilitation of a comfortable transport to and from the simulation facilities. Playing a role that you do

ISBN: 1-60132-479-0, CSREA Press ©

not understand or have not experienced is challenging, and for that reason we recommend having real nurses and physicians playing the associated roles to have a reliable and valid outcome.

This study had some limitations, such as including data from one single research project. However, several end-user groups were represented in the simulation, which provided useful experiences on how the two-test room infrastructure worked. The empirical data from the simulation is not in the scope of this paper, as it targets the technical and physical laboratory infrastructure for telemedicine simulation.

5 Conclusion

This paper was made within the project *Telemedicine Agder* to share experiences from laboratory simulation of telemedicine. The main contribution lies on how the technical and physical infrastructure was used in the simulations of cardiac telemedicine monitoring, and the lessons learned may be transferable and applicable in other contexts of health informatics. As telemedicine technology is used by multiple user groups, there is a need to test both technical functionalities and how the technology would be used in a clinical workflow before final implementation. The physical and technical laboratory infrastructure enabled studying the user interactions with the technology and provided an environment for carrying out clinical work processes. Future research agenda should target simulation of other telemedicine scenarios, with an extension of the clinical user group.

6 Acknowledgement

The research team would like to thank all participants and informants for their disinterested contribution in the study. Thanks to Åsmund Rodvig Somdal for technical assistance in the clinical laboratory. The Research Council of Norway provided financial support with Grant number 247929.

7 References

[1] World Health Organization (WHO), "Telemedicine. Opportunities and developments in member states," [retrieved: May, 2018]. Available from: http://www.who.int/goe/publications/goe_telemedicine_2010.pdf

[2] D. A. Perednia and A. Allen, "Telemedicine technology and clinical applications," JAMA, 273(6), pp.483-488, 1995, doi:10.1001/jama.1995.03520300057037.

[3] R. L. Bashshur, "On the definition and evaluation of telemedicine," Telemed J, 1(1), p. 19-30, 1995, doi:10.1089/tmj.1.1995.1.19.

[4] J. Craig and V. Patterson, "Introduction to the practice of telemedicine," J Telemed Telecare, 11(1), pp. 3-9, 2005.

[5] Norwegian Ministry of Health and Care Services. "The Coordination Reform, Proper treatment – at the right place and right time"; Report No. 47 (2008-2009) to the Storting. [retrieved: May, 2018]. Available from: https://www.regjeringen.no/contentassets/d4f0e16ad32e4bbd8d8ab5c21445a5dc/no/pdfs/stm200820090047000dddpdfs.pdf

[6] B. Smaradottir, R. Fensli, E.B. Sundby and S. Martinez. "Infrastructure for health care simulation- recommendations from the Model for Telecare Alarm Services project"; In proceedings of the 3rd International Conference on Health Informatics and Medical Systems (HIMS'17), p. 64-69, July 17-20, 2017 in Las Vegas, USA, CSREA press.

[7] Telemedicine Agder. [retrieved: May, 2018]. Available from: http://www.telma.no/

[8] B. Smaradottir, R. Fensli and C.E. Moe. "Recommendations of a laboratory infrastructure for simulation of telemedicine services" (diabetes); In press, IEEE, 2018.

[9] Open TeleHealth. [retrieved: May, 2018]. Available from: http://opentelehealth.com/

[10] Siemens healtineers. [retrieved: May, 2018]. Available from: https://www.healthcare.siemens.no/

[11] Tricaster. [retrieved: May, 2018]. Available from: https://www.newtek.com/tricaster/

[12] The Norwegian Centre for Research Data. [retrieved: May, 2018]. Available from: http://www.nsd.uib.no/nsd/english/index.html

Using Matching Algorithm on Rehabilitation Therapy

Lun-Ping Hung[1], Chien-Liang Chen[2], Yi-Pin Du[1] and Chia-Ling Ho[3]

[1]Department of Information Management, National Taipei University of Nursing and Health Sciences, Taiwan
[2]Department of Computer Science and Information Engineering, Aletheia University, Taiwan
[3]Department of Marketing and Logistics Management, Taipei City University of Science and Technology, Taiwan
Email: lunping@ntunhs.edu.tw

Abstract - *With the rapid growth of the elderly population, the prevalence of chronic disease dysfunction has increased. The number of elderly rehabilitation service demanders has also increased, leading to failure for professional caretaking manpower and existing medical resources to timely cope with the rapid aging development. From a traditional mindset, solving the supply and demand problem in rehabilitative medicine is an utterly inadequate measure. In this study, an application model with theory and practice combined was proposed. Using a mixed matching algorithm, a home rehabilitation service platform was constructed; under long-term care was collected, computed, and analyzed. In addition, a two-way automatic computing model, a medical-professional service system with disabled elders as individuals and rehabilitation therapists will be set up. Through the collaboration of the government, families and rehabilitation medical teams, seamless rehabilitation services can be achieved, thereby enhancing the quality of medical care.*

Keywords: Matching Algorithm, Home Rehabilitation, Information and Communication Technology: Cloud Computing

1 Introduction

Taiwan became an aging society in 2018 when chronic disease and dysfunction increased yearly and elderly needing long-term care services increased, resulting in the inability of professional caretaking manpower and medical resources to cope with the rapid aging development. In order to meet the needs of the increasing number of elderly in need of long-term care, the Taiwan government has proposed a 10-year long-term care plan. Depending on the elderly's varied care needs, relevant agencies offering care by specially-assigned persons are available, such as a nursing home serving as a transfer station between hospital and home and providing technical care and daily care, or an elderly care center accommodating conscious elderly needing daily assistance, providing them with a space for rehabilitation activities and leisure and recreation. Despite the availability of multiple long-term care related services, service units often operate independently without affiliation. Moreover, the strict application qualifications, inadequate professional caretaking manpower and overly concentrated medical resources have resulted in promotion difficulties, unable to cope with the problem of a great medical professional manpower demand that arises from an aging society.

On the other hand, with the economic development of the data technology platform, the traditional healthcare information and medical service business model has changed. The platform economy is supported by digital technologies, big data drives, and transaction platforms, while the funding platforms integrate consumers[1][2], service providers and money supply end to form a highly collaborative platform economy. A matching platform is defined as a platform that meets home rehabilitation medical needs, allowing people from all sides with specific needs and specific suppliers to achieve interaction and transactions (exchanges) through the identification and screening of mutual data.

In addition, the first and foremost purpose of the platform is to link products and services from both sides. With the construction of a "technical" platform as the basis, the basic framework that links the supply end (RT) and the demand end (the case) is established, and the complete rules governing use and interaction are proposed. Through the matching calculation method, fast and effective matching of specific linked groups will be conducive to the improvement of medical service quality[3].

Home rehabilitation applications must be reviewed by the care center. After passing the review, it will take about 7-14 days for a therapist to administer treatment at home. Obviously, home rehabilitation application processes are tedious and time consuming. As far as PAC patients are concerned, the need for rehabilitation needs is urgent and impossible to wait for. Therefore, through home rehabilitation and assistive device related literature analysis, this study designed a matching platform that meets the PAC service needs to provide both sides with asymmetrical dynamic matching algorithms. Through this platform, the best rehabilitation therapist can be found, while the most suitable splints can be recommended for people in need, thus solving the problem of uneven distributions of medical resources and professionals.

2 Methodology

2.1 The Main Concept of Matching between Two Sides

The home rehabilitation matching service designed in this study consists of two aspects: Parameters must be collected, including the basic conditions and personal preferences of the demander, the basic conditions and personal preferences of the supplier end, in order to match services for both sides. In the matching condition interface design, it can be divided into two user interfaces: one is to divide the matching condition interface design into two user interfaces, one of which is the case user interface at the demander end; the other is the user interface for rehabilitation therapists at the supplier end.

In the user interface at the demander end, home rehabilitation application process, whether one applies for services personally or the hospital discharge preparation team assists in carrying out an evaluation, review filing at the care center must be done. The cases' basic information is to be filled out in corresponding columns[4] in order for follow-up therapists to obtain the cases' personal information after completing matching. These columns mainly include: basic information, date and time of a home rehabilitation service applied for, etc. Then, according to the matching preferences in sequence, rehabilitation therapists at the supply end are matched.

On the other hand, the supplier (rehabilitation therapist) user interface includes filling of basic information and conditions, checking of service areas the supplier is willing to serve in, and establishment of available hours for the supplier to offer services. Finally, personal matching preferences in sequence and the cases at the demand end are matched. However, in terms of information filling at the demand end and supplier end, common information should be screened. However, in the information filled out by the demand end and supply end, common information must be screened and which key matching columns needed by the cloud platform should be defined to complete matching between both sides.

This study consists of four items, which are preferences to be filled out by both sides, which in sequence are: gender, region, service date, hours (time) and fees. In the succeeding chapter, how to give key matching conditions sores will be explained in detail and candidates from both sides will be sequenced to find the most suitable candidates.

2.2 Matching Items and Operational Steps

The improved matching algorithm of the Gale-ShaPley Algorithm was proposed in this study. The method can be divided into two step: Step 1: Establish key columns in the preference list. As for its mode of operation, which key matching columns are needed by the system are first discussed. Additionally, the supplier and the demander can freely choose contents of their preference; Step 2: The matching algorithm was computed. According to the preference sequence proposed by each case, the matching algorithm was computed for each rehabilitation therapist to find the most suitable candidate and until every case was matched with one rehabilitation therapist.

(1) Step 1: Establish a preference list and key columns.

As is mentioned in the key matching columns above, the key matching columns are divided into gender, region, service date, hours, and fees. These four items are the required preference items to be filled out by both sides (the case and the rehabilitation therapist).

(2) Step 2: Matching Algorithm Computing

According to the key matching conditions compiled above, four items, namely, gender, region, service date and hours (time), and fees, were cited as examples for matching algorithm computing. As shown in Table 1, supposing the cases are $\mathbf{P} = \{\mathbf{P}_1, \mathbf{P}_2, \mathbf{P}_3, \mathbf{P}_4\}$, the preference levels are ranked from left to right, (For $\mathbf{P}_1$, the preference levels in sequence are: gender>fees>region>time).

Table 1: Table of case preference sequence.

Case	Preference sequence			
$\mathbf{P}_1$	gender	fee	region	time
$\mathbf{P}_2$	region	time	fee	gender
$\mathbf{P}_3$	fee	gender	time	region
$\mathbf{P}_4$	fee	region	time	gender

As shown in Table 2, supposing the rehabilitation therapists are: $\mathbf{C}=\{\mathbf{C}_1, \mathbf{C}_2, \mathbf{C}_3, \mathbf{C}_4\}$, the preference levels are ranked from left to right. (For C_1, the preference levels in sequence are: region>fee>time>gender).

Table 2: Table of rehabilitation therapist preference.

Rehabilitation therapist	Preference sequence			
$\mathbf{C}_1$	region	fee	time	gender
$\mathbf{C}_2$	gender	fee	time	region
$\mathbf{C}_3$	fee	region	time	gender
$\mathbf{C}_4$	region	gender	fee	time

Take Case $\mathbf{P}_1$ for example, the basic conditions of rehabilitation therapists were compared according to the sequence relationship between $\mathbf{P}_1$ vs. $\mathbf{C}_1$, $\mathbf{C}_2$, $\mathbf{C}_3$, $\mathbf{C}_4$ compiled in Table 4. When the basic conditions and the preference conditions of $\mathbf{P}_1$ are the same, a score of A is given; when they differ, a score of B is given, and so on and so forth to compute the respective scores.

The way the key matching conditions are scored is first defined: gender→boy/girl; when $\mathbf{P}_1$ and $\mathbf{C}_1$ are the same gender, the score is A; if they are not, the score is B. Region→ When the correspondence address of P_1 matches the service region range of C_1, the score is A; otherwise, it is B. Fees→ government subsidies, self-paid; When P_1 meets the service type C_1 is willing to offer (government subsidies or self-paid), the score is A; if not, it is B. Hours→Monday ~Sunday and morning, noon, evening; When the hours of service applied by P_1 and the available service hours of $C_1$are the same, the score is A; if not, it is B. Therefore, when it is 4A(AAAA), the rehabilitation therapist is the most suitable candidate. When the sequence is: 3A1B(AAAB, AABA, ABAA, BAAA)>2A2B(AABB, ABAB, BBAA, BABA, BAAB, ABBA)>1A3B(ABBB, BABB, BBAB, BBBA)>4B(BBBB), 4B is the least suitable candidate (The preference sequence of $\mathbf{P_1}$ is $X_1 > X_3 > X_4 > X_2$(X_1=gender, X_3=fees, X_4=region, X_2=hours)

The matching scores of four rehabilitation therapists $\mathbf{C_1}$, $\mathbf{C_2}$, $\mathbf{C_3}$, $\mathbf{C_4}$ vs. P_1 cases are: $\mathbf{C_1}$: the score of 1A3B (BABB), $\mathbf{C_2}$: the score of 2A2B (AABB), $\mathbf{C_3}$: the score of 4B (BBBB), $\mathbf{C_4}$: the score of 1A3B (BBBA). At this time, $\mathbf{C_1}$ and $\mathbf{C_4}$ are found to have the same score. Therefore, the sequence of scores must be taken into account. $\mathbf{C_1}$ is BABB and $\mathbf{C_4}$ is BBBA. In the matching algorithm, the higher the preference sequence of score A, the faster the matching will be completed. Therefore, score A of $\mathbf{C_1}$ is ranked second; score A of $\mathbf{C_4}$ is ranked fourth. The degree of matching between $\mathbf{C_1}$ and $\mathbf{P_1}$ is greater than that of $\mathbf{C_4}$.

It can be found that the degrees of matching between rehabilitation therapists $\mathbf{C_1}$, $\mathbf{C_2}$, $\mathbf{C_3}$, $\mathbf{C_4}$ and $\mathbf{P_1}$ are $\mathbf{C_2} > \mathbf{C_1} > \mathbf{C_4} > \mathbf{C_3}$, with $\mathbf{C_2}$ being the most suitable candidate. Based on this matching algorithm, the same algorithm was applied to cases $\mathbf{P_2}$, $\mathbf{P_3}$, and $\mathbf{P_4}$, which derived at the priority sequence of $\mathbf{C_1}$, $\mathbf{C_2}$, $\mathbf{C_3}$, and $\mathbf{C_4}$. $\mathbf{P_1}$, $\mathbf{P_2}$, $\mathbf{P_3}$, and $\mathbf{P_4}$ also had their own basic conditions, which derived at the priority sequence of cases $\mathbf{P_1}$, $\mathbf{P_2}$, $\mathbf{P_3}$, and $\mathbf{P_4}$ versus rehabilitation therapists. Based on this, the objective of finding the most suitable candidates for both sides can be achieved (The preference sequence of $\mathbf{C_1}$ is $X_4 > X_1 > X_3 > X_2$(X_4=region, X_1=fees, X_3=time, X_2=gender)

2.3 Solving the Problem of Matches with Same Score

However, when the score is the same and the preference sequence of is the same, the above method cannot be used for sequencing, thus resulting in troubled matching. In order to solve this problem, scholar Irving engaged in extended study and proposed the Hospitals/Residents problem with Ties, HRT to solve the problem of having the same score [6].

To find solutions using the HRT algorithm execution, the example of the therapists and cases was substituted into the problem. Supposing for case $\mathbf{P_1}$, the scores of four therapists $\mathbf{C_1}$, $\mathbf{C_2}$, $\mathbf{C_3}$, $\mathbf{C_4}$ in sequence are: $\mathbf{C_1}$: the score of 2A2B (AABB), $\mathbf{C_2}$: the score of 2A2B (AABB), $\mathbf{C_3}$: the score of 4B (BBBB), $\mathbf{C_4}$: the score of 1A3B (BBBA), the supplier conditions and case demand conditions that can be mutually provided in sequence derive at the best matches of $\mathbf{C_1}$ and $\mathbf{C_2}$, while $\mathbf{C_4}$ is in third place and $\mathbf{C_3}$ is in fourth place. When $\mathbf{C_1}$ and $\mathbf{C_2}$ have the same sequence, the problem of a priority right should be resolved. This problem is solved using HRT below to find hyper-stable matching.

P_1:((C_1)(C_2)) C_4 C_3	C_1 : P_3 (P_2(P_1))P_4
P_2 :(C_2) C_4 C_3 C_1	C_2 :(P_2)(P_1)(P_3 P_4)
P_3 :(C_3) C_2 (C_1 C_4)	C_3 : P_1 P_2 ((P_3)P_4)
P_4 :(C_4) C_2 C_3 C_1	C_4 :(P_1 P_3)((P_4)P_2)

Fig. 1 HRT Step 1

Fig. 1 shows the hypothetical preference sequence of four cases ($\mathbf{P_1}$, $\mathbf{P_2}$, $\mathbf{P_3}$, $\mathbf{P_4}$) versus four rehabilitation therapists ($\mathbf{C_1}$, $\mathbf{C_2}$, $\mathbf{C_3}$, $\mathbf{C_4}$). $\mathbf{C_1}$ and $\mathbf{C_2}$ of case $\mathbf{P_1}$ have the same score. Therefore, both are bracketed as a common priority right (left side of Fig. 1). When performing provisional assignment of therapists and cases, both must be assigned at the same time. Step 1: with cases as the orientation, rehabilitation therapists undergo provisional assignment. The four cases and the first-priority therapists underwent provisional matching.

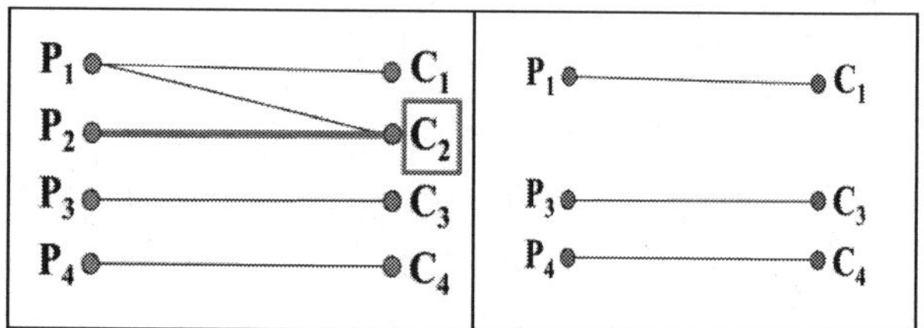

Fig. 2 HRT Step 2

The matches from the provisional assignment were sketched into a provisional assignment diagram (Fig. 2). It can be seen that $\mathbf{C_2}$is selected by both $\mathbf{P_1}$ and $\mathbf{P_2}$ in the provisional assignment. At this time, a look back on $\mathbf{C_2}$ shows that $\mathbf{P_2}$ is the first priority in the preference sequence. Hence, ($\mathbf{P_2}$, $\mathbf{C_2}$) are an ultra-stable match.

As shown in Fig. 3, since ($\mathbf{P_2}$, $\mathbf{C_2}$) were successfully matched, the original provisional distribution of $\mathbf{P_1}$ and $\mathbf{C_2}$ was removed, and the bonded match was deleted, forming the provisional assignment diagram in Fig. 4. Additionally, the ($\mathbf{P_1}$, $\mathbf{C_1}$), ($\mathbf{P_3}$, $\mathbf{C_3}$), ($\mathbf{P_4}$, $\mathbf{C_4}$) matches were the key candidates.

P_1:(C_1 ~~C_2~~) C_4 C_3	C_1 : P_3 (~~P_2~~ P_1) P_4
P_2 :(C_2) C_4 C_3 C_1	C_2 (P_2) P_1 (P_3 P_4)
P_3: C_3 ~~C_2~~ (C_1 C_4)	C_3 : P_1 ~~P_2~~ (P_3 P_4)
P_4: C_4 ~~C_2~~ C_3 C_1	C_4 :(P_1 P_3) (P_4 ~~P_2~~)

Fig. 3 HRT Step 5

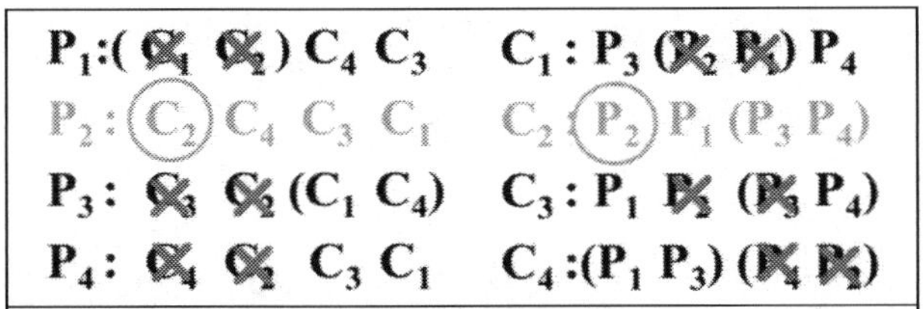

Fig. 4 HRT Step 5

Since (P_2, C_2) are an ultra-stable match, P_2 and C_2 were deleted from the sequence of other candidates. The key candidates set in Step 4 were deleted until the key set was empty. The remaining people underwent a second provisional assignment.

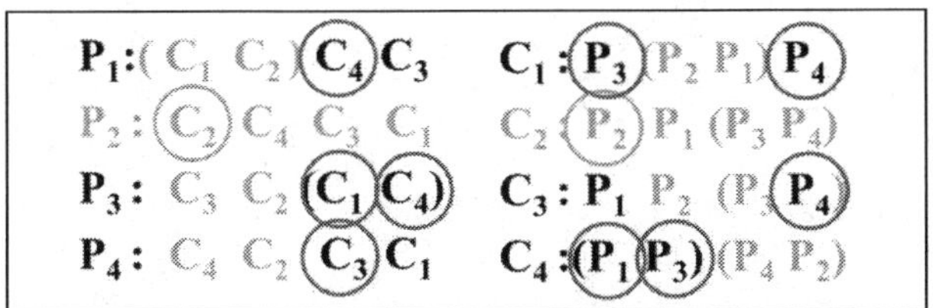

Fig. 5 HRT Step 6

As shown in Fig. 5, a second provisional assignment was carried out (the part circled in blue). Similarly, when two candidates are bracketed (C_1 and C_4 of P_3), there is common priority right, meaning they must simultaneously be chosen to carry out provisional assignment.

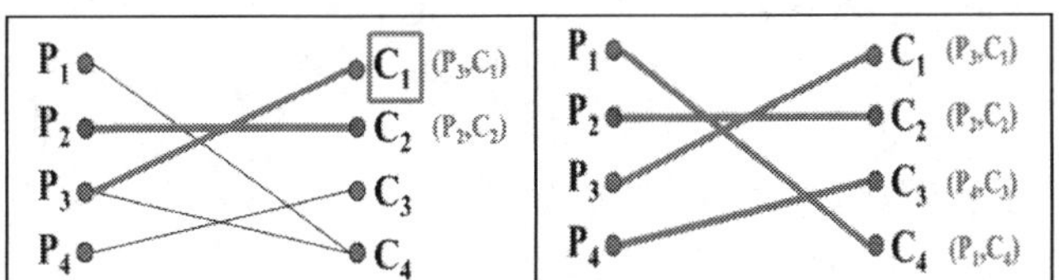

Fig. 6

As shown on the left side of Fig. 6, with the cases as the starting point, in the preference list of P_3, C_1 and C_4, there is common priority right. Therefore, the most suitable candidate for P_3 cannot be determined at this point. On the contrary, from the preference list of C_1 and C_4, it can be found that P_1 and P_3 also have common priority right. Therefore, determination cannot be made from C_4 but from C_1. From the preference list of C_1, it can be found that in the second provisional assignment, P_3 is the first priority of C_1 and thus (P_3, C_1) are a stable match.

C_4 was originally chosen by P_1 and P_3, but (P_3, C_1) had been matched into a stable match. Hence, P_1 only chose C_4 to match. Only P_1 was left as the first priority of C_4, both completing a stable match (P_1, C_4). As shown on the right side of Fig. 6, finally, P_4 and C_3 completed a stable match. Therefore, in the above examples of therapists and cases, the HRT algorithm resolved the problem of many people sharing a common priority right. The matching results obtained are: M=(P_1, C_4), (P_2, C_2), (P_3, C_1), (P_4, C_3).

3 Conclusions

This study set up the PAC service matching platform to help cases and rehabilitation therapists to quickly and effectively find suitable candidates according to their own personal needs and conditions, thereby improving the traditional tedious processes of home rehabilitation applications, substantially reducing the burden of families, enhancing the willingness of rehabilitation therapists to seek employment, enabling cases to have better quality home rehabilitation services, and implementing the vision of home care.

4 Acknowledgment

This research was supported by the Ministry of Science and Technology of Taiwan, R.O.C. under grant No. MOST106-2221-E-227-001.

5 References

[1] Foster Provost and Tom Fawcett. "Data Science and its Relationship to Big Data and Data-Driven Decision Making". Big Data. February 2013, 1(1): 51-59.

[2] Kickstarter.Available at: https://www.kickstarter.com/

[3] Geoffrey G. Parker, Marshall W. Van Alstyne, Sangeet Paul Choudary(2016), "Platform Revolution: How Networked Markets Are Transforming the Economy--and How to Make Them Work for You". W. W. Norton & Company

[4] Ministry of Health and Welfare-Long-term care application.https://www.mohw.gov.tw/cp-189-208-1.html

[5] Gale and L. S. Shapley, "College admissions and the stability of marriage," American Mathematical Monthly, 69:9-15, 1962.

[6] Irving, R. W and Manlove, D.F and Scott, S., "The hospitals /residents problem with ties," Lecture Notes in Computer Science Vol 1851, pages 259-271, 2000.

ARMStrokes: A Mobile System for Customized Everyday Upper Limb Rehabilitation

Yahya M Alqahtani
Dept.Computer and Information Sciences
Towson Univeristy
Towson, US
yalqah1@students.towson.edu

Sonia Lawson
Dept. Occupational Therapy and Occupational Science
Towson Univeristy
Towson, US
slawson@towson.edu

Ziying Tang and Jinjuan Heidi Feng
Dept.Computer and Information Sciences
Towson University
Towson, US
ztang,jfeng@towson.edu

Abstract— **Adherence to a home exercise program (HEP) is a recurring issue impacting the outcomes of therapies or personal goals, which rely on the individual to perform exercises regularly to obtain optimal results. It is important to provide an exercise program that is motivating and easily accessible to promote self-efficacy and long term participation. We developed a low-cost, mobile system that allows stroke survivors to conduct rehabilitation exercises through their smart phones. A re-design allows the system to support a much broader population through automated calibration, multiple storylines that appeal to patients from different age groups, and a reward system. Individuals with upper limb problems or limited physical activity due to chronic conditions may benefit from the increased activity and targeted movement patterns provided through using the application.**

Keywords—Mobile application, upper extremity injury, rehabilitation

I. Introduction

A large number of medical conditions can result in upper extremity injuries that require rehabilitation exercises. An estimation based on the National Electronic Injury Surveillance System (NEISS) data suggests an estimated total of 3,468,996 upper extremity injuries presented to the emergency department in the USA per year, which corresponds to an incidence of 1,130 such injuries per 100,000 persons per year [1]. Stroke and arthritis are other common causes for upper extremity dysfunction. The Centers for Disease Control and Prevention (CDC) in the US recognizes that stroke is a major public health issue: in the US 795,000 people sustain a stroke annually, and stroke costs the nation $34 billion each year [2]. From 2013 to 2015, an estimated 54.4 million US adults (22.7%) annually had ever been diagnosed with some form of arthritis, rheumatoid arthritis, gout, lupus, or fibromyalgia [3].

Research suggests that performing regular rehabilitation exercises (high intensive and repetitive for neurological problems) is critical for recovery. However, The recovery and rehabilitation of the arm and hand after injury or disease is often slow and difficult. It was estimated that only 31% of those recovering from a stroke actually follow therapists' suggestions and perform the recommended exercises due to a variety of factors including lack of motivation [4]. A growing number of research projects have been conducted on how to use commercial or specially designed games or haptic-based virtual rehabilitation systems to make in-home rehabilitation fun and engaging. Those studies confirm the potential of using gaming systems and haptic devices in the rehabilitation process. They also suggest challenges such as high cost, technical complexity, and difficulty to adapt to patients with poor postural control.

To address those challenges, we developed ARMStrokes, a novel approach to support interactive rehabilitation exercises via mobile games in a distributed environment. This low-cost, easily accessible solution allows the user to conduct rehabilitation exercises through smart phones under supervision of a health care professional. ARMStrokes was originally designed for and evaluated by stroke survivors. In this paper, we describe our recent effort to re-design ARMStrokes to support a much broader population. Through newly added functions such as automated calibration, multiple enriched storylines and rewards, ARMStrokes 2.0 can support general upper extremity rehabilitation for individuals with upper limb problems or limited physical activity due to chronic conditions.

II. Related Work

Substantial research has been conducted in the therapy area to examine the potential of existing commercial games and virtual reality environments for rehabilitation. For example, commercial PlayStation and console games have been used to improve rehab motivation [5, 6]. However, most of the commercial games are designed for users with a full range of motion without cognitive and physical limitations. A large number of patients who need upper limb rehabilitation require modifications to these gaming systems to enable performance. In addition, most of those games require hardware set up and can only be conducted in home environment.

Robotic and mechanic devices have also been used for rehabilitation. For example, Colombo et al. [7] proposed a robot-aided arm rehabilitation solution, while Jack et al. [8] examined the use of a haptic glove to improve finger flexion and extension. More recently, Jiang et al. [9] developed a haptic device specifically for wrist and elbow rehabilitation that supports the following motions: opposition, rotation, translation, pitch and yaw. Guneysu Ozgur, A. et al [10] developed a game with a robotic layout to help in upper limb rehabilitation and evaluated it with 18 patients with Cerebral Palsy and 7 therapists. In the majority of those studies, participants who incorporated haptic games into their rehabilitation improved more than those who only used traditional rehab exercises [11]. However, those devices can be expensive and requires technical expertise to set up. They can also be bulky and heavy, making them difficult to access in a mobile environment that makes up today's society.

Mobile applications for rehabilitation have drawn increasing attention recently [12]. However, most of them aren't able to detect and record the quality of the user's physical movement, which is crucial for health care professionals to monitor and adjust the rehabilitation program.

III. ARMStrokes 1.0 and Pilot Study

ARMStrokes was designed and developed through close collaboration with stroke survivors and therapists. Rather than use specialized sensors to track user movements, we focused on developing an approach on top of existing mainstream technology without the need for any additional hardware. Movement speed and position information (e.g., pitch, roll and yaw value) are detected through the built-in sensors (accelerometer, gyroscope, and device orientation sensor) of common smartphones.

Because 66% of stroke survivors have a weak upper limb (arm and hand), we focused on improving upper extremity functions in the game design. Eight exercises for different muscles and joints of upper limbs were selected by occupational therapists, namely forearm rotation, elbow flexion, elbow raise to front, elbow raise to side, shoulder flexion, shoulder rotation, shoulder horizontal adduction, and shoulder abduction. Two games were developed using different metaphors: a monkey picking bananas and an astronaut exploring the space. When a specific body movement that meets the desired measures is detected by the built-in sensors, the monkey or the astronaut rotates or jumps on the screen to signal the completion of one movement. Feedback about the quality of the movement is provided to patients both during the exercise through audio, visual and haptic cues. A graphical chart illustrating the movement pattern was generated at the completion of each exercise.

ARMStrokes can be customized to fit each stroke survivor's specific functionalities in different recovery stages. It also provides an online platform where the patients, physicians, therapists and caregivers can review the exercise data at different levels. Adjustments to the rehabilitation program can be made based on the data.

The system architecture of ARMStrokes is illustrated in Figure 1. Implementation details of the system was reported in Tang et al. 2016 [13].

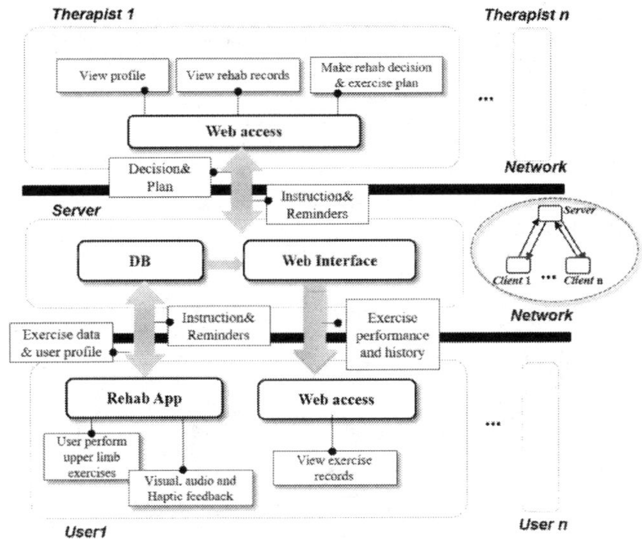

Fig. 1. System architecture of ARMStrokes

We conducted a pilot study to evaluate the efficacy of the ARMStrokes system [14]. Data were collected from pre- and posttest assessments of stroke survivors during a 6 week protocol. During the pre-assessment, the therapists calibrated the app to the participant's performance level for target movement goals, time, and intensity based on manual test results. The participants then used the app for 6 weeks before the post assessment. The user feedback was highly positive. Improvements were observed in accuracy of movements, decreased fatigue, and increased passive range of motion and passive range of motion. Participants also reported improved ability to perform daily activities and ease with using the app.

The pilot study also identified several challenges that need to be addressed. First, the manual calibration conducted by therapists was time consuming and required an in-person visit to establish settings on the app. Patients who were not seeing a therapist would not be able to calibrate the app based on their capabilities and needs. Second, although the app provided a more engaging experience than rehabilitation without any technological support, the motivation component of the design was rather primitive. Both the monkey and the astronaut scenario only supported simple, repetitive motion for visual feedback. Some patients also suggested adding a reward system to provide further motivation for rehabilitation. The identification of these challenges was very helpful for the re-design of ARMStrokes to serve a much broader population.

IV. ARMStrokes 2.0: Supporting Upper Limb Rehabilitation for a Broader Population

After the pilot study with stroke survivors, we decided to re-design ARMStrokes to support general upper extremity rehabilitation for individuals with upper limb problems or limited physical activity due to chronic conditions. Examples include children with cerebral palsy, brain injury or other conditions, patients with arthritis, seniors with diabetes or other chronic conditions that need more physical exercise. Since many patients may not have a therapist or other health professional readily accessible, an automatic calibration function is needed to acquire the patient's personal movement profile including range of motions (ROMs) and moving speed without involving therapists or physicians. . With the goal of serving this diverse population, it is also highly important to engage and motivate the patient so that they can complete the exercises with the desired quality. We focused on those two challenges in the re-design of the ARMStrokes system.

A. *Automatic Calibriation*

The automatic calibration acquires user data through a mobile phone's built-in sensors. For example, users' pronation and supination angles (shown in Fig. 3) are needed to evaluate the "Forearm Rotation" exercise (shown in Fig. 2). To assess the unique pronation and supination angles for a user, the app asks the user to complete the "Forearm Rotation" exercise several times. The related movement parameters are tracked through the phone's gyroscope change and recorded every time the user completes the movement. The data is used to calculate the maximum pronation and supination angles the user can rotate (Range of Motions (ROMs)).

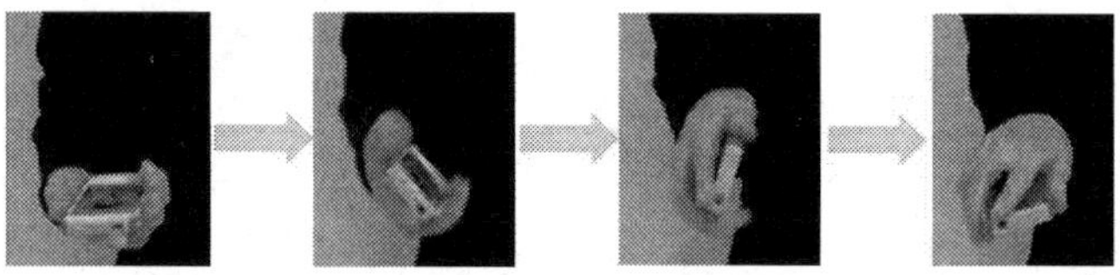

Figure 2. Movement sequence for the "Forearm rotation" exercise

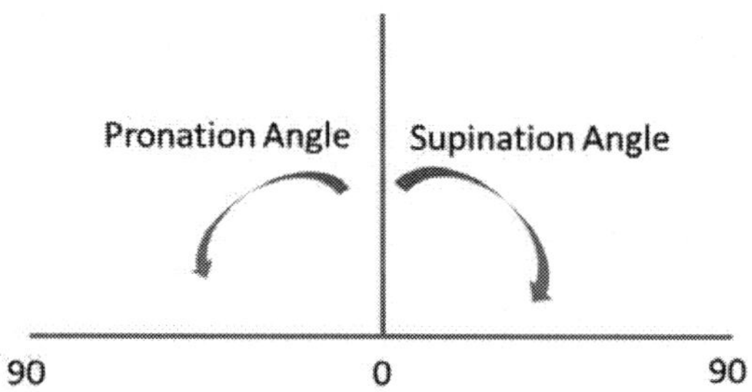

Figure 3. Related angles for the "Forearm rotation" exercise demonstrated in Figure 2.

Fig 4(a) illustrates the instruction page of the automatic calibration function. Fig 4(b) shows the automatic calibration page for the "Shoulder Rotation" exercise as an example. This page includes a video that demonstrates the movement of the exercise. Once a patient starts the calibration, the built in sensors will capture 10 repetitions of the movement and calculate the desired value for related motion measures. Noticing our user's movements are normally limited and not perfectly aligned, which implies gyroscope change happens at more than one direction, the ROMs are recorded in all direction for each exercise.

In addition, we introduced a buffer angle or buffer speed to provide flexibilities when a user performs the exercises. Specifically, we set the maximum and minimum angles or speed as a set of numbers instead of two fixed numbers to offer maximum and minimum ranges. For example, if one patient's maximum and minimum angles for "Forearm Rotation" exercise are 145 degree and 25 degree respectively based on the results from automatic calibration and the buffer angle is set to be 10 degree, the range will be [135-155] and [15-35]. In this case, if the patient's maximum rotation angle falls between 135 and 155 degrees and minimum angle falls between 15 and 35 degrees, the system will record that movement as one valid movement that meets the desired requirement.

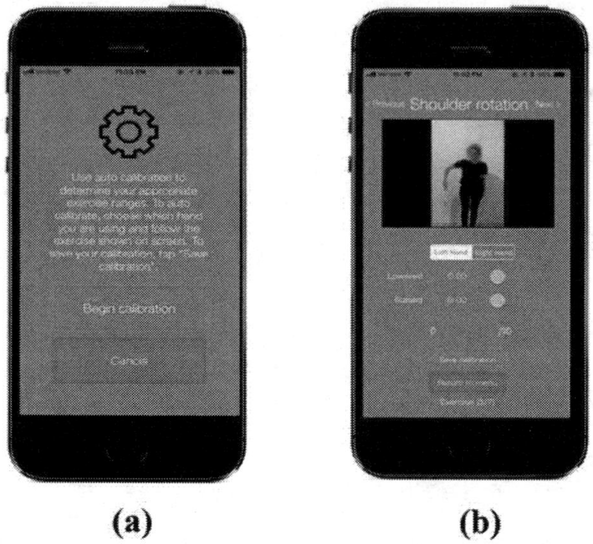

Figure 4. Demonstration of calibration pages. 4(a) shows the page presenting instructions of the calibration process. 4(b) shows the automatic calibration page for the "Shoulder Rotation" exercise.

B. *Storylines*

In order to make the app appealing and engaging to a diverse population potentially including all age groups and a variety of conditions, we decided to implement multiple storylines into the app. The first two storylines being implemented are the farm scenario and the auto shop scenario. Both storylines were chosen based on user feedback collected through the pilot study with stroke survivors and interviews with patients with the targeted conditions. The farm storyline was developed specifically for young children. It features a child walking around a farm engaging in a variety of activities such as helping small animals, playing with animals, or completing farmer chores. As summarized in Tables I, each exercise was mapped to a specific activity that involved similar types of movement. The sound used for audio feedback was also correlated with the specific action or activity.

The auto shop storyline was developed specifically for adults and the seniors. It features a technician working in an auto shop to fix a variety of mechanical problems. Table II summarizes the mapping between each rehabilitation exercise and activity in the auto shop storyline. Other storylines that we plan to implement include kitchen tasks and space travel.

TABLE I. MAPPING BETWEEN THE EXERCISES AND THE ACTIVITIES IN THE FARM STORYLINE

Exercise	Farm Activity
Forearm rotation	Planting a seed/ feeding animals
Elbow flexion	Chop logs
Elbow raise to front	Raising a falling bird back to the nest
Elbow raise to side	Ringing a bell
Shoulder rotation	Throwing a banana to a monkey
Shoulder Abduction	Waving to cows
Shoulder flexion	Rolling a ball with a dog
Shoulder Horizontal Adduction	Open a fence

TABLE II. MAPPING BETWEEN THE EXERCISES AND THE ACTIVITIES IN THE AUTO SHOP STORYLINE

Exercise	Auto Shop Activity
Forearm rotation	Unscrew a spark plug
Elbow flexion	Hammering
Elbow raise to front	Getting supply from top shelf
Elbow raise to side	Pulling hose from the ceiling
Shoulder rotation	Throwing rags to a basket
Shoulder Abduction	Signaling stop
Shoulder flexion	Opening car hood
Shoulder Horizontal Adduction	Washing/waxing car hood

C. *Reward System*

To further motivate the users to be fully committed, a reward system is introduced to track and celebrate the patient's accomplishments. After completing a set of exercises, the patient will be rewarded with stars. The number of stars awarded will be determined based on the quality of the movements. The patient can be promoted to a higher level (e.g., from Bronze to Silver) once a specific number of stars have been accumulated. We are also adding functions that will allow patients to, with permission, connect to other patients and track each other's high level accomplishment statistics. This function will create a collaborative and competitive environment in which patients can motivate each other to complete the exercises.

V. CONCLUSIONS

We have re-designed ARMStrokes to support upper extremity rehabilitation for a broad patient population. The newly added functions will allow the patients to automatically calibrate the app for customized exercises. The system also provides better motivation mechanisms through featured storylines and rewards. We are collaborating with multiple community healthcare providers and support groups to evaluate the system. The first two user studies will focus on seniors with chronic conditions and young children who need upper limb rehabilitation.

ACKNOWLEDGMENT

The project was supported by the Aetna Foundation under grant No. 13-06691, and the School of Emerging Technologies at Towson University.

REFERENCES

[1] Ootes, D. Lambers, K., and Ring, D. (2012). "The epidemiology of upper extremity injuries presenting to the emergency department in the United States". Hand (N Y). v. 7(1): 2012, 18-22.

[2] Centers for Disease Control and Prevention. "Stroke facts". https://www.cdc.gov/stroke/facts.htm

[3] Barbour, E., Helmick, G., Boring, A., Brady. J. "Vital signs: prevalence of doctor-diagnosed arthritis and arthritis-attributable activity limitation — United States, 2013—2015". Morb Mortal Wkly Rep. 2017;66:246–253.

[4] Shaughnessy, M., Resnick, B.M., and Macko, R.F. "Testing a model of post-stroke exercise behavior". Rehabilitation Nursing: The Official Journal of the Assoc. of Rehabil. Nurses 31, 1 (2006), 15- 21.

[5] Alankus, G., Proffitt, R., Kelleher, C., and Engsberg, J. "Stroke Therapy through Motion-Based Games: A Case Study". ACM Transactions on Accessing Computing, 2011,vol. 4.

[6] Chang, Y.-J., Kang, Y.-S., Chang, Y.-S., Liu, H.-H., Wang, C.-C., & Kao, C. C. (2015). "Designing Kinect2Scratch games to help therapists train young adults with Cerebral Palsy in special education school settings". In Proceedings of the 17th International ACM SIGACCESS Conference on Computers & Accessibility - ASSETS '15 (pp. 317–318). New York, New York, USA: ACM Press

[7] Colombo, R., Pisano, F., Mazzone, A. Delconte, C., Micera S., Carrozza,M. C., Dario,P., and Minuco, G. "Design strategies to improve patient motivation during robot-aided rehabilitation". Journal of Neuroengineering and Rehabilitation, 2007, vol. 4:3.

[8] Jack, D., Boian, R., Merians, A.S., et al. "Virtual Reality- enhanced stroke rehabilitation". Neural Sys. And Rehab. Engr., IEEE Trans. 2001, vol. 9: 3, 308-318.

[9] Jiang, J., Xie, L., Li, G. (2015). "A haptic device for wrist and elbow rehabilitation". Digital Medicine, Vol. 1 (2).

[10] Guneysu Ozgur, A., Wessel, M. J., Johal, W., Sharma, K., Özgür, A., Vuadens, P., Dillenbourg, P. (2018). "Iterative design of an upper limb rehabilitation game with tangible robots". In Proceedings of the 2018 ACM/IEEE International Conference on Human-Robot Interaction - HRI '18 (pp. 241–250). New York, New York, USA: ACM Press

[11] Turolla, A., Daud Albasini, O. A., Oboe, R., Agostini, M., Tonin, P., Paolucci, S., Sandrini, G., Venneri, A., and Piron, L. "Haptic-based neurorehabilitation in poststroke patients: A feasibility prospective multicentre trial for robotics hand rehabilitation". Computational and mathematical methods in medicine, vol. 2013, 2013.

[12] Lee, B.C., Kim, J., Chen, S., and Sienko, K.H. "Cell phone based balance trainer". Journal of NeuroEngineering and Rehabilitation, 2012, 9:10.

[13] Tang, Z., Lawson, S., Messing, D., Guo, J., Smith, T., & Feng, J. (2016). "Collaborative rehabilitation support system: A comprehensive solution for everyday rehabilitation". In *Proceedings - 2015 IEEE International Symposium on Multimedia, ISM 2015* (pp. 61–64). Institute of Electrical and Electronics Engineers Inc.

[14] Lawson, S., Tang, Z., & Feng, J. (2017). "Supporting Stroke motor recovery through a mobile application: A pilot study". American Journal of Occupational Therapy, 71(3).

SpeakMore: A Mobile App towards Better Stuttering Awareness to Improve Speech Therapy

Man-Ching Yuen[1], Shin Ying Chu[2], and Normah binti Che Din[2]
[1] Department of Computer Science and Engineering,
The Chinese University of Hong Kong, Sha Tin, Hong Kong
[2] Centre of Rehabilitation & Special Needs,
Universiti Kebangsaan Malaysia, Malaysia
[1] mcyuen@cse.cuhk.edu.hk, [2] {chushinying, normahcd} @ukm.edu.my

Abstract - *Generalization of treatment is a challenging task for speech therapists and adult who stutter (AWS), and it can contribute a barrier to long-term treatment success. Given that AWS often are aware of their speech problems at different speaking situations, self-evaluation of their own speech performance in real-life communication situations could be used to control their stuttering. This project aims to develop a mobile application for smartphones,* SpeakMore, *directed to AWS and speech therapist usage. This software will allow the AWS to register their stuttering related situations, self-evaluate their anxiety level and fluency level. It could help to promote daily self-monitoring of speech as a means of controlling stuttering. This system also allows speech therapists to monitor, receive report, and score their client's speech performance. This collected data could use to improve the therapeutic process using their client's personalized real-life communication situations.*

Keywords: Stutter, Speech Therapy, Mobile Application

1 Introduction

Stuttering is a speech disorder which affects the capacity to communicate effectively. Anxiety has been recognized as a significant concomitant of stuttering [9], [10]. Adults who stutter (AWS) frequently reported increased stuttering in real-life communication in comparison with clinical setting [1], which is why standardized assessment and treatment is vital element in treatment plans to track the progress of AWS in both within and beyond clinical setting. For individuals with stuttering, the existence of speech associated negative emotion and anxiety is often the reason why they seek for speech therapy [11]. In fact, stuttering behaviors can vary across situations, listeners, time, making the process of obtaining a valid measurement complicated [2]. Therefore, repeated assessment (before, during, and after treatment) are important for stuttering treatment [3], [4]. Many speech therapists (STs) faced an issue of continuously assessing the patients due the lack of tools that allow STs to analyze their client's stuttering situations recorded immediately after a real-life communication situation, so it hampers the therapeutic process.

Because of the increasing popularity of mobile apps and social games, many researchers use them to solve problems [5]. Many mobile apps are currently available for delivering advice and therapy. Some apps, like *Optimism*, *PTSD Coach*, *SuperBetter*, are designed for people with depression and anxiety. Some apps, like *Gottman Apps*, offer relationship advice. Some apps, like *MediSafe*, offer medication management service. Besides, a number of previous studies examined the content of apps for mental health management [6], [7]. In 2014, Lee Ventola pointed out that "Mobile devices and apps provide many benefits for Health Care Professionals, perhaps most significantly increased access to point-of-care tools, which has been shown to support better clinical decision-making and improved patient outcomes" [8]. To the best of our knowledge, there is no previous work on developing mobile apps for stuttering treatment.

One of the intervention techniques that has potential to improve current speech treatment for AWS but has not been incorporated into speech therapy, is the self-monitoring strategy. In this paper, we propose "*SpeakMore*", which is a mobile app for better stuttering awareness to improve speech therapy. The mobile app can be used by both STs and AWS to assess and self-monitoring (aka self-evaluating) the fluency of speech for individuals with stuttering. The STs who are familiar with smartphones can strengthen ties with clients and extend treatment to their daily lives using the proposed mobile app.

2 Mobile App: SpeakMore

In this section, we present the design overview and system implementation of the app, *SpeakMore*.

2.1 Design Overview

The purpose of the app, *SpeakMore*, is to (1) assess stuttering severity and 2) assess speech-anxiety levels during real-life situations by AWS themselves (self-evaluating). This application for smartphones could provide a platform for AWS to register their stuttering related situations and record the anxiety level that they faced when stutter. The ability to self-monitor their stuttering events, rate their fluency level, and anxiety level towards the real-life daily communication provides a chance for the AWS to self-reflect their communication abilities. This could guide them to use the fluency techniques that they have learned at the clinic and generalize to the daily life. Additionally, this application provides a platform for the STs to provide real-time assessment of their client's speech performance, understand their client's anxiety level at different speech situations, track their client's speech performance, and provide feedbacks to the client.

Fig. 1 shows the system's architecture, which consists of 2 parts: (1) Android app for collecting input from patients and STs; (2) system server for storing input from patients and therapists in a centralized database. Besides, the data analysis can also be done at the system server. All patients, therapists and system administers have an Android phone with our app installed. The system server is based on MYSQL as central data storage for ease of communications between the patient and the therapist.

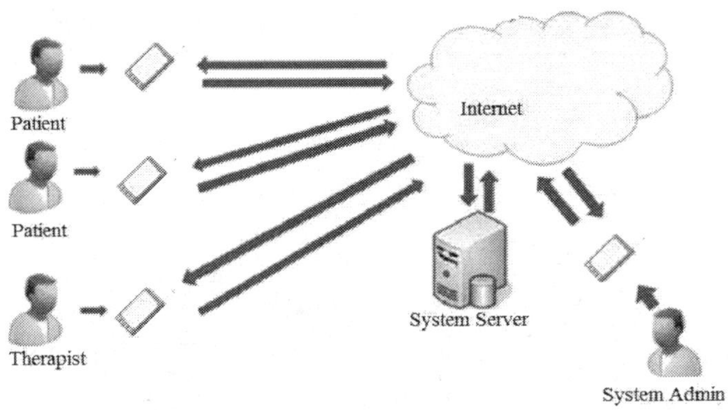

Fig. 1. System architecture

This is a 2-way system: (1) Patients use an Android phone to record video/speech and send the conversation (in different situations) to the server for storage. Patients will rate their fluency of speech, and anxiety level by themselves, and these ratings are also stored in the data server. (2) STs use an Android phone to download the video/speech (3 minutes) from the data server and judge the percentage of stuttering, fluency rating, and feedback. All these data will be sent to the centralized data server and then sent to the patient later.

2.2 How to Communicate using SpeakMore

Therapists (STs) can continuously assess the patients after a real-life communication situation by using our app *SpeakMore*. Fig. 2 shows how *SpeakMore* and its server help patients and therapists to communicate. By using *SpeakMore*, patients can record a real-life communication situation and upload to the server via *SpeakMore*. Once the server receives a new record, it will send out a notification to therapist. Since each therapist have many patients, therapists can download the record at any time they like. Once therapists send their feedback to the server, the server will send out a notification to patient.

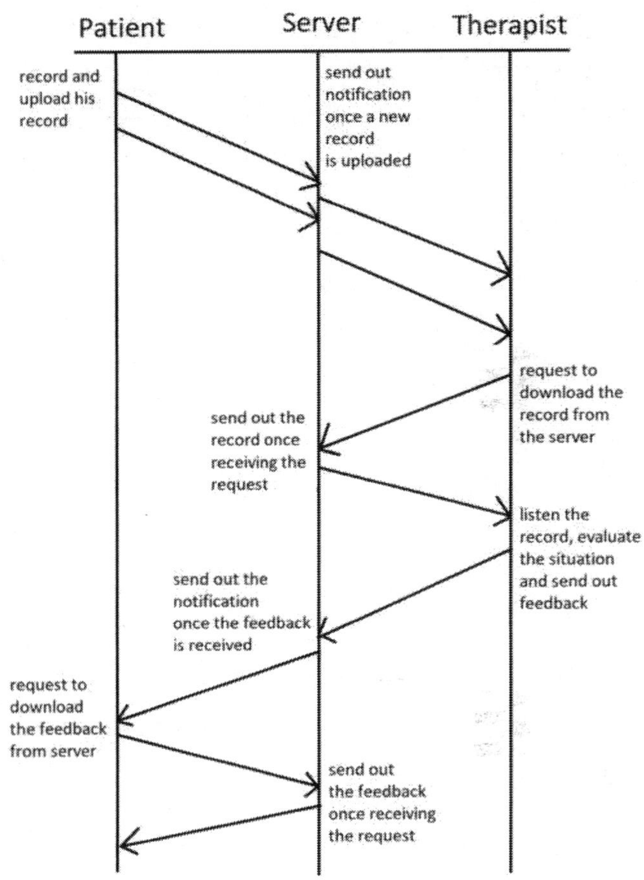

Fig. 2. How to communicate using SpeakMore

2.3 Implementation of SpeakMore

Before using *SpeakMore*, users need to register and log in as either patient or therapist. The functions offered to patients and therapists are different. Fig. 3 shows the interfaces of *SpeakMore* for patients. First, a patient chooses the situation of his recording as shown in Fig. 3(a). Suppose the patient selects the first option, which is "face-to-face conversation with a family member or a close friend". The patient needs to rate his speech anxiety before recording as shown in Fig. 3(b). Once finish recording, the patient needs to rate his anxiety and also listen back his recorded speech to self-evaluate on the level of stuttering as shown in Fig. 3(c). When save button is pressed, all data are sent back to the system server.

Fig. 4 shows the interface of *SpeakMore* for therapists. Once a pop-up message is received by the therapist, he can use *SpeakMore* to download the client's speech and rate the level of stuttering as shown in Fig. 4, and the rating input by the therapists is also stored in the system server.

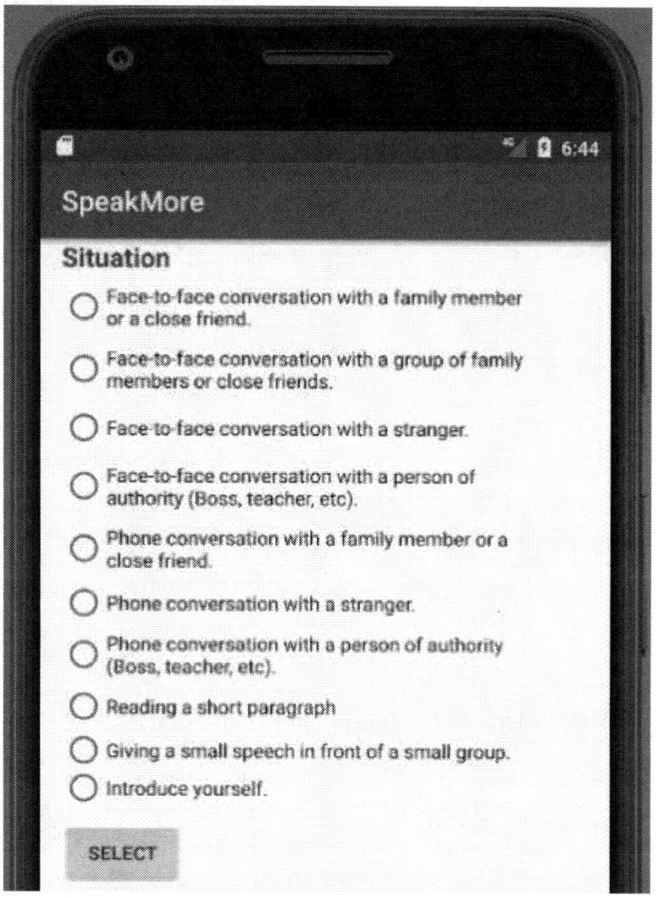

(a)

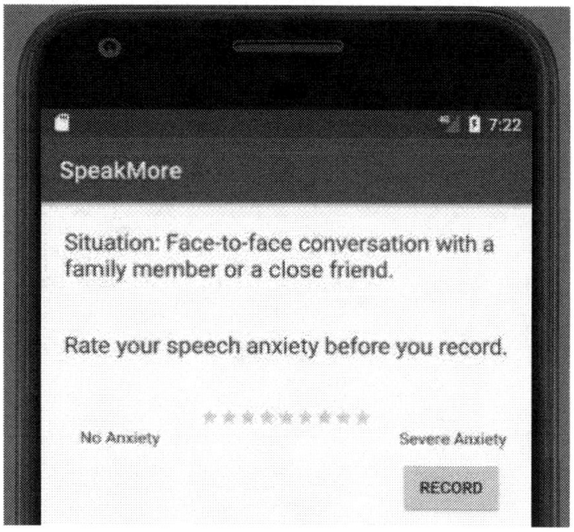

(b)

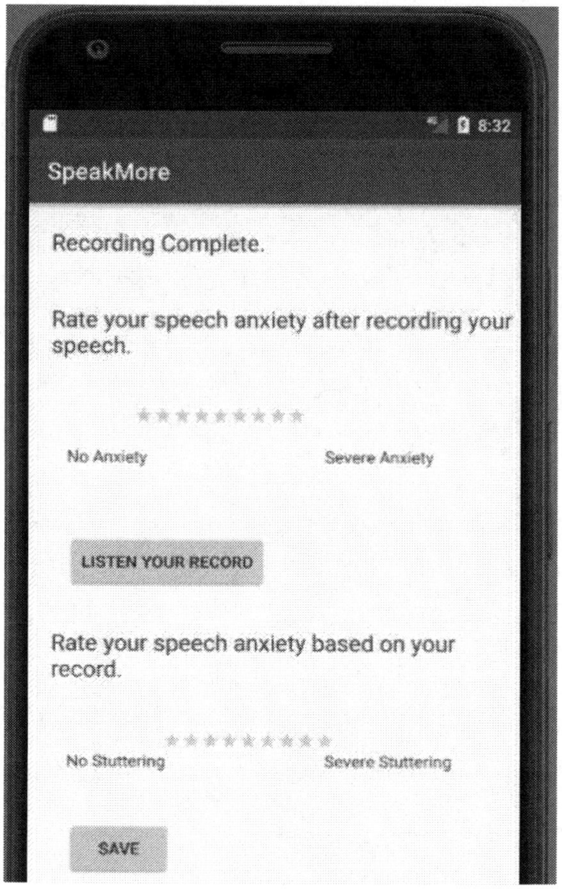

(c)

Fig. 3. Overview of the interface of adults who stutter

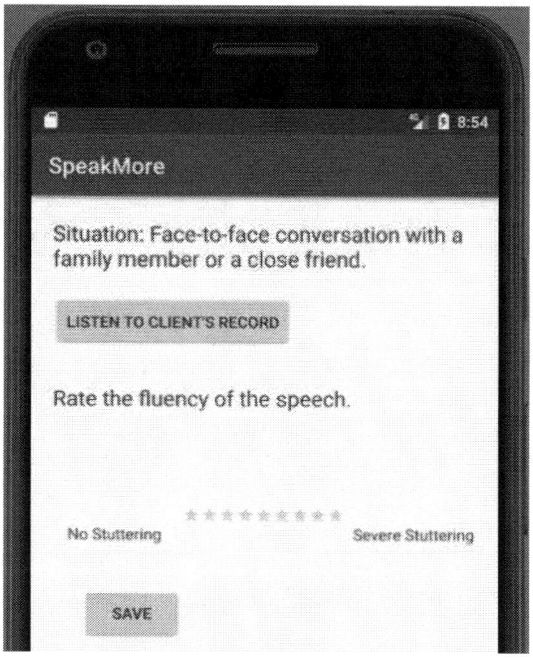

Fig. 4. The interface of the therapist

3 Conclusions

In this paper, we build a mobile app, *SpeakMore*, towards better stuttering self-evaluation in order to improve speech therapy. This mobile app could benefit both STs and AWS because it offers a module for the ST, which can monitor and receive reports related to their clients continuously. This collected data could improve therapeutic process. It could help to promote daily self-monitoring of speech as a means of controlling stuttering. Besides, the mobile app will allow users to self-monitor their stuttering related general condition, and eventually realize how they are evolving throughout treatment. In the future, we will carry out user experience evaluation in real clinical situations to evaluate the content of the mobile app.

Acknowledgments. We thank the anonymous reviewers for their careful reading of our manuscript and their many insightful comments.

4 References

[1] Finn, P.: Self-regulation and the management of stuttering. Seminars in Speech and Language, 24 (2003), 27–32.

[2] Manning, W. H.: Clinical decision making in fluency disorders (2nd ed.). San Diego, CA: Thomson Learning, Inc. (2001).

[3] Chu, S.Y., Sakai, N., Mori, K., & Iverach, L.: Japanese normative data for the Unhelpful Thoughts and Beliefs about Stuttering (UTBAS) Scales for adults who stutter. Journal of Fluency Disorders, 51 (2017), 1-7.

[4] Ingham, J.C., Riley, G.: Guidelines for Documentation of Treatment Efficacy for Young Children Who Stutter. Journal of Speech, Language, and Hearing Research, 41 (1998), 753-770.

[5] Yuen, M. C., Chen, L. J., King, I.: A Survey of Human Computation Systems, Proceedings of IEEE International Symposium on Social Computing Applications (SCA09), Vancouver, Canada, August 2009.

[6] Breton, E., Fuemmeler, B., Abroms, L.: Weight loss—There is an app for that! But does it adhere to evidence-informed practices? Translational Behavioral Med. 2011; 1(4):523-529.

[7] Abroms, L.C., Padmanabhan, N., Thaweethai, L., Phillips, T.: iPhone apps for smoking cessation: A content analysis. American Journal of Preventive Medicine. 2011; 40(3):279-85.

[8] Lee Ventola, C.: Mobile Devices and Apps for Health Care Professionals: Uses and Benefits, P T. 2014 May; 39(5): 356-364.

[9] Iverach L., et al.: Social anxiety disorder and stuttering: current status and future directions. American Journal of Speech-Language Pathology 40 (2014): 69-82.

[10] Langevin M., et al.: Peer responses to stuttering in the preschool setting. American Journal of Speech-Language Pathology 18.3 (2009): 264-276.

[11] Chu, S. Y., "Speech-Language Services for Individuals Who Stutter: Consideration of Anxiety". EC Psychology and Psychiatry 5.6 (2017): 167-168.

SmartCarb: An Intelligent Mobile System to Assist Diet Control for Gestational Diabetes Patients using Deep Learning Neural Networks

Yujie Hu[1], Yu Sun[2], Fangyan Zhang[3], Bo Guo[4]

[1]Northwood High School, Irvine, CA 92620
[2]California State Polytechnic University, Pomona, CA 91768
[3]Mississippi State University, Mississippi State, MS 39762
[4]Meizu Inc., Beijing, China 100871

***Abstract*— Gestational Diabetes, only developed during female pregnancy, is just like other types of diabetes which are caused by excessive amount of glucose intake and could be harmful to both the mother and the baby. For gestational diabetes patient, it is essential to control the serving size of their daily diet, particularly the amount of carbohydrates. For instance, it is recommended that the amount of carbohydrates for each food should not be exceed 17g per serving. In order to help patients to effectively control the diet and know the right amount of serving, a number of diet rules have been developed to specify the recommended amount to eat for different types of the food.**

***Index Terms*— Neural Networks, Machine Learning, Mobile Computing, Diet Control.**

I. Introduction

Gestational Diabetes [1] [2], only developed during female pregnancy, is just like other types of diabetes which are caused by excessive amount of glucose intake. For women above 25 years old who do not pay much attention to their diet and spend time on exercising during their pregnancy, they will have a higher chance of adapting gestational diabetes which can lead to severe consequences to their children. First, excessive birth weight is a common risk that these women with gestational diabetes will face. Due to the excessive amount of sugar across the mother's bloodstream which crosses the placenta, it will trigger the baby's pancreas to produce more insulin.

This will cause the baby to grow larger than the normal size (about 9 pounds or more than normal babies) which will likely cause these large babies to become wedged in the birth canal, sustain birth injuries or require a C-section birth. Second, a mother's high blood sugar may increase the risk of early delivering of the baby before the baby's original due date. Then the early born baby has a chance of experiencing respiratory distress syndrome which makes breathing difficult. If a baby develops this syndrome, they will need breathing aid until their lungs are fully developed. Moreover, babies can also develop low blood sugar (hypoglycemia) after birth for a short period due to their high insulin production by their pancreas; once hypoglycemia is severe, it will provoke seizures in babies. Lastly, when the baby finally grows up and gets older, they will have a higher risk of developing obesity and type 2 diabetes.

All the above are potential threats to the baby when the mother has gestational diabetes. Fortunately, it is not difficult to avoid adapting this type of diabetes. During the mother's pregnancy, eating health foods containing high fiber and low fat and calories will always help. Fruits, vegetables, and whole grains are not a bad choice, however, always be careful about the serving sizes to make sure that the nutrients do not exceed the doctor's prescription.

Nevertheless, eating healthy without exercising will not show much benefits. According to specialists, being moderate active for 30 mins a day for most days of the week will prevent pregnant women from developing gestational diabetes. Since pregnant women cannot do certain exercises, walking, riding a bike and swimming slowly are all optional ways to exercise. In addition, doctors strongly suggest that during pregnancy, it is necessary to not lose too much weight. However, losing weight before wanting to get pregnant may help having a healthier and easier pregnancy.

Thus, having a healthy diet and keep exercising will provide a healthier pregnancy. However, keep exercising only requires personal perseverance, but keeping a healthy diet is difficult to control. For example, different food has different nutrition elements, which requires different rules and guidance. It is very challenging to accurately remember the specific numbers and portions to eat for each type of food or diet plan. In this paper, we propose a solution to this problem by developing a mobile-based automated food recognition and diet suggestion application that helps patients to follow the diet plan. The interface is shown in Figure 1.

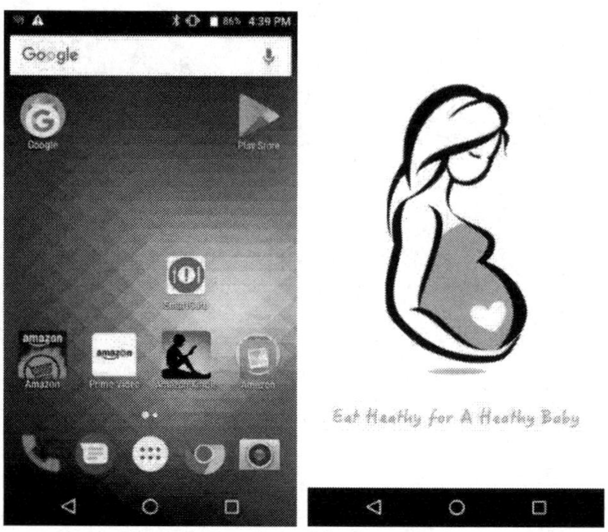

Figure 1: Interface of the SmartCarb app

The rest of the paper is organized as follows: Section 2 discusses the challenges in this research project; one solution is presented in Section 3, followed by showing the experiment and configuration in Section 4; we compare the related works in Section 5, and Section 6 offers the conclusion remarks and future work directions.

II. CHALLENGES

During this project, there are many challenges regarding the advanced technology and countless failures throughout the process.

Challenge 1: recognizing foods from camera

The first challenge that we need to address is the varying amount of carbohydrates for different types of food. Each type of food usually contains different amount of carbohydrates, thus gestational diabetes need to be aware of what amount of food they need to take at one time. Since the entire program relies on the front camera of the device to capture images, it is important to let computers or smartphones accurately recognize the wide variety of food computers or smartphones.

Challenge 2: real-time recognition and processing

The second challenge that we need to address is real-time recognition and suggestion executed in the same device. Due to the limit in the device's capacity and the speed of the device in general, it is not an easy task to process images from camera and offer some reasonable informative suggestions.

Furthermore, since the program's result will be a digital report which analyzes the user's meal, it is difficult for the language to be straightforward to integrate the healthy diet plans and suggestions into the regular mobile application.

III. SOLUTION

To address these issues, a detailed solution was proposed specially to solve all these problems. We have designed and implemented an intelligent mobile system to assist diet control for gestational diabetes patients using deep learning neural networks [3] [4]. This system can provide flexibility and convenience to gestational diabetes patients while eating.

TensorFlow [5] [6] was chosen in the project to make the source input accepted by the system. TensorFlow is an open source library for numerical computation, specializing in machine learning applications. Since this application mainly relies on the software itself to process and analyze the images captured by the front camera, Tensorflow does this perfectly by training a simple classifier using the deep learning branch of machine learning.

To get everything started, we used transfer learning [7] [8]. Transfer learning is basically reusing a model that has been trained on one problem and then retraining it on a similar problem. We chose transfer learning because, unlike deep learning, transfer learning can be done in a short period of time while deep learning usually takes days when starting from scratch. First, it is necessary to install tensorflow on the computer that most of the coding will be at. Then, before any training of the computer, we gathered a large set of pictures to represent the one class that we want the device to recognize.

Last thing before starting the training is launching TensorBoard in the background. TensorBoard [9] is a monitoring and inspection tool included with Tensorflow which keeps track of the training and eliminate any outliers. After all these prerequisites are met, we can finally start the training by executing the following command:

```
python -m scripts.retrain \
  --bottleneck_dir=tf_files/bottlenecks \
  --how_many_training_steps=500 \
  --model_dir=tf_files/models/ \
  --
summaries_dir=tf_files/training_summaries/"${ARCHITEC
TURE}" \
  --output_graph=tf_files/retrained_graph.pb \
  --output_labels=tf_files/retrained_labels.txt \
  --architecture="${ARCHITECTURE}" \
  --image_dir=tf_files/flower_photos
```

This script will download a pre-trained model while adding a new layer where the training will be taken place with the large number of pictures gathered previously. Since the training has started, it will be going through its first phase-analyzing all images on the disk as well as calculating the bottleneck values for each of them. A bottleneck is an informal term used for the layer before the final output layer which actually does the classification. In this case, bottleneck is not implying that the layer is slowing down the entire network; instead, this term is used to describe the representation which is much more compact than in the main body of the network.

In this project, we defined a class: *ClassifierActivity*, which extended from *CameraActivity* by implementing *OnImageAvailableListener*. The most important function is the *onImageAvailable,* which will trigger event while an image is available form camera. The following source code shows the details.

```
public onImageAvailable(final ImageReader reader) {
    Image image = null;
    try {
      image = reader.acquireLatestImage();
      if (image == null) {
        return;
      }
      if (computing) {
        image.close();
        return;
      }
      computing = true;
      Trace.beginSection("imageAvailable");
      final Plane[] planes = image.getPlanes();
      fillBytes(planes, yuvBytes);

      final int yRowStride = planes[0].getRowStride();
      final int uvRowStride = planes[1].getRowStride();
      final int uvPixelStride = planes[1].getPixelStride();
      ImageUtils.convertYUV420ToARGB8888(
          yuvBytes[0],
          yuvBytes[1],
          yuvBytes[2],
          previewWidth,
          previewHeight,
          yRowStride,
          uvRowStride,
```

```
            uvPixelStride,
            rgbBytes);
        image.close();
    } catch (final Exception e) {
        if (image != null) {
            image.close();
        }
        LOGGER.e(e, "Exception!");
        Trace.endSection();
        return;
    }
    rgbFrameBitmap.setPixels(rgbBytes, 0, previewWidth, 0, 0,
previewWidth, previewHeight);
    final Canvas canvas = new Canvas(croppedBitmap);
    canvas.drawBitmap(rgbFrameBitmap,
frameToCropTransform, null);
    if (SAVE_PREVIEW_BITMAP) {
        ImageUtils.saveBitmap(croppedBitmap);
    }
    runInBackground(
        new Runnable() {
            @Override
            public void run() {
                final long startTime = SystemClock.uptimeMillis();
                final List<Classifier.Recognition> results =
classifier.recognizeImage(croppedBitmap);
                lastProcessingTimeMs =
SystemClock.uptimeMillis() - startTime;

                cropCopyBitmap =
Bitmap.createBitmap(croppedBitmap);
                resultsView.setResults(results);
                requestRender();
                computing = false;
            }
        });
    Trace.endSection();
}
```

Since each image is used multiple time during the training, calculating the bottleneck behind each of them will take a significant amount of time. Therefore, after the script finishes generating all the bottleneck files, the final training of the final layer of the network begins. "The training operates efficiently by feeding the cached value for each image into the Bottleneck layer. The true label for each image is also fed into the node labeled GroundTruth. Just these two inputs are enough to calculate the classification probabilities, training updates, and the various performance metrics".

After the training, there will be a series of outputs generated by the system including training accuracy, validation accuracy, and cross entropy. The training accuracy demonstrates the percent of pictures that are categorized in the right class out of the all the pictures that were uploaded during the training. Validation accuracy, similarly, shows the precision in a randomly selected set of pictures. Lastly, cross entropy is a loss function that shows how well the learning process is (lower number is better).

IV. Configuration

In order to adjust some parameters to see if we can increase the final validation accuracy. We can do some related configurations. For example, the *--learning_rate* parameter controls the magnitude of the updates to the final layer during training. So far, we have left it out, so the program has used the default *learning_rate* value of 0.01.

The *learning_rate* can be set other values to increase or decrease the accuracy, for example, if we set *learning_rate* at 0.005, the training will take longer, but the overall precision might increase. If we set *learning_rate* at higher values. For example, 1.0, then the system could train faster, but definitely reduces precision, or even makes training unstable.

It is very helpful for this type of work if we give each experiment a unique name, so they show up as separate entries in TensorBoard.

It's the *--summaries_dir* option that controls the name in TensorBoard. For an instance that we used in the experiment,

--summaries_dir = training_summaries/basic

TensorBoard is monitoring the contents of the training summaries directory, if the *training_summaries* or any subdirectory of *training_summaries* is configured for *summarys_dir,* which works fine.

Also, we are also allowed to set the following two options together, so our results are clearly labeled:

--learning rate=0.5

--summaries_dir=training_summaries/LR_0.5

After seeing the script working on the flower example images, we can start looking at teaching the network to recognize different categories. In theory, all we need to do is run the tool, specifying a set of sub-folders. Each sub-folder is named

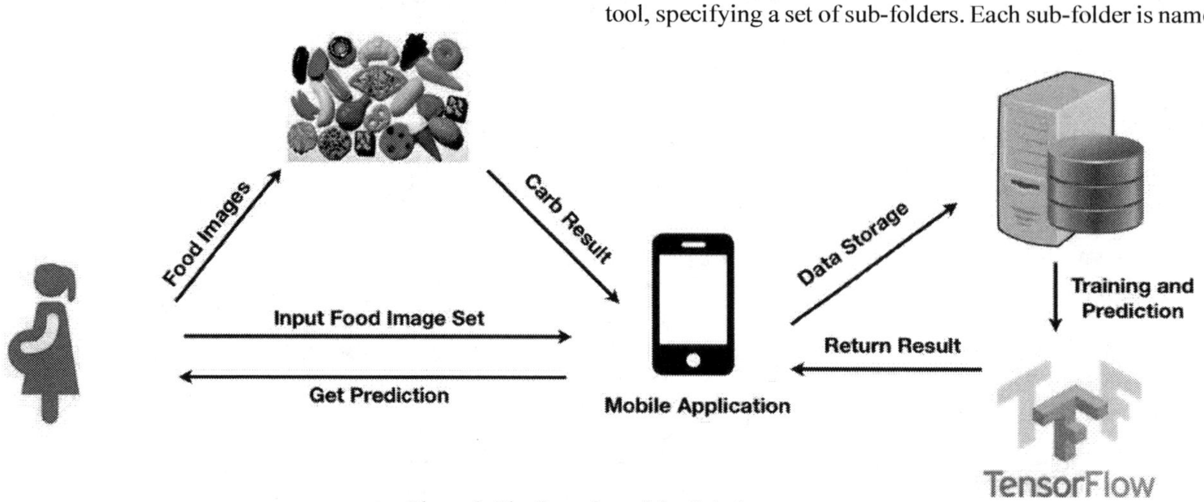

Figure 2. The Overview of the Solution

after one of categories and contains only images from that category.

After we finish this step and pass the root folder of the subdirectories as the argument for the --*image_dir* parameter, the script should train the images that we have provided, just like it did for the flowers. The classification script uses the folder names as label names, and the images inside each folder should be pictures that correspond to that label, as we can see in Figure 2.

V. Evaluation and Configurations

To measure the performance with these three outputs, a specialized system of evaluation is developed. The performance is measured mainly on the validation accuracy. For instance, if only the training accuracy is high, but other indexes are not, that means the network is outfitting, and the network is memorizing features that do not help classifying images generally. In other words, the training object is to make the cross entropy as low as possible.

According to TensorFlow, the script runs 4,000 training steps with each step choosing 10 images from a set of pictures and analysis them: finding the bottleneck from the cache and then feeding them into the layer to get predictions. Finally, when the final accuracy value is between 85% and 99%, the training is successful, and the model is fully trained.

After training, it is time to move everything to the developing mobile. By using Android studio as the developing station, we successfully created an application that stores all the training detail and can identify all the classes that are trained. Figure 3 shows two examples on fires and hamburger.

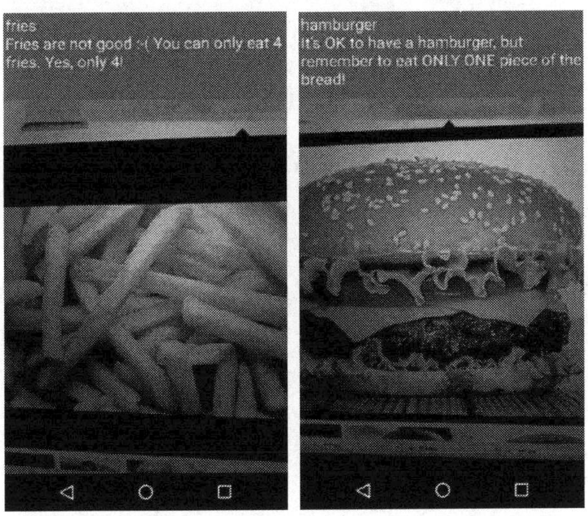

Figure 3: Two examples of usage of the App

VI. Related Work

Similar work also applied machine learning to eating behavior. Li and Ko [10] applied the food ontology technique to construct the food care diet car. Although they enabled an automated approach to construct the ontology, their approach is based on the knowledge base, without using machine learning algorithms. Kourou et al. [11] presented a survey of machine-learning-based approaches to predict cancer and understand the growth and development of cancer.

Polat el atl. [12][13] applied the Generalized Discriminant Analysis and Least Square Support Vector Machine to assist the diagnosis of diabetes disease. However, it is more data-driven approach without using the images. In addition, they focus on the general diabetes patient, rather than the specific group of gestational diabetes that requires a different type of assistance.

VII. Conclusion and Future Work

To summarize, this project had aimed to help gestational diabetic patients to follow the recommended diet plan in an easy and effective way. To save the trouble for gestational diabetic patients to figure out carbohydrate in each food, this projected used deep learning to identify the amount of carbohydrate in each kind of food and to provide valuable suggestions for users.

Furthermore, to allow the diet control system to adjust accordingly to different kinds of food, this project used input data to constantly update the diet control system.

As for the future work, we will investigate other deep learning algorithms and other new technologies to keep improving the accuracy.

Furthermore, from studying related works, we plan to also integrate more machine learning into project. This can be done by predicting details about diet based on data ingredients.

References

[1] Kim, Catherine, Katherine M. Newton, and Robert H. Knopp. "Gestational diabetes and the incidence of type 2 diabetes: a systematic review." Diabetes care 25, no. 10 (2002): 1862-1868.

[2] American Diabetes Association. "Gestational diabetes mellitus." Diabetes care 27 (2004): S88.

[3] Specht, Donald F. "Probabilistic neural networks." Neural networks 3, no. 1 (1990): 109-118.

[4] Schmidhuber, Jürgen. "Deep learning in neural networks: An overview." Neural networks 61 (2015): 85-117.

[5] Abadi, Martín, Paul Barham, Jianmin Chen, Zhifeng Chen, Andy Davis, Jeffrey Dean, Matthieu Devin et al. "TensorFlow: A System for Large-Scale Machine Learning." In OSDI, vol. 16, pp. 265-283. 2016.

[6] Rampasek, Ladislav, and Anna Goldenberg. "Tensorflow: Biology's gateway to deep learning?." Cell systems 2, no. 1 (2016): 12-14.

[7] Pan, Sinno Jialin, and Qiang Yang. "A survey on transfer learning." IEEE Transactions on knowledge and data engineering 22, no. 10 (2010): 1345-1359.

[8] Bengio, Yoshua. "Deep learning of representations for unsupervised and transfer learning." In Proceedings of ICML Workshop on Unsupervised and Transfer Learning, pp. 17-36. 2012.

[9] TensorBoard: https://www.tensorflow.org/programmers_guide/summaries_and_tensorboard

[10] Li, Huan-Chung, and Wei-Min Ko. "Automated food ontology construction mechanism for diabetes diet care." Machine Learning and Cybernetics, 2007 International Conference on. Vol. 5. IEEE, 2007.

[11] Kourou, Konstantina, et al. "Machine learning applications in cancer prognosis and prediction." Computational and structural biotechnology journal 13 (2015): 8-17.

[12] Polat, Kemal, Salih Güneş, and Ahmet Arslan. "A cascade learning system for classification of diabetes disease: Generalized discriminant analysis and least square support vector machine." Expert systems with applications 34.1 (2008): 482-487.

[13] Mani, Subramani, et al. "Type 2 diabetes risk forecasting from EMR data using machine learning." AMIA annual symposium proceedings. Vol. 2012. American Medical Informatics Association, 2012.

Cancer Specific Imaging

Philippos Costa[1], Anielle Almeida[2], Noelio Dantas[2], Luciano Lima[3], Eduardo Costa[3], Anderson Santos[4], Guilherme Fernandes[3], Antonio Basile[5], Marcus Santos[6], Marcelo Silva[7]

[1]Harrington Training Programs, University of Miami, Miami, FL, U.S.
[2]Institute of Physics, Federal University of Alagoas, Maceio, Brazil
[3]School of Engineering, University of Uberlandia, Uberlandia, Brazil
[4]Computer Science, University of Uberlandia, Uberlandia, Brazil
[5]Computer Science, University of Uberlandia, Uberlandia, Brazil
[6]Computer Science, Ryerson University, Toronto, Ontario, Canada
[7]Laboratory of Immunology, University of Uberlandia, Uberlandia, MG, Brazil

Abstract— *This paper discusses the design of intelligent nanomaterials for building biosensors and cancer-specific imaging, and how such a technology could impact the healthcare system of a developing country. One can utilize a capacitive field effect biosensor for detecting bacterial antigens. On the other hand, for cancer-specific imaging, the authors propose the use of magic-sized quantum dots, since they noted through their own experience that quantum dots can preserve luminescent properties for many years, while traditional cancer-specific dyes last at most a few months. In the main body of this article, the interested reader will find case studies that he or she can follow in order to grow nanomaterials that interact with tell-tale proteins selected from the genome of a microorganism or cancer.*

Keywords: cancer imaging CAD nanotechnology AI

Type of the submission: LATE BREAKING PAPER

1. Introduction

As is commonly the case in bioinformatics, the reader will find three kinds of contribution in the present paper: Computer algorithms used for mathematical modelling, molecular biology processes and nanotechnology. The authors will provide enough information about such algorithms, in order that the interested reader may recreate them with little effort and without the need of help from computer scientists. However, the reader will need to find collaborators from the fields of nanotechnology and experimental biology, in order to build the biosensors and luminescent compounds described on the pages that follow. In both cases, the authors aim at providing details for researchers with adequate resources to reproduce most results published in the present paper, and complete the experiments that they could not finish for lack of time or expertise.

Today's advances is Artificial Intelligence (AI) make one wonder if researchers in AI could be considered stage magicians rather than scientists, since their work appears to create an illusion of intelligence, instead of real intelligence. One could generalize this assessment to most scientists, but not because they create illusions instead of something real, but because they do not reveal key elements of their research for someone interested in reproducing their results. One of the main goals of the present paper is to make a small contribution to change this situation, by providing a head start for other researchers and professionals.

The body manufactures protein complexes, called antibodies. These bind themselves to a specific protein of a particular pathogen, such as bacteria or cancer cells. A scientist can conjugate a luminescent material to such an antibody, and in this way produce a cancer-specific dye. The surgeon applies this dye to the affected tissue and then flashes a laser beam on it. The result is that the luminescent material will emit light, illuminating the malign cell to which it is bound, while the healthy anatomy will remain dull [9], [10], [1]. Using a surgical robotic system, external beam radiotherapy or sealed source radiation therapy, the physician can eliminate the cancer revealed through such techniques in a minimally invasive surgery.

2. Measurement theory

Measurement theory was proposed for evaluating those attributes that do not yield to direct observation. One must be careful to note that the measurement theory discussed in the present paper is a branch of statistics developed by Georg Rasch to deal with hidden aspects of complex systems, such as skill, efficiency or competence. It should not be confused with Measure Theory, which is a field of mathematical analysis.

When one is intent upon measuring something, a choice of measurement scales has to be made. Scales are always based on comparison. In the case of hidden entities, it is advisable that such comparisons be based on ratios, as the reader will see in the next paragraphs.

Let us consider two technologies c and v, and a problem r that they are intent on solving. The first problem is to compare the skills of c and v based on their performance in dealing with r. Let us ignore those results where both c and v hit or both of them fail together.

The probability of c succeeding in solving the problem r is given by P_{cr} and the probability of it failing to solve the same problem can be calculated by $(1 - P_{cr})$. On the other hand, the probabilities of v succeeding and failing at solving the same problem are given by P_{vr} and $(1-P_{vr})$ respectively.

If researchers wish to compare c with r, they can ignore the number of occasions where both hit and the number of cases where both miss. Let N_{10} be the notation of how many items c hits and v misses in N trials. On the same token, let N_{01} denote the number of c misses and v hits in N trials. The probability of c hitting and v missing can be estimated through the ratio between N_{10} and N for N_{10} very large. The probability of c missing and v hitting can be estimated through the ratio between N_{01} and N, for N very large.

$$P_{cr} \times (1 - P_{vr}) = \frac{N_{10}}{N}$$

$$P_{vr} \times (1 - P_{cr}) = \frac{N_{01}}{N}$$

From the equations above, one can calculate the ratio between N_{10} and N_{01}, which is given below

$$\frac{N_{10}}{N_{01}} = \frac{P_{cr} \times (1 - P_{vr})}{(1 - P_{cr}) \times P_{vr}}$$

Probability is estimated as the relative ratio of success to the number of trials, where the number of trials tends to infinity.

One can say that c is better at performing a task than v if its superior results do not depend on the problem. This property is called specific objectivity. Let us consider two variations r and s of a given problem. For performing a statistical comparison between c and v, the researcher must require that the ratio N_{10}/N_{01} does not change when one changes the item. In this case, one has the equality given below.

$$\frac{P_{cr} \times (1 - P_{vr})}{(1 - P_{cr}) \times P_{vr}} = \frac{P_{cs} \times (1 - P_{vs})}{(1 - P_{cs}) \times P_{vs}}$$

Odds can be described as the ratio of the probability of an event occurring to the probability of it not occurring. One can rewrite this equality in order to obtain the odds of success for c performing task r.

$$\frac{P_{cr}}{(1 - P_{cr})} = \frac{P_{cs}}{(1 - P_{cs})} \times \frac{(1 - P_{vs})}{P_{vs}} \times \frac{P_{vr}}{(1 - P_{vr})}$$

2.1 Origin

The next step is to choose the origin for the measurement scales that one intends to introduce. Let us consider a technology o with an efficiency that matches the difficulty of a problem o. In this case, the technology will solve the problem in half of the trials, and the problem will defeat the technology in the other half. This technology is said to be at the origin of the efficiency scale, and the problem is at the origin of the difficulty scale. Since the technology solves the item half of the times, the probability of success is $P_{oo} = 0.5$. Let us compare c with the technology at the origin. The efficiency of a technology at the origin ties with the difficulty of the problem at the origin.

For the problem discussed in this work, when a technology discriminates cancer cells from normal peripheral tissue, the technology is said to overcome the problem, on the contrary, the problem defeats the technology.

When the technology and the problem are tied in strength, the probability of the technology at the origin solving the problem at the origin is 0.5, and the probability of the problem persisting is also 0.5. To provide a quick reference, the formula for calculating the odds of c solving problem r is reproduced below.

$$\frac{P_{cr}}{(1 - P_{cr})} = \frac{P_{co}}{(1 - P_{co})} \times \frac{(1 - P_{oo})}{P_{oo}} \times \frac{P_{or}}{(1 - P_{or})}$$

Since P_{oo} is 0.5, one has that $(1-P_{oo})/P_{oo} = 1$. Therefore

$$\frac{P_{cr}}{(1 - P_{cr})} = \frac{P_{co}}{(1 - P_{co})} \times \frac{P_{or}}{(1 - P_{or})}$$

Let's take the logarithm from both sides of this equation

$$\ln(\frac{P_{cr}}{(1 - P_{cr})}) = \ln(\frac{P_{co}}{(1 - P_{co})} \times \frac{P_{or}}{(1 - P_{or})})$$

$$\ln(\frac{P_{cr}}{(1 - P_{cr})}) = \ln(\frac{P_{co}}{(1 - P_{co})}) + \ln(\frac{P_{or}}{(1 - P_{or})})$$

$$\ln(\frac{P_{cr}}{(1 - P_{cr})}) = \ln(\frac{P_{co}}{(1 - P_{co})}) - \ln(\frac{(1 - P_{or})}{P_{or}})$$

Then if one defines

$$A_c = \ln(\frac{P_{co}}{(1 - P_{co})})$$

$$D_r = \ln(\frac{(1 - P_{or})}{P_{or}})$$

the equation becomes:

$$\ln(\frac{P_{cr}}{(1 - P_{cr})}) = A_c - D_r$$

From the definition of logarithm, one has:

$$\frac{P_{cr}}{(1 - P_{cr})} = e^{A_c - D_r}$$

$$P_{cr} = e^{A_c - D_r} - P_{cr} \times e^{A_c - D_r}$$

$$P_{cr} \times (1 + e^{A_c - D_r}) = e^{A_c - D_r}$$

$$P_{cr} = \frac{e^{A_c - D_r}}{1 + e^{A_c - D_r}} \quad \text{Logistic equation} \quad (1)$$

Note that A_c does not depend on the problem r and D_r does not depend on the technology c. This finding is the greatest contribution made by Georg Rasch to the Measurement Theory. Therefore, A is a measurement of the technology, and does not depend on any problem in particular; D is the measurement of the problem, and does not depend on any particular technology.

In Equation 1, one often refers to parameters A_c and D_r as the efficiency of the technology and problem difficulty respectively.

The present section uses binomial probability distribution to explain the basic concepts of measurement. For a perspective using different distributions, the interested reader may consult the excellent tutorial by Benjamin Wright [2].

3. What should one measure?

In order to measure different technologies for tumor recognition and extirpation, one often uses criteria such as five or ten year age-standardised net survival rates. Medical care is often ranked through life expectancy and child mortality rate. These indexes are heavily influenced by factors that do not stem from medical technology, such as nutrition, physical activities and simple prophylactic or prevention measures. It is easy to show that the aforementioned indexes are not good for measuring technology. For instancy, in 2017, according to an organization called World Life Expectancy [3], life expectancy in Cuba was practically the same as in the United States, although American Medical Care is arguably better than in Cuba. The only explanation for this kind of data is that economical hardships force Cubans to eat less meat and walk more than Americans.

Therefore, lifespan and survival rates should not be the only variable that researchers take into account. Let us consider four other variables, acceptance of treatment, healthy survival rates, disability-free survival rates, and lifespan without any lasting discomfort.

In order to demonstrate the Rasch method, the authors of the present paper estimated the damage on the healthy anatomy caused by surgery and radiation therapy guided by cancer specific biomarkers. Since it is not possible to perform actual guided surgeries and radiation therapy, one can say that their estimations are little more than an educated guess. In any case, a researcher who adopt this new imaging technology could hope to increase the probability of disability-free life during a period of five years from something around 0.6 to somewhat above 0.7.

Calibration of the Rasch method produces the difficulties of solving each of the aforementioned four problems. The tools and technologies that will solve these problems are traditional and guided surgery, robotic surgery, external beam radiotherapy and sealed source radiation therapy. Besides the difficulty parameters of the model, the Rasch calibration also calculates the efficiency of technologies in solving the four problems.

The only index that traditional technologies seem to beat technologies guided by cancer specific staining is acceptance of treatment. As one should expect, most people shun experimental treatments.

The authors want to make the statement that all experiments were made with tissues from tumor banks or biopsy samples.

4. Immune system

In this section the reader will find a short analysis of the immune systems that one can find in living organism.

The advances made through nanotechnology and molecular biology allowed engineers and biologists to tinker with the molecular machinery of living beings. Examples of such are pattern recognition receptors (PRRs), which are considered part of the non-specific immune system, as they detect molecules common to a large array of pathogens.

In order to arrive at an adequate understanding, one can visualize PRRs as proteins expressed by macrophages, monocytes, and other cells of the non-specific immune system. These are able to identify pathogen-associated molecular patterns, as well as damage-associated molecular patterns. Biologists believe that pattern recognition receptors and the non-specific immune system as a whole evolved before the acquired immune system.

The acquired immune system is highly specific to a given pathogen. One can say that the acquired immune system prepares the organism for a second showing of the same pathogen, by learning how to combat it through exposure to the corresponding disease.

Since the reader already knows that living organisms perform molecular pattern recoginition, he or she can understand that there are at least three methods of tinkering with immune systems. The first one is to reverse engineer Nature, and learn how to build artificial molecular pattern recognition sensors and drug delivery nanobots. The second one is to design molecular nanorobots that complement the natural defenses of a living being. Finally, one could use a natural pattern recognition molecule as part of a sensor or imaging system. The authors of the present paper are not stating that any of these proposals of improving Nature are easily implemented, or even possible. In any case, Marcelo Silva, Anielle Almeida and Noelio Dantas, who are co-authors of the present paper, have shown that nanostructures called magic-sized quantum dots could be used in order to create highly stable luminescence in human tissue [9]. They have also shown how to control the cytotoxicity of CdSe, a key component of their magic-sized quantum dots [8]. The resulting nanostructure can create a stable luminescence in animal tissue that lasts more than 36 hours after the insertion of the magic-sized quantum dots. The luminescence of a traditional cancer specific biomarker would start waning 2 hours after its application. Unfortunately, magic-sized quantum dots produce positive luminescence on normal tissue as much as on cancer tissue. Therefore, this nanomaterial cannot be used as a cancer biomarker per se. The conclusion reached through the prior discussion is that magic-sized quantum dots must be guided by molecular pattern recognition.

Figure 1 shows a magic-sized quantum dot coupled with a cancer-specific antibody.

An antibody, also known as an immunoglobulin[1] is a large Y-shaped protein produced mainly by plasma cells that is used by the immune system to neutralize pathogens such as bacteria and viruses.

One can envisage many applications to the long lasting luminescence of magic-sized quantum dot molecular probes. For instance, a researcher would be able to follow tumor

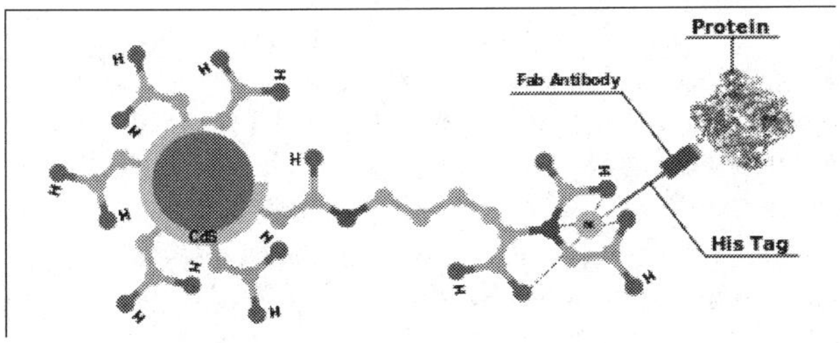

Fig. 1
QUANTUM DOT COUPLED TO ANTIBODY

cell migration in vivo or intracellular exchange of proteins. Another exciting application would be building fluorescent staining for differentiating malign in contrast with healthy tissue during cancer surgery. The interested reader has certainly learned about quantum dots, since manufacturers of consumer electronics use these nanostructures to create high dynamic range (HDR) TVs. These quantum dots that revolutionized TV by providing unheard-of color purity range between 6 to 20 nanometers in diameter, which is equivalent to 50 atoms. The magic-sized quantum dots that the Anielle Almeida and Noelio have used in cancer-specific markers go below 3 nanometers.

The physicists among the readers know that quantum dots are very small semiconductor pellets. In fact, they are so small that their sizes are comparable to the wavelength of the electron; as consequence, the motion of the electron is confined to a tiny 3D box. Electrons respond to these constraints by adjusting their energy emitting light, which leads to highly tuneable optoelectronic properties: Quantum dots of radius between 5 and 6 nanometers emit longer wavelengths, while smaller ones can produce colors from blue to green.

To close this discussion about specific immune-luminescence, the figure on the left hand side picture of Figure 2 was taken 24 hours after the staining, while the right hand side shot was taken 36 hours after the insertion of the magic-sized quantum dots.

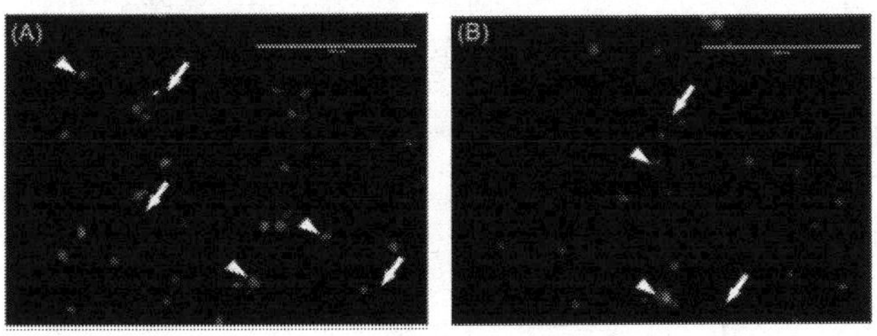

Fig. 2
CANCER SPECIFIC LUMINESCENCE

Besides imaging applications, the engineer can also use antibodies as part of sensors for detecting pathogens. However, before delving in such complex endeavor, let us examine the viability of creating molecular pattern recognition sensors for simple biochemical compounds. Figure 3 shows a sensor that can recognize biochemical molecules, such as nucleic acids, proteins and prosaic chemicals like β-D-glucose and urea.

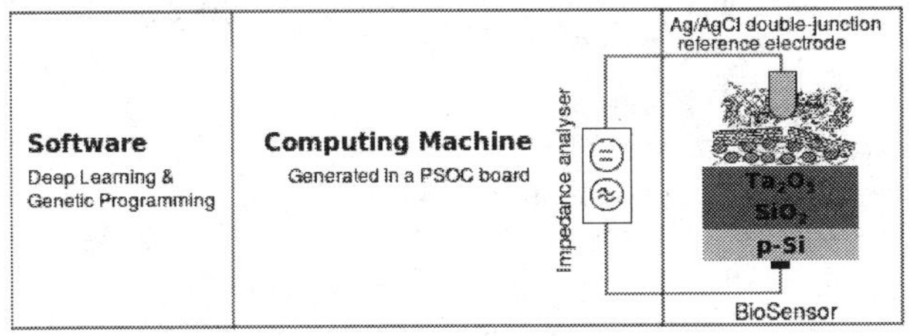

Fig. 3
CAPACITIVE FIELD-EFFECT BIOSENSOR

A clinical mobile laboratory can be used to perform blood tests, urinalysis and even biopsies in the very place where a doctor or nurse is diagnosing the patient. As one can see on Figure 3, these semiconductor based lab-on-chips have three stages. The first stage contains the sensor, which will use physical and chemical interactions with the world to carry out pattern recognition, i. e., it will identify proteins, DNA strands, particulates, chemicals, etc. Also in the first stage one finds the transducer, which transforms the measured phenomenon into an electrical signal.

Most researchers build biosensors based on a field-effect transistor, which is a FET gated by surface potential changes induced by the binding of biomolecules to the molecular pattern recognition nanomaterial. The authors of the present paper adopted a slightly different design. Their field effect biosensor produces a change in the capacitance of the mounting, when ions that characterize the analyte are captured in a $PAH - ZnO/CNTs$ matrix. The capacitance variation is detected by an impedance analyzer, which an electronic CAD Haskell compiler assembles onto a programmable System on Chip microprocessor (SoC). Finally, the software stage contains intelligent programs that interpret the results.

A biosensor can be based on a broad range of magnetic, metallic, isolating, semiconductor, semi-magnetic and core shell nanostructures. Figure 3 shows a diagram for a capacitive field effect sensor based on an Electrollite Insulator Semiconductor (EIS), therefore it is a controlled isolating nanostructure. The EIS was built in a cleanroom at the Fachhochschule Aachen by José Roberto Siqueira Junior. The mounting was performed by Noelio Dantas and Anielle Silva at the University of Uberlandia [41]. This experiment proves that one can build the semiconductor layer in a place with advanced facilities for building semiconductor devices, and mount the rest of the sensor in the point of care, i. e., where it will be used by people who know which problem must be solved.

5. The tell-tale protein

Before proceeding, let us learn a few acronyms that one often finds when dealing with nanotechnology. MEMS means Micro-Electro-Mechanical System. In the modern world, MEMS are everywhere, for instance, in vibrating gyroscopes that detect error states in an automobile yaw, inkjet printers, car tire pressure sensors, etc. Bio-MEMS, such as the ones embedded in medical devices, such as stents, are of special interest to this work.

SoC means *System on Chip*. A programmable SoC device is composed of a Computer Processing Unity (CPU), which can be configured through analog and digital blocks, and programmable routing. These configurable blocks in programmable SoCs set them apart from traditional microcontrollers.

The first stage of Figure 3 represent traditional application programs. These programs may rely on Artificial Intelligence technology, such as genetic programming or deep learning.

Let us assume that a engineer put together all technology necessary for building a machine, such as the one described on Figure 3, which can detect a given protein. How can this lab-on-chip be used to identify a pathogen, for instance, a bacteria? A microorganism produces proteins that are unique to it, or is shared with very few other living beings. Anderson Santos, who is one of the authors of the present paper, belives that he can discover these tell tale proteins.

In living beings, proteins are synthesized through a process denominated gene expression. Genomics is the study of genomes, i.e., the complete set of genetic material of a given organism. By examining the genome of a bacteria or a virus, Anderson Santos can figure out the best protein for identifying it. Once they know the protein, Noelio Dantas and Anielle Almeida can fabricate the nanomaterial that interacts with it and can be used in a biosensor that detects it and identifies the pathogen associated with it.

6. Lisp and Biobike

Let us assume that a team created a CAD system to develop nanomaterials to detect a protein associated with a pathogen, such as bacteria, virus or even cancer cells. The question is: How to discover the target protein? Consider, for instance, human tuberculosis, which is caused by the Mycobacterium tuberculosis (Mt). The Mt genome contains more than four thousand protein expressions. Indeed, it is not an easy task to decide which one of these one should use as the target for diagnosis. Fortunately, Anderson Santos [11], [12], one of the authors of this paper, devised an algorithm that chooses a good identifier from the genome of the pathogen.

For the time being, Anderson's algorithm is written in a main stream computer language. However, Marcus Santos is porting it to BioBIKE [13], an automatic reasoning system on big data that people use to make inferences about genomes.

7. Building prototypes

A very important facet of engineering is the building of a prototype. Computer Engineering from its inception was divided into two branches: Computer Hardware Engineering and Software Engineering. Until the end of the nineteen seventies, both computers, peripherals and programming tools were expensive. This fact made it difficult to train young engineers in the development of both software and hardware. During these early years of the trade, all branches of Computer Engineering were centralized within a few large American and Russian Corporations, such as IBM, Control Data, Cray Research and IPMCE (Institute of Precision Mechanics and Computer Engineering). Sometime around 1977, inexpensive hardware became widely available, which allowed for the training of people in computer programming to be carried out in small colleges, technical institutions, high schools and even at home by self taught individuals. Therefore, Software Engineering experienced a large innovative influx.

The Bureau of Labor Statistics [22] claims that *a limited number of engineers will be needed to meet the demand for new computer hardware because more technological innovation takes place with software than with hardware.* Until recently, in order to build a prototype of an Integrate Circuit, one needed a silicon foundry that requires billions of dollars in investment. However, due to advances in Electronic CAD, one can say that creating hardware is almost as easy today as writing a computer program.

In order to develop a computer like the one in Figure 3, the reader needs to learn how to program in a functional language. This paper argues that high productivity and correcteness can be achieved by describing circuits with programs written in a functional language, such as Scheme, Racket, SKILL, Haskell or OCAML. In particular, Clash [4] is a Haskell based hardware programming language that permits the design and implementation of Domain Specific Machines, such as a biosensor. Programming in Clash is not more difficult than programming in Haskell itself.

Besides Haskell programming, the researcher that wants to replicate the results of this paper should also acquire proficiency in the use of emacs, a display text editor. It helps to have some experience in electronics, in order to build docks for providing power, input and output interfaces for ASIC, SoC or FPGA circuits. By the way, the acronym ASIC stands for Application Specific Integrated Circuit. SoC (System-on-a-chip) refers to an integrated circuit, where all the components of an application, such as a mobile phone, are on a single substrate.

To make a long story short, in 2007, programmable SoC became widely available, which permits that engineers build prototypes of VLSI by combining standard cells onto inexpensive development boards. The prototypes can be manufactured by providing a machine specification. The specification is given in a high level functional language, such as Haskell, Scheme or Ocaml.

8. Atomic Force Microscope

Ideally, one should use a tunneling microscope in this kind of work. However, an Atomic Force Microscope (AFM) is less expensive.

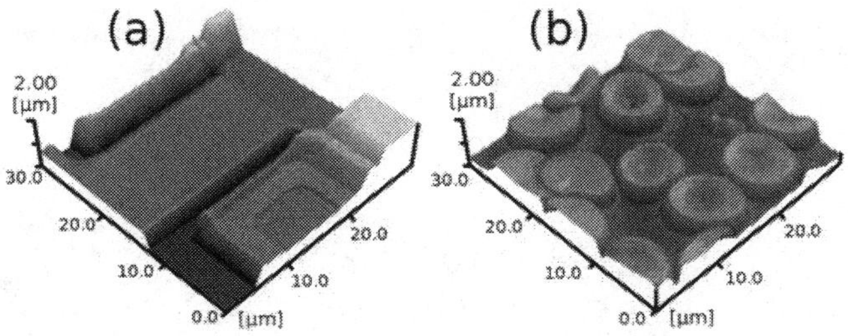

Fig. 4
MICROSCAN

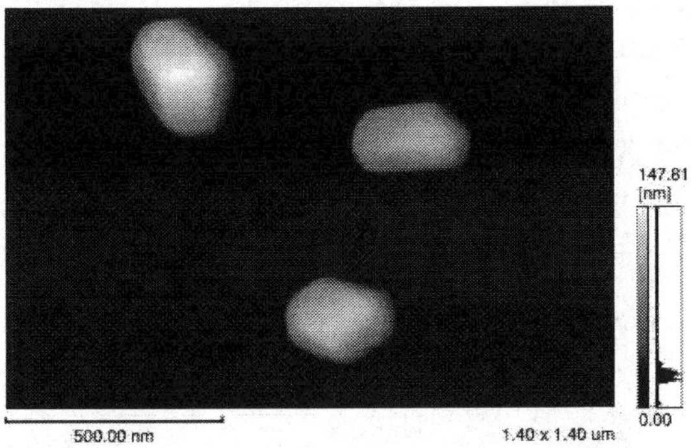

Fig. 5
VIRUS

The authors of the present paper used an AFM to obtain images from cells, virus, integrated circuits and quantum dots. As an example of the output of this AFM, Figure 4 shows a region of an integrated circuit side by side with a blood sample.

Figure 5 shows the AFM image of a virus that the authors believe to be a bacteriophage. Bacteriophages are nanoorganisms with a size that does not exceed 100 nm.

9. Quantum dots

The reader has seen that the authors of this work use quantum dot generated images for evaluating cancer treatments. One of the collaborators of the authors of the present work grew quantum dots in a matrix of borosilicate glass and used an Atomic Force Microscope to make an image of these tiny structures [38], [39], [40], as shown in Figure 6.

The atomic force microscope can find many medical applications, such as performing a cancer biopsy. In fact, another collaborator of the author of the present work is a physician, and the first application that he envisaged for the atomic force microscope (AFM) is cancer diagnosis. The difficulty with medical applications is that they require a lot of legal red tape and care for details. For instance, a physician needs to obtain permission to use histological tissue samples from a tumor. Besides this, traditional analysis of biopsied material is not appropriate for the AFM. The researcher should develop an entirely new method of biopsy. A surgeon told the authors

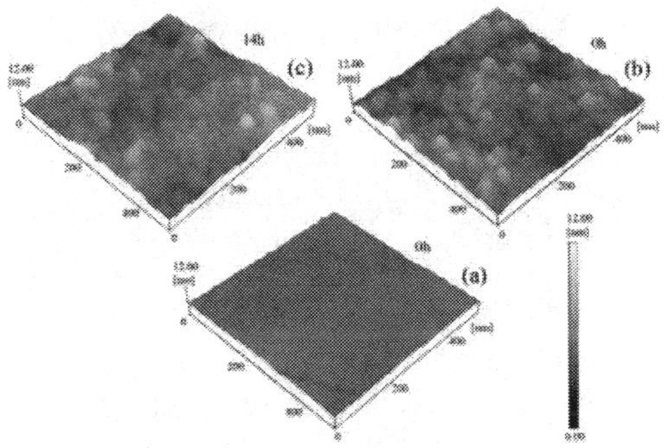

Fig. 6
QUANTUM DOTS

that if not collected correctly, an excisional biopsy could damage the cells, making diagnosis based on AFM images very difficult. The branch of medicine that deals with biopsy is called pathology. Most physicians develop clinical skills, not the habilities required of a pathologist. Therefore, even if the authors had developed the techniques necessary to perform biopsies with the AFM, physicians and AI programs would need to learn how to determine whether a lesion is benign or malignant from the images.

The authors of the present paper intends on returning to the problem of using the AFM for biopsies in a future study.

10. Conclusion

One of the main applications of Artificial Intelligence is pattern recognition, a technology that focuses on the recognition of patterns and regularities in data, in order to classify and recognize objects. Image processing and artificial vision relies heavily on pattern recognition. In order to perform automatic pattern recognition, researchers often collect images from samples of the objects that he or she wishes to classify. The next step is to use the images to train a neural network or a genetic programming algorithm to perform the classification. The machine learning system usually is a program that runs in a General Purpose Computer. This approach, however, does have its problems.

1) People and animals search actively for features that they need in order to classify an object. Let us assume that one desires to find a court house. The person moves to the location where the court house is supposed to be, chooses a better position to find striking features, like Greek columns, signs and street names, etc. Most machine learning programs work with snapshots of the objects they want to classify, and are not able to perform an active search for features.
2) Machine learning programs often work on fields where they are not very useful. A program to check banana plants for frost damage is not very useful, since few individuals need a computer to inspect a platation.
3) A neural network is a simulation of the neuron networks found in the brain and nevous system. One can expect

that tiny Domain Specific Machines play the role of a neuron better than processing an array of numbers with a Matlab program.

The authors of this paper believe that they have addressed at least the second of these problems: Their system performs a classification task that physicians consider hard to do.

Disclaimer

All the experiments of this work were carried out in Brazil with samples of a tumor bank (tissue bank). No Canadian or American institutions were involved in the experiments. Philippos Costa is at the Harrington Program Miller School of Medicine just as an observer. All standards of Brazilian, international and traditional bioethics were observed. No animals were harmed in this work.

References

[1] Yongjun Cheng, Jinhua Zhao, Wenli Qiao, and Kai Chen. Recent advances in diagnosis and treatment of gliomas using chlorotoxin based bioconjugates. American Journal of Nuclear Medicine and Molecular Imaging. 2014; 4(5): pages 385-405

[2] Wright, Benjamin D., MOK, Magdalena M. C.. An Overview of the Family of Rasch Measurement Models. In Introduction to Rasch Measurement, pp.1-24, 2004.

[3] www.worldlifeexpectancy.com

[4] Martijn Bakker. Numerical mathematics on FPGAs using CλaSH. BSc thesis, University of Twente, Enschede, The Netherlands, 2015. Rule-Based Expert Systems: The MYCIN Experiments of the Stanford Heuristic Programming Project. Reading, MA: Addison-Wesley, 1984.

[5] Antoine Italiano. Prognostic or Preditive? It's Time to Get Back to Definitions. Journal of Clinical Oncology, V. 29, no. 35, December 2011, pp. 4718-4718.

[6] Azriel Rosenfeld, Picture Processing by Computer, New York: Academic Press, 1969

[7] Janeway, C.A.; Travers, P.; Walport, M.; Shlomchik, M.J. (2005). Immunobiology (6th ed.). Garland Science.

[8] Almeida Silva, Anielle Christine, Silva, Marcelo José Barbosa, Da Luz, Felipe Andrés Cordero, Silva, Danielle Pereira, De Deus, Samantha Luara Vieira, Oliveira Dantas, Noelio. Controlling the Cytotoxicity of CdSe Magic-Sized Quantum Dots as a Function of Surface Defect Density. Nano Letters (Print), v. 14, 2014.

[9] Silva, Anielle Christine Almeida; Deus, Samantha Luara Vieira De; Silva, Marcelo José Barbosa; Dantas, Noelio Oliveira. Highly stable luminescence of CdSe magic-sized quantum dots in HeLa cells. Sensors and Actuators. B, Chemical, v. 191, p. 108-114, 2014.

[10] Silva, Anielle Christine Almeida; Freschi, Ana Paula Peres; Rodrigues, Cláudia Mendonça; Matias, Bruna França; Maia, Larissa Prado; Goulart, Luiz Ricardo; Dantas, Noelio Oliveira. Biological analysis and imaging applications of $CdSe/CdS_xSe_{1-x}/CdS$ core-shell magic-sized quantum dot. Nanomedicine, v. 12, p. 1421-1430, 2016.

[11] A. R. Santos, V. B. Pereira, E. Barbosa, J. Baumbach, J. Pauling, R. Röttger, M. Z. Turk, A. Silva, A. Miyoshi and V. Azevedo. Mature Epitope Density – a strategy for target selection based on immunoinformatics and exported prokaryotic proteins. BMC Genomics, vol. 14 Suppl 6, p. S4, 2013.

[12] A. F. Rezende, A. A. Brum, C. G. Reis, H. R. Angelo, K. S. Leal, M. T. Silva, S. Simionatto, V. Azevedo, A. Santos, R. W. Portela, O. Dellagostin and S. Borsuk. In silico identification of Corynebacterium pseudotuberculosis antigenic targets and application in immunodiagnosis. Journal of Medical Microbiology, v. 65, p. 521-529, 2016.

[13] Jeff Shrager. BioBIKE – Biological Integrated Knowledge Environment. http://biobike.csbc.vcu.edu

[14] Caio Cesar de Lima França, Emanuella G. da Silva Terto, Marcus V. Dias-Vermelho, Anielle Christine A. Silva, Noelio O. Dantas, Fabiane Caxico de Abreu. The electro chemical behavior of core-shell CdSe/Cds magic-sized quantum dots linked to cyclodextrin for studies of the encapsulation of bioactive compounds. Journal Solid State Electrochemistry, v. 20, p. 2533-2540, 2016.

[15] Marquis de Condorcet Essai de Lánalyse à la probabilité des décisions. Paris, Imprimerie Royale.

[16] Briscoe, T., Buttery, P., Carroll, J., Medlock, B., Watson, R. Open Source RASP 3.1 – Robust Parsing System for English. http://ilexir.co.uk

[17] Nielsen, Jakob Information Pollution. Available in `http://www.nngroup.com/articles/information-pollution/` on August 11, 2003. Accessed at July 03, 2015.

[18] Garside, R. The CLAWS Word-tagging System. In: R. Garside, G. Leech and G. Sampson (eds), The Computational Analysis of English: A Corpus-based Approach. 1987. London: Longman. http://ucrel.lancs.ac.uk/claws/

[19] Koza, John. Genetic Programming: On the Programming of Computers by Means of Natural Selection. The MIT Press, 1992.

[20] Wright, Benjamin D., MOK, Magdalena M. C.. An Overview of the Family of Rasch Measurement Models. In Introduction to Rasch Measurement, pp.1-24, 2004.

[21] Seibel, Peter Practical Common Lisp. Apress, First Edition, 2005.

[22] computer-and-hardware-engineers.htm, Bureau of Labor Statistics. Consulted in 18 May 2017. https://www.bls.gov/ooh/architecture-and-engineering

[23] Steel Bank Common Lisp. Available in `www.sbcl.org`.

[24] Beane, Zach. quicklisp Beta. Available in `www.quicklisp.org`

[25] SLIME: The Superior Lisp Interaction Mode for Emacs. Available from `https://common-lisp.net/project/slime/`

[26] Fernando C. N. Pereira and Stuard M. Shieber. Prolog and Natural-Language Analysis.

[27] Peter Norvig. Paradigms of Artificial Intelligence Programming: Case Studies in Common Lisp.

[28] Stonebank, M. UNIX Tutorial for Beginners. http://www.ee.surrey.ac.uk/Teaching/Unix/

[29] Mark Kantrowitz. Infix. http://www.cliki.net/infix

[30] Doug Hoyte. Let Over Lambda. Hoytech, 2008. ISBN: 978-1-4357-1275-1

[31] A. Church, A set of postulates for the foundation of logic, Annals of Mathematics, Series 2, 33:346–366 (1932).

[32] Alonzo Church. The Calculi of Lambda Conversion. Princepton University Press, 1986.

[33] Arlo J. Miller; Martin C. Mihm Junior. Melanoma. The New England Journal of Medicine, Massachusetts, v. 355, p. 51-65, 2006.

[34] Crayston Toby Charles William. Textrazor. https://www.textrazor.com

[35] Eric Schulte. Neutral Networks of Real-World Programs and their Application to Automated Software Evolution. University of New Mexico.
https://github.com/eschulte/netgear-repair
Retrieved on April, 13, 2017.

[36] Rod Canion. Open: How Compaq Ended IBM's Domination and Helped Invent Modern Computing. Ben Bella Books, Inc. 2013. ISBN 978-1-936661-92-3

[37] Boris Chertok. Rockets and People. There are three English editions of this book. Progressive Management has a carefully typesetted edition for epub ereaders. NASA published a pdf edition, on which the Progressive Management edition is based. Finally, there is also a Kindle edition that is almost illegible due to layout and OCR errors. ISBN 0-16-073239-5.

[38] Dantas, N. O., Fernandes, G. L., Anielle, C. A. Controlling the growth of ultrasmall CdTe quantum dots and the diffusion of cadmium vacancies: Thermal annealing. Journal of Alloys and Compounds, v. 637, p. 466-470, 2015.

[39] Dantas, N. O., Fernandes, G. L., Baffa, O. Controlling Densities of Manganese Ions and Cadmium Vacancies in Cd 1-x Mn x Te Ultrasmall Quantum Dots in a Glass Matrix: x-Concentration and Thermal Annealing. Journal of Physical Chemistry, v. 119, p. 17416-17420, 2015.

[40] Dantal, N. O., de Lima Fernandes, G. Cd1-xMnxTe ultrasmall quantum dots growth in a silicate glass matrix by the fusion method. Applied Physics Letters, v. 105, p. 13410, 2014.

[41] Morais, P. V. ; Gomes, V. F. ; Silva, A. C. A. ; Dantas, N. O. ; Shoning, M. J. ; Siqueira, J. R. . Nanofilm of ZnO nanocrystals/carbon nanotubes as biocompatible layer for enzymatic biosensors in capacitive field-effect devices. Journal of Materials Science, v. 52, p. 12314-12325, 2017.

SESSION

TOOLS AND MODELS FOR DECISION MAKING, SUPPORT SYSTEMS AND DIAGNOSTICS

Chair(s)

TBA

ISBN: 1-60132-479-0, CSREA Press ©

Modeling of Clinical Practice Guidelines for an Interactive Decision Support Using Ontologies

P. Philipp[1], M. Bommersheim[2], S. Robert[2], D. Hempel[3], and J. Beyerer[1,2]
[1]Karlsruhe Institute of Technology KIT, Vision and Fusion Laboratory IES, Karlsruhe, Germany
[2]Fraunhofer Institute of Optronics, System Technologies and Image Exploitation IOSB, Karlsruhe, Germany
[3]Steinbeis-Transfer-Institut Klinische Hämatoonkologie, Donauwörth, Germany

Abstract— *Modern medicine typically offers a diverse set of treatment options, rapidly evolving over time. In this context, Clinical Practice Guidelines (CPGs) are able to provide recommendations for actions and by that a frame of reference for medical experts during various treatment processes. To facilitate the implementation of these recommendations, we propose an interactive decision support system (DSS). For this reason, the CPGs of Chronic Myeloid Leukemia, Myelodysplastic Syndromes, Mantle Cell Lymphoma, and Multiple Myeloma are formalized using ontologies. The resulting models serve as an exemplary basis for a DSS, providing patient-specific as well as CPG compliant recommendations.*

Keywords: Clinical Practice Guidelines, Treatment, Interactive Assistance, Decision Support, Ontology

1. Introduction

Curse and blessing of modern medicine can be seen in the variety and number of treatment options rapidly changing over time. Furthermore, the steady growth of published findings makes it almost impossible for an individual to keep their knowledge up-to-date [1]. Clinical Practice Guidelines (CPGs) can help to condense knowledge into recommendations for actions. Thereby, CPGs rely on consolidated medical knowledge for providing state-of-the-art care [2].

Although, this should bring scientific findings into practice, the use of CPGs at the point of treatment still represents a challenge. That is, because there is a gap between theoretical knowledge on the one side – which is typically given by lengthy documents written in prose [2] – and practical as well as patient-specific treatment solutions on the other side [3], [4], [5]. As a consequence, a passive dissemination of CPGs (e.g. by print media) has proven to have only little effect on the actual practitioners behavior [2], [6].

Therefore, we propose an interactive decision support facilitating the treatment process by bridging the gap between CPG recommendations and the actual treatment delivered to patients. Following this idea, in this contribution we elaborate an exemplary formalization of CPGs concerning Chronic Myeloid Leukemia (CML), Myelodysplastic Syndromes (MDS), Mantle Cell Lymphoma (MCL) and Multiple Myeloma (MM) using Ontologies. Thereby, the following main requirements of a decision support system (DSS) based on these models have been determined with the help of medical experts. Firstly, performed examinations and treatment action have to be stored. Secondly, warnings have to be issued in case examinations are missing or, thirdly, if abnormal results are observed. Finally, suitable examinations and treatment actions have to be proposed by the DSS.

2. Related Work

How ontological formalization can be leveraged in context of medical applications is elaborated in [7], [8], [9]. Thereby, an ontology-based decision support system is presented that allows to assess the risk factors of diabetic patients and provide appropriate treatment suggestions [7]. In [8] an ontology for cancer therapy is used to discover possible problems of data consistency in electronic patient records. In [9], a disease-specific ontology for the treatment of colon cancer using information found in medical abstracts is developed.

In this work, we focus on ontologies to formalize knowledge embodied in CPGs of complex cancerous diseases. Therefore, CML [10], [11], MDS [12], [13], MCL [14], [15], and MM [16], [17] are exemplary modeled. The developed ontology is basis of an interactive decision support for medical practitioners, providing patient-tailored recommendations during treatment. The use of ontologies for this application example has many advantages. One of them is that ontologies can encapsulate CPGs as classes and relationships. That means, in contrast to, e.g. graphic modeling languages, they allow to represent and facilitate the semantics of knowledge using relations and axioms. Given this formalized knowledge base, conclusions can then be drawn automatically.

Moreover, the formal representation of this knowledge base can be expanded, adapted and reused at any time [7] which is especially important in the given context. E.g. in clinical trials, new drugs and treatment options are being tested or drug side-effects and drug interactions are under investigation.

ISBN: 1-60132-479-0, CSREA Press ©

This leads to a knowledge base that is continuously subject to change. While new knowledge can be incorporated by extending the existing ontology, changes in knowledge can also be dealt with efficiently. E.g. if clinical trials show that limits of drug doses must be changed, it is sufficient to adjust the ontology in one place (i.e. there is no need for redundant adjustments).

Due to their high level of semantic expressiveness, ontologies are a suitable tool for modeling complex knowledge representations [18]. Furthermore, their use as foundation of knowledge-based decision systems are widely adopted [19].

3. Basics and Terminology of Ontologies

An ontology consists of a set of concepts, i.e. the classes and relations of the universe of discourse, as well as formal axioms which limit the semantics and guarantee a correct application of these concepts [20]. There is also a lexical level to describe the meaning of the concepts in natural language terms. Formally, an ontology is a tuple [20]

$$T = (O, L) \ ,$$

whereby O is the structure of the ontology and L is the lexicon. The latter is a set of human-readable term definitions. The ontologies structure is given by

$$O = \{A, K\} \ ,$$

where A is set of axioms that limit the semantics and guarantee a correct application of the concepts. K is the set of concepts, i.e. the union of the set of classes and the set of relations:

$$K = C \cup R \ .$$

Thereby C is the set of classes which contains the instances of the universe of discourse

$$C = \{c_1, \ldots, c_n\} \ ,$$

and R is the set of relations between the classes of the universe of discourse [21], so that

$$R : C \times C \ .$$

These classes and their relations can also be represented by a graph

$$G = (V, E) \ ,$$

where the set of vertices V is given by the set of classes C and the set of edges E is given by the set of relations R.

4. Modeling Approach

For modeling the cancerous diseases CML, MDS, MCL and MM, the methodology elaborated in [22] has been utilized. The process comprises several steps starting with (e.g.) the assessment of requirements. Furthermore, building and evaluating the ontology, e.g. by checking the fulfillment of requirements, is necessary. Finally, establishing a suitable documentation is important since inadequate documentation has been identified as one of the main barriers for effective use of ontologies [22].

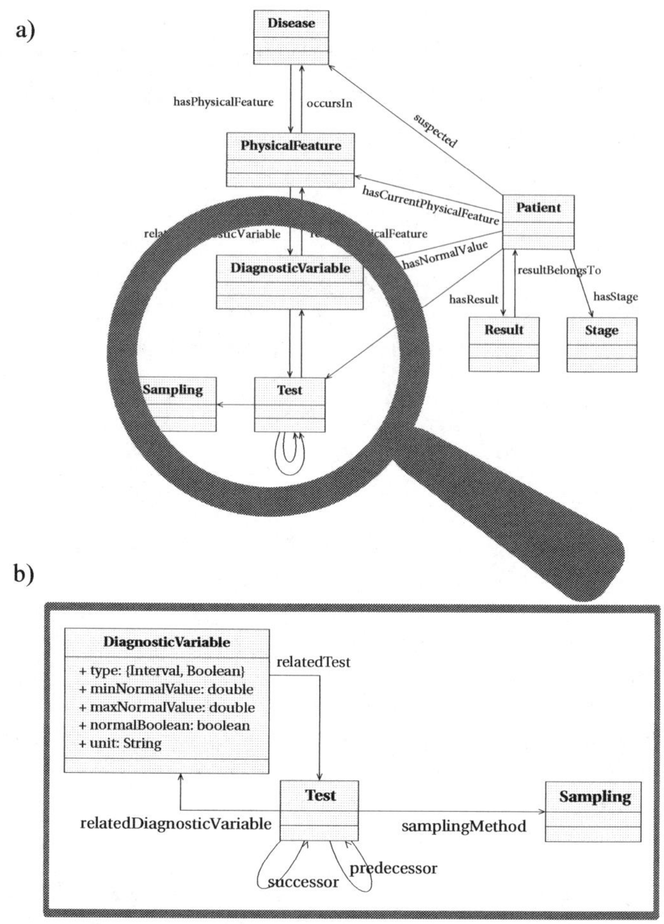

Fig. 1: Subfigure 1a) shows an overview of the classes and relations used for modeling test results. In Subfigure 1b), several classes and their relations are shown in more detail (magnifier). The class "DiagnosticVariable" incorporates, i.e., a reference range limited by "minNormValue" and "maxNormValue" (e.g. $[4 \cdot 10^9, 10 \cdot 10^9]$) as well as a unit (e.g. $1/L$). To model a sequence of tests, the functional relations "successor" and "predecessor" are used for class "Test". Furthermore, "Sampling" specifies how a test sample is obtained.

4.1 Examinations

During the treatment of cancerous diseases, examination values have to be collected continuously to check whether the treatment is effective or not. Subfigure 1a) gives an overview of the classes involved in the proposed modeling approach.

Thereby the class "Disease" contains information on the diagnosis as well as the treatment of the specific cancerous disease. A disease is characterized by a set of specific physical features – e.g. leukopenia (lack of leukocytes). For this purpose, the class "PhysicalFeature" is created which is linked to a disease via the relation "hasPhysicalFeature".

The class "DiagnosticVariable" depicted in Subfigure 1b) incorporates a reference range, a unit and a type for each component of a test. For instance, the reference range of leukocytes using the unit $1/L$ is given by $[4 \cdot 10^9, 10 \cdot 10^9]$. Therefore this variable is stored as type "Interval" using a "minNormalValue" of $4 \cdot 10^9$ and a "maxNormalValue" of $10 \cdot 10^9$ with "unit" $1/L$.

The class "Test" models different medical examinations like fine-needle aspiration biopsy or complete blood count (CBC). The latter has several related diagnostic variables such as hemoglobin or leukocytes. In order to represent this connection in the ontology, the class "Test" is connected to the class "DiagnosticVariable" via the relations "relatedTest" and "relatedDiagnosticVariable" – see Subfigure 1b).

To model a sequence of different tests, the functional relations called "successor" and "predecessor" are defined. Each test can also be assigned to one or more instances of the class "Sampling". Thereby, class "Sampling" specifies how a test sample is obtained. E.g., a sample for hematopathological analysis of a tumor tissue can be obtained by fine needle biopsy or a more invasive incision biopsy.

To model the order of examinations, an axiom of the Semantic Web Rule Language is used:

$$\text{Patient}(?p) \land \text{suspected}(?p, \text{MCL}) \quad (1)$$
$$\rightarrow \text{hasTestSuggestion}(?p, \text{HistoryAndPhysicalMCL})\,. \quad (2)$$

In (1) it is checked if there is an instance of class "Patient" suspected of suffering from MCL[1]. If this is the case, the relation "hasTestSuggestion" is added to the ontology, whereby variable $?p$ is replaced by the corresponding instance (2). By doing this, history and physical examination is proposed initially. The class "Result", cf. Subfigure 1a), is used to store patient specific examination values. These results are assigned to the patient via the relation "hasResult".

Finally, in order to determine the progress of the disease, disease-specific axioms are defined. E.g., in case of MCL, a patient is assigned to stages "I" to "IV" via the relation "hasStage". The corresponding relation is shown in Subfigure 1a).

4.2 Treatment

Subfigure 2a) shows an overview of the classes and relations involved in the treatment of the diseases CML, MDS, MCL, and MM. Thereby, the central class is "Treatment", from which subclasses can be formed, each representing a therapeutic option, cf. Subfigure 2b). There are three treatment approaches: radiation therapy, chemotherapy and treatment with drugs. Depending on the patient's age and

[1]Please note: Variables in SWRL axioms are prefixed by a question mark.

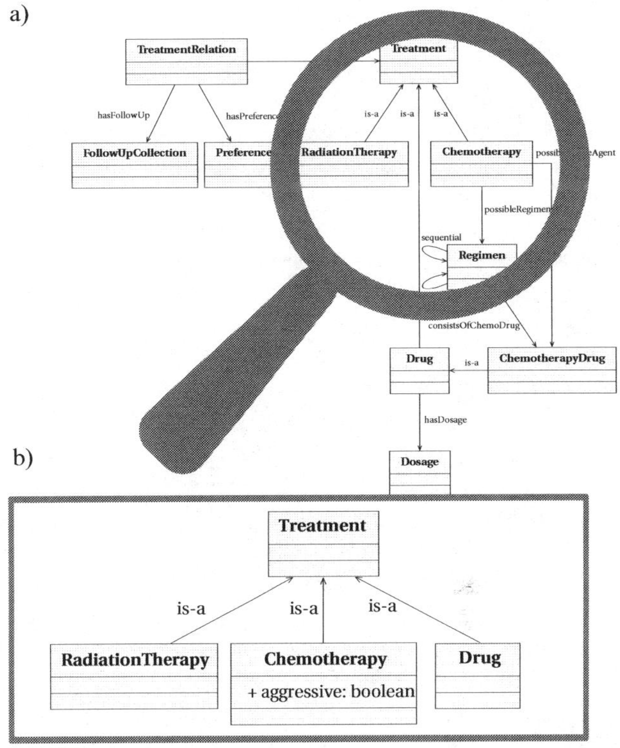

Fig. 2: Subfigure 2a) shows an overview of the classes and relations used for modeling the treatment. Subfigure 2b) depicts a detailed view of the class "Treatment" and its subclasses representing different treatment options. For simplification the classes "Surgery", "TKI" and "BloodCellGrowthFactors" are not shown.

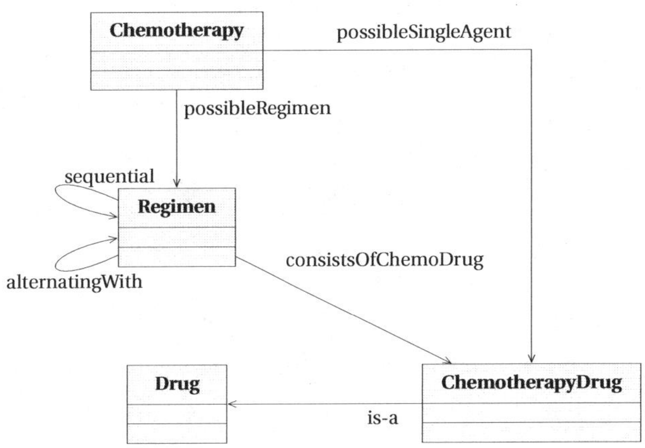

Fig. 3: Figure depicts the classes used for modeling a chemotherapy. Single chemotherapeutic drugs (single agents) or combinations of drugs can be used (regimens). The latter can be carried out sequentially or in alternation with other regimens.

preferences, chemotherapy can be carried out either low-intensity or high-intensity. This is represented by the boolean attribute aggressive of class "Chemotherapy" – iff the intensity of chemotherapy is high, this attribute is given the value "true". To cover a wider range of diseases, further subclasses such as "Surgery", "TKI" or "BloodCellGrowthFactors" are added. For simplification they are not depicted in Figure 2.

There are different types of chemotherapy drugs, acting in different ways to kill existing cancer cells or prevent the formation of new ones [15]. Often more than one drug is used – in this case the treatment is called a combination regimen (cf. Figure 3).

Otherwise, if exactly one drug is used, it is called a single agent. In order to map this assignment of chemotherapy to an associated medication, the relation "possibleSingleAgent" between the class "Chemotherapy" and "Chemotherapy-Drug" is used. Thus, chemotherapies that consist only of one single drug can be represented.

If a chemotherapy consists of two or more medications, the class "Regimen" can be used. The relation "consistsOfChemoDrug" relates a combination regimen to any number of chemotherapy drugs. A combination regimen is assigned to chemotherapy via the relation "possibleRegimen". Different combination regimes can be given alternately or sequentially (cf. e.g. MCL [14]). For their representation the relations "alternatingWith" and "sequential" for the class "Regimen" were created.

To facilitate extensions of the ontology regarding further details on chemotherapy cycles, four relations have been added to class "Drug" (cf. Figure 4). The first relation is "hasDosage" from class "Drug" to class "Dosage". The latter contains the attributes "value" and "unit" for storing information about the dosage of a medication.

The second relation is given by "administrationDays" of the class Drug. It represents the fact that in a chemotherapy cycle, treatment days are followed by specific number of rest days (cf. e.g MCL [15]). To indicate the type of drug administration of a cancer treatment (i.e. subcutaneous, oral or intravenous), the third relation "administrationMethod" of class "Drug" is used. The frequency of drug administration can be specified using the fourth relation "administrationFrequency". Possible values are QD or BID, whereby QD stands for "quaque die", every day. BID stands for "bis in die", twice a day. Further frequencies can be added to the range.

4.3 Multiple Treatment Options

To provide suitable treatment options, the class "Treatment" is not sufficient. That is because generally, a treatment may consist of several approaches. E.g for MCL in stage I or II, radiation therapy can be combined with chemotherapy. In addition, different treatment options can depend on the physical condition and preferences of a patient.

Moreover, for some treatments the CPG recommends tests to verify their efficacy. In order to implement these aspects a quinary relation is necessary to link a patient with two or more treatments and (depending on the treatment) a preference as well as a possibly large number of examinations. Therefore a design pattern is used [23]. Thereby, a n-ary relation is represented by a new class and n new relations. An instance of the relation that connects n individuals is an instance of this new class – e.g. the class "TreatmentRelation" is used to propose different treatment options for a patient (cf. Figure 5). The main treatment option is specified via the relation "mainTreatment". E.g., for MCL in stage I or II, the main treatment is radiation therapy. If this treatment is combined with other approaches (e.g. chemotherapy), this information is added via the relation "inCombinationWith".

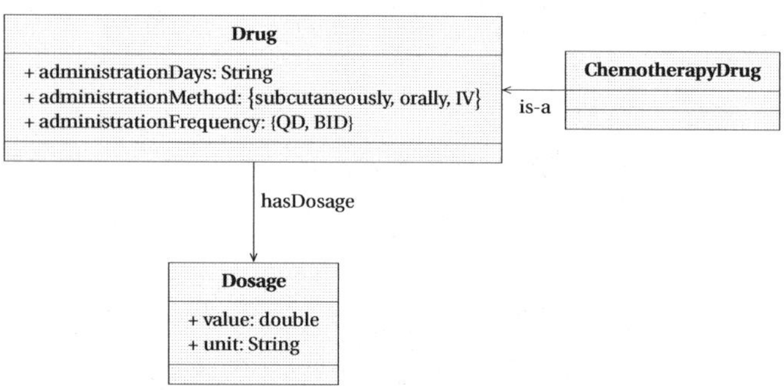

Fig. 4: Detailed view of the classes "Drug", "Dosage" and subclass "ChemotherapyDrug". The former incorporates several relations. Thereby, e.g., "administrationDays" represents the fact that a chemotherapy is typically carried out in cycles of treatment- and rest days. Furthermore, the frequency of drug administration (e.g BID, i.e. "twice a day") is represented by "administrationFrequency".

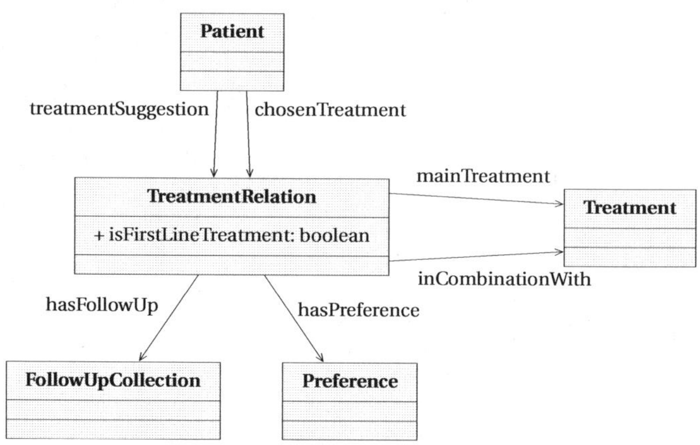

Fig. 5: Detailed view of the classes "TreatmentRelation", "FollowUpCollection", "Preference", "Treatment", and "Patient". Thereby, e.g., "mainTreatment" specifies the primary treatment (e.g. radiation therapy) and combined approaches are specified by "in CombinationWith" (e.g. chemotherapy).

To be able to represent treatment preferences, the relation "hasPreference" is used. E.g. for MCL, depending on the stage, age and preference of the patient different treatment options can be chosen. This comprises, e.g. radiation therapy in combination with aggressive or less aggressive chemotherapy or radiation therapy without chemotherapy. Whereby a patient should be offered one of these three options, medical experts prefer specific treatments. E.g., radiation therapy without chemotherapy for MCL stage I patients or radiation therapy with less aggressive chemotherapy for older patients in stage II, and radiation therapy with aggressive chemotherapy for younger patients in Stage II. An instance of the class "TreatmentRelation" can be assigned to one of the instances "Preferred" and "Alternative" of class "Preference". This can be used to express whether medical experts prefer the current treatment for a patient or consider it as an alternative. In order to propose treatment options for a patient, the relation "treatmentSuggestion" is used. Which treatment options are actually proposed is determined by axioms. The medical expert can select one of the treatments by specifying the desired treatment option for the relation "chosenTreatment".

4.4 Follow-Up

Generally, CPGs recommend examinations to evaluate the treatment success. These so called follow-ups usually take place regularly over a longer period of time. E.g., after radiation therapy in combination with chemotherapy, complete blood counts are carried out every three months for a period of two years. However, the assignment of an examination to a regularly recurring period is not generally unique. E.g. for MM, every 3 to 6 months a complete blood count is carried out each year. To represent follow-up examinations, the design pattern for n-ary relations was used (cf. class $FollowUp$ in Figure 6). The scheduled examination is determined by the relation "requiredTest". The relation "followUpMapping" connects the class "FollowUp" to the class "Mapping".

The latter allows for capturing the time periods in which the specified examination has to be repeated. Using the relations "everyXMonths" and "years" of the class "Mapping", a typical statement such as "The examination is carried out every three months for two years" can be represented. In order to structure the information about the follow-up examinations, the class "FollowUpCollection" is used. Therby, the relation "consistsOfFollowUp" connects the classes "FollowUpCollection" with the class "FollowUp" in order to bundle the multitude of possible follow-up examinations. The class "FollowUpCollection" can be reached via the relation "hasFollowUp" of class "TreatmentRelation", because generally, different combinations of follow-up examinations are needed depending on the type of treatment.

After the follow-up examinations have been performed, results are stored in instances of class "Result" (cf. Section 4.1). The medical expert can then decide if the treatment has been successful. The class "TreatmentResponse" contains the subclasses "CompleteResponse", "PartialResponse", "StableDisease", and "ProgressiveDisease". Therby, the physician determines which of these subclasses represent the patient's outcomes. Patients who have achieved complete remission will typically receive a special follow-up treatment. For this purpose, the relation "isComplete" is used, which is set to "true" by an axiom for instances of the class "CompleteResponse". Naturally, it is set to "false" for any instances of any other subclasses of "TreatmentResponse" – which facilitates the suggestion of subsequent treatments.

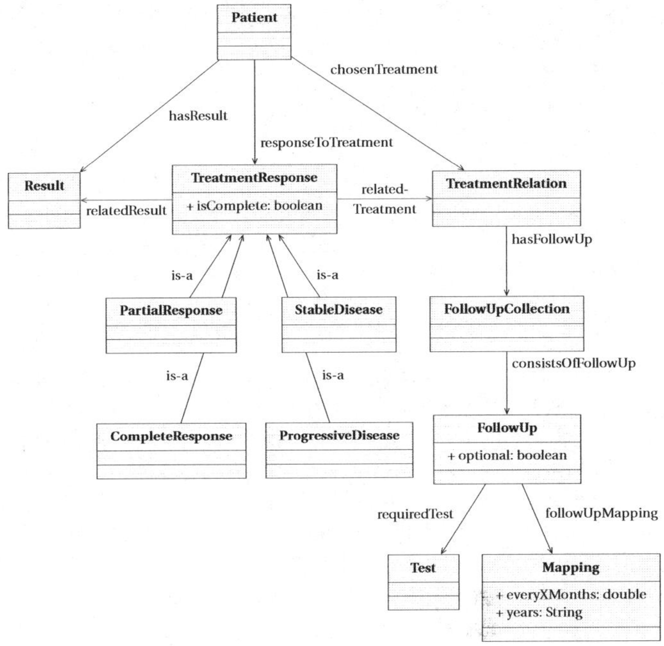

Fig. 6: Overview of the classes related to the treatment of a disease. The class "FollowUp" models an n-ary relation which is necessary to generally represent combinations of involved examinations. The class "FollowUpCollection" bundles these examinations.

5. Verification

To verify the modeled ontologies for CML, MDS, MCL and MM, typical patients regarding cancer statistics are generated [24], [25]. These statistics document e.g. the number of newly diagnosed cancer diseases in Germany in 2012 as well as the mean age of onset. For the model implementation, the open-source ontology framwork Protégé [26] was used.

According to [24], 16,150 people were newly diagnosed with a non-Hodgkin's Lymphoma in Germany in 2012, which also includes MCL [14]. Among them are 8,580 men and 7,570 women. The average age of men being newly diagnosed with MCL is 70 years whereas the average age

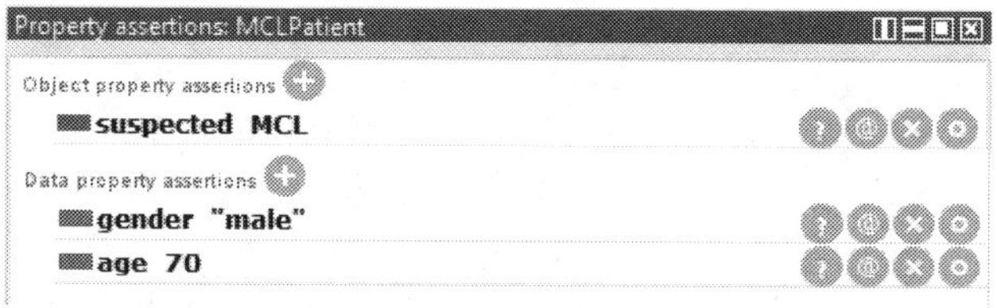

Fig. 7: Property assertions of a sampled MCL patient created on basis of cancer studies [24]. Screenshot of the Protégé ontology editor [26].

of newly diagnosed woman is 72 years. As a consequence, in a first step, a 70 year old male patient is sampled for verification (cf. Figure 7). To issue warnings if examinations are missing (cf. requirements in Section 1), corresponding tests to assess the missing values can be proposed by the DSS. To avoid inconsistencies by conflicting information at the same time, we do not model explicitly which values are missing but focus on the suggestion of tests in order to assess the corresponding values. Therefore, for the example patient, the diagnosis starts with a suggested test for the assessment of history and physical examination. This is represented by the object property assertion "hasTestSuggestion(MCLPatient, HistoryAndPhysicalMCL)", cf. Figure 8.

Please note, that the NCCN guidelines cite a variety of diagnostic tests, needed to confirm the suspicion of the disease under consideration. However, medical experts carry out tests in a patient-specific order – i.e. starting from non-invasive test to invasive tests. Therefore the DSS correctly proposes the non-invasive test of history and physical which includes e.g. the non-invasive palpation of the number of involved lymph nodes as well as the involvement of the spleen.

After carrying out the test, corresponding results are stored in the ontology (cf. requirement 1 in Section 1). For this, the ontology enables the creation of an instance of class "Result". For the sample patient, an instance of "LymphNodeResult" is used to store the corresponding result of the test (cf. Figure 8). Furthermore, it is specified to which patient the result belongs and which diagnostic variable has been tested. That means in effect that "resultBelongsTo(LymphNodeResult,MCLPatient)", "testedDiagnosticVariable(LymphNodeResult, LymphNodes)" and "resultValue(LymphNodeResult, 3.0)" are set. Please note that every diagnostic variable is associated with a test and therefore the latter has to be specified explicitly as shown in Section 4.1.

To verify requirements 3 and 4 (cf. Section 1), the instance "SpleenSizeResult" is created (cf. Figure 8). Furthermore, "resultBelongsTo(SpleenSizeResult, MCLPatient)", "testedDiagnosticVariable(SpleenSizeResult, SpleenSize)" and "resultBoolean(SpleenSizeResult, true)" are added. The true value given in the relation "resultBoolean" means that the spleen is affected. Please note that the connected diagnostic

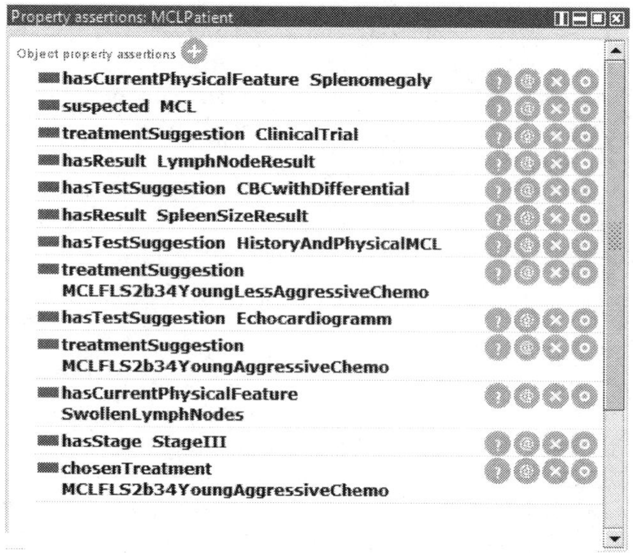

Fig. 8: Property assertions of a sampled MCL patient created on basis of cancer studies [24] after several steps of diagnoses and treatment. Screenshot of the Protégé ontology editor [26].

variable specifies the information of how the relation should be structured in order to indicate the result (cf. Section 4.1).

Given the information about the patient, conclusions can be drawn: e.g., that the example patient has swollen lymph nodes as well as splenomegaly. By this, the medical practitioner is warned in case of abnormal values of the patient, which satifies requirement 3. After completion of history and physical examination, a complete blood count (CBC) is proposed (cf. Figure 8). This corresponds to the judgment of involved medical experts and does not contradict the corresponding CPG [14], also. From this and also from subsequent tests, results can be added (as described above).

For the verification of requirement 4, the stage of the disease present has to be determined. The CPG provides guidance on the determination of the stage – the ontology incorporates this information by axioms which are evaluated as soon as necessary test results are available. Since multiple lymph nodes and the spleen are affected, the example patient is assigned to MCL Stage III (cf. Figure 8).

In accordance to the CPG and medical judgment, the treatment options for MCL Stage III are: aggressive chemotherapy or less aggressive chemotherapy or participation in a clinical trial. These options are proposed to the physician according to requirement 4 (cf. Figure 8). Please note that the sample patient is counted among the younger patients since his age is ≤ 70 years.

In a first step, the medical expert can specify the chosen treatment (e.g. aggressive chemotherapy) by setting the relation "chosenTreatment" accordingly (cf. Figure 8). In further steps the response of the treatment can be specified and treatment suggestions are proposed correspondingly –

this can also involve additional recommendations for examinations which are also part of the treatment process.

Overall, this demonstrates that for the treatment of MCL the requirements 1, 2, 3, and 4 are fulfilled, given an examplary patient. Please note that MM, CML and MDS have also been modeled and verified with similar results. This does not only show that the four modeled complex cancerous diseases can be represented in a suitable manner. We are convinced, because of their prototypical character, the results obtained can also be useful in context of other diseases.

6. Conclusion and Outlook

In this work, Clinical Practical Guidelines of the cancerous diseases Chronic Myeloid Leukemia, Myelodysplastic Syndromes, Mantle Cell Lymphoma, and Multiple Myeloma are modeled.

Their formalization is used for enabling a Decision Support System bridging the gap between theoretical knowledge and practical solutions at the point of treatment. Thereby, ontologies are utilized to represent the incorporated knowledge of the considered guidelines. Because of their prototypical character, the presented modeling approach can also provide valuable insights into the modeling of other cancerous diseases. Verification shows that the requirements for the proposed Decision Support System are fulfilled. For this, exemplary patients are generated which are based on cancer statistics. In this contribution we exemplary presented a verification based on a patient suffering from Matle Cell Lymphoma.

Developing a DSS for daily use requires close collaboration with medical experts who regularly use CPGs. Therefore, we plan to bring our findings into a currently developed software system [27] for further investigation.

References

[1] C. D. Mulrow, "Rationale for systematic reviews." *BMJ: British Medical Journal*, vol. 309, no. 6954, p. 597, 1994.

[2] E. Steinberg, S. Greenfield, M. Mancher, *et al.*, *Clinical Practice Guidelines We Can Trust*. National Academies Press, 2011.

[3] P. Philipp, Y. Fischer, D. Hempel, and J. Beyerer, "Modeling of clinical practice guidelines for interactive assistance in diagnostic processes," in *HIMS 2015, International Conference on Health Informatics and Medical Systems, july 27-30, Las Vegas, USA*, 2015, pp. 3–9.

[4] P. Philipp, Y. Fischer, D. Hempel, and J. Beyerer, "Framework for an interactive assistance in diagnostic processes based on probabilistic modeling of clinical practice guidelines," *in Emerging Trends in Applications and Infrastructures for Computational Biology, Bioinformatics, and Systems Biology, Elsevier*, pp. 371–390, 2016.

[5] P. Philipp, Y. Fischer, D. Hempel, and J. Beyerer, "Framework for an Interactive Assistance in Diagnostic Processes Based on the Translation of UML Activities into Petri Nets," in *Proceedings of ISHI 2015 – International Symposium on Health Informatics and Medical Systems: CSCI 2015. International Conference on Computational Science and Computational Intelligence*. IEEE Conference Publishing Services, 2015, pp. 732–737.

[6] E. Field and K. Lohr, *Guidelines for Clinical Practice: From Development to Use*. National Academies Press, 1992.

[7] P. C. Sherimon and R. Krishnan, "Ontodiabetic: An ontology-based clinical decision support system for diabetic patients," *Springer*, 2015.

[8] C. Eccher, A. Scipioni, A. A. Miller, A. Ferro, and D. M. Pisanelli, "An ontology of cancer therapies supporting interoperability and data consistency in eprs," *Elsevier Computers in Biology and Medicine*, vol. 43, pp. 822–832, 2013.

[9] C. S. G. Khoo, J.-C. Na, V. W. Wang, and S. Chan, "Developing an ontology for encoding disease treatment information in medical abstracts," *DESIDOC Journal of Library and Information Technology*, vol. 31, no. 2, pp. 103–115, March 2011.

[10] National Comprehensive Cancer Network, "NCCN clinical practice guidelines in oncology, chronic myeloid leukemia," January 2017, Version 2.2017.

[11] *NCCN Guidelines For Patients, Chronic Myelogenous Leukemia*, 1st ed., National Comprehensive Cancer Network, 2016.

[12] National Comprehensive Cancer Network, "NCCN clinical practice guidelines in oncology, myelodysplastic syndromes," November 2016, Version 2.2017.

[13] *NCCN Guidelines For Patients, Myelodysplastic Syndromes*, 1st ed., National Comprehensive Cancer Network, 2016.

[14] National Comprehensive Cancer Network, "NCCN clinical practice guidelines in oncology, b-cell lymphomas," March 2017, Version 3.2017.

[15] *NCCN Guidelines For Patients, Mantle Cell Lymphoma*, 1st ed., National Comprehensive Cancer Network, 2016.

[16] National Comprehensive Cancer Network, "NCCN clinical practice guidelines in oncology, multiple myeloma," November 2016, Version 3.2017.

[17] *NCCN Guidelines For Patients, Multiple Myeloma*, 1st ed., National Comprehensive Cancer Network, 2016.

[18] C. Feilmayr and W. Wöß, "An analysis of ontologies and their success factors for application to business," *Data & Knowledge Engineering*, vol. 101, pp. 1–23, 2016.

[19] M. A. Musen, B. Middleton, and R. A. Greenes, "Clinical decision-support systems," in *Biomedical informatics*. Springer, 2014, pp. 643–674.

[20] B. M. Konopka, "Biomedical ontologies - a review," *Elsevier Biocybernetics and Biomedical Engineering*, vol. 35, pp. 75–86, 2014.

[21] Z. E. Jerroudi, *Eine interaktive Vorgehensweise für den Vergleich und die Integration von Ontologien*. EUL Verlag, 2010.

[22] M. Uschold and M. King, "Towards a methodology for building ontologies," in *In Workshop on Basic Ontological Issues in Knowledge Sharing, held in conjunction with IJCAI-95*, 1995.

[23] N. Noy and A. Rector, "Defining n-ary relations on the semantic web," https://www.w3.org/TR/swbp-n-aryRelations/, 2006, accessed: 2017/11/08.

[24] Robert Koch-Institut, "Zentrum für Krebsregisterdaten – Krebs in Deutschland," October 2015, Accessed: 2017/11/23. [Online]. Available: http://www.krebsdaten.de/Krebs/DE/Content/Publikationen/

[25] P. D. U. Germing and P. D. N. Gattermann, "Myelodysplastische Syndrome - Informationen für Patienten und Angehörige," November 2015, Accessed: 2017/11/23. [Online]. Available: https://www.leukaemie-hilfe.de/nc/broschuerenangebot.html

[26] J. H. Gennari, M. A. Musen, R. W. Fergerson, W. E. Grosso, M. Crubézy, H. Eriksson, N. F. Noy, and S. W. Tu, "The evolution of protégé: an environment for knowledge-based systems development," *International Journal of Human-computer studies*, vol. 58, no. 1, pp. 89–123, 2003.

[27] D. Hempel, "Oncoguide system: A computerized interactive assistance system for the diagnosis and treatment of cml/mpn and mds d." *Journal of Clinical Oncology*, vol. 34, no. 15_suppl, pp. e18 545–e18 545, 2016.

Prediction of Glaucoma through Convolutional Neural Networks

Marco A. Espinoza[1], Germán H. Alférez[1], and Javier Castillo[2]
School of Engineering and Technology[1], Instituto de la Visión del Hospital La Carlota[2]
Universidad de Montemorelos
Apartado 16-5 Montemorelos, N.L. Mexico
E-mails: 1120631@alumno.um.edu.mx[1], harveyalferez@um.edu.mx[1], oftalmo@um.edu.mx[2]

***Abstract*—Glaucoma is a disease that damages the optic nerve and becomes chronic as time progresses. Its early detection is vital for treatment. Although there are tools to carry out the analysis of the optic nerve, they do not automatically detect this illness. For this reason, the objective of this research is to carry out experiments with convolutional neuronal networks to achieve the automatic detection of this disease. The experiments performed obtained an average accuracy of 99%.**

***Index Terms*—Glaucoma, convolutional neuronal networks.**

I. Introduction

One of the most important and complex aspects for glaucoma treatment is an early diagnosis to prevent permanent structural damage and irreversible loss of vision [1], [2]. Moreover, the proper diagnosis of glaucoma is key due to the fact that it occurs without symptoms and can lead to irreversible loss of sight [3].

There are tools for taking pictures of the fundus of the eye, such as Visucam NNM/FA[1] and Kevork[2]. These kind of tools are useful for detecting glaucoma by means of Ocular Coherence Tomography (OCT), Heidelberg Retina Tomography II (HRT II), Optical Coherence Tomography (Stratus OCT), and Scanning Laser Polarimetry with Variablecorneal Compensation (GDx VCC), and Confocal Scanning Laser Ophthalmoscopy. However, these tools lack the automatic early detection of glaucoma.

The contribution of this research work is to use convolutional neural networks implemented in TensorFlow for the automatic early detection of glaucoma by means of analyzing pictures of the fundus of the eye. To this end, pictures were taken at the Instituto de la Visión, an ophthalmologic clinic that belongs to Universidad de Montemorelos, Mexico. Within a period of three months, 22 pictures of the fundus of the eye with confirmed diagnosis of glaucoma and 14 pictures of healthy people were taken. These pictures were used for training a convolutional neuronal network. To this end, TensorFlow was used for extending the pre-trained model Inception v3 with the new pictures. The results of the classification were compared with medical diagnosis.

This paper is organized as follows. The second section presents how glaucoma has become a public health problem. The third session presents the state of art. The fourth section presents the underlying concepts of our approach. The fifth section presents the results. The last section presents conclusions and future work.

[1]http://www.medicalexpo.es/prod/carl-zeiss-meditec/product-67959-801991.html

[2]http://kevork-instruments.com/productos/nexy

II. Glaucoma - A Public Health Problem

According to the National Eye Institute (NEI) [4], glaucoma is a group of diseases that can lead to damage to the eye's optic nerve and ends in blindness. Glaucoma usually has no early symptoms. Moreover, by the time people experience problems with their vision, they usually have lost a significant amount of their sight. According to NEI, increased pressure inside the eye is a key cause of open-angle glaucoma.

Since glaucoma has no symptoms, the only way to detect its progression is by conducting studies based on the internal structure of the eye. The risk of blindness depends on the intraocular pressure, the severity of the disease, the age of glaucoma onset, as well as family history of this disease [5].

Glaucoma is a global health problem. In fact, it is the second leading cause of blindness worldwide, affecting approximately 6.7 million people [6]. Several population-based epidemiological studies have reported that more than 50% of glaucoma cases remain undiagnosed even in developed countries [7]. Most importantly, glaucoma is the main cause of irreversible blindness, being cataract the prime reversible cause. Glaucoma is the main cause of irreversible blindness in people older than 60 years. In fact, blindness due to glaucoma can be prevented if treated early [5]. Although this is true, there are no symptoms of glaucoma. Therefore, the early detection is primarily done by observing structural changes in the exploration of the head of the optic nerve.

Over the years, technology has made great progress in the creation and modification of instruments used for different diagnoses within the medical area. In the field of ophthalmology, there is a wide variety of tools for taking pictures that stand out for their image quality, cost, and easy interaction [8]. Nevertheless, these machines lack the necessary software for the automatic detection of glaucoma.

The use of artificial neural networks in recent years has given solutions to a wide variety of pattern recognition problems, such as computer vision, image recognition, and speech recognition [9]. Currently, the most used tool in the construction of convolutional neural networks is TensorFlow[3]. TensorFlow is an open source software specialized in speech, text, and image recognition. Its flexible architecture allows to implement algorithms in one or more CPUs or GPUs. TensorFlow was developed by Google. Its great impact on artificial intelligence has led companies such as Intel, Nvidia, and Twitter to use this tool [10]. Through the flexibility offered by TensorFlow, models based on previously trained convolutional neural networks can be extended such in the case of the Inception v3 model. Inception v3 has been trained with images from ImageNet [11]. This model can be retrained in order to save computing time in the generation of a new classification model. We believe that by extending the Inception v3 model with pictures of the fundus of the eye, the glaucoma detection process could be automated.

III. State of the Art

Ophthalmologists would like to achieve the detection and diagnosis of glaucoma in the shortest possible time [12]. To this end, in [13] different machine learning algorithms were compared to evaluate the performance of each one of them for detecting glaucoma. In that research work, the authors used multilayer perceptron, support vector machines, among other algorithms. These algorithms had a high performance during classification [13].

In [14] the results of comparing different classifiers for the diagnosis of glaucoma were presented. In that research work, artificial neural networks and other image processing methods were used to compare them with the Stratus OCT that is frequently used for the detection and diagnosis of glaucoma or other eye diseases. The result was successful with a sample of 89 images of eyes of patients with glaucoma using feed-forward backpropagation.

Other research works also used feed-forward backprogation. For example, in [15], pictures of fundus of eye were collected and used to train a feed-forward backpropagation neural network. To this end, Matlab was utilized to process the images and thus obtain the features to be used in training. In [16], the gradient method was used for detecting the presence of glaucoma using an artificial neural network that is trained with the processed images. As a result it was possible to detect the different stages of glaucoma using backpropagation. In [17], the gradient method was used to detect the presence of glaucoma using artificial neural networks. In that research work, photo editing methods were used to eliminate the noise of each image. The artificial neural network was based on feed-forward backpropagation and the mathematical morphology was used for the analysis of the extraction of the features necessary for training.

In [16], an approach based on support vector machines was proposed to detect glaucoma. The objective of that research work was to use pictures of the fundus of the eye processed by techniques such as noise elimination, contrast enhancement, and principal component analysis. By means of analyzing 40 images, an accuracy of 85% was obtained.

[3]https://www.tensorflow.org/about/uses

Although the approaches above based on feed-forward backpropagation or other classical classifiers are interesting, recent advances in computer vision indicate that the trend has turned to the use of convolutional neural networks for the recognition of patterns in images [18].

IV. Underpinning of Our Approach

In this section the underlying concepts of our approach are presented. The relationship of these concepts is shown in Figure 1.

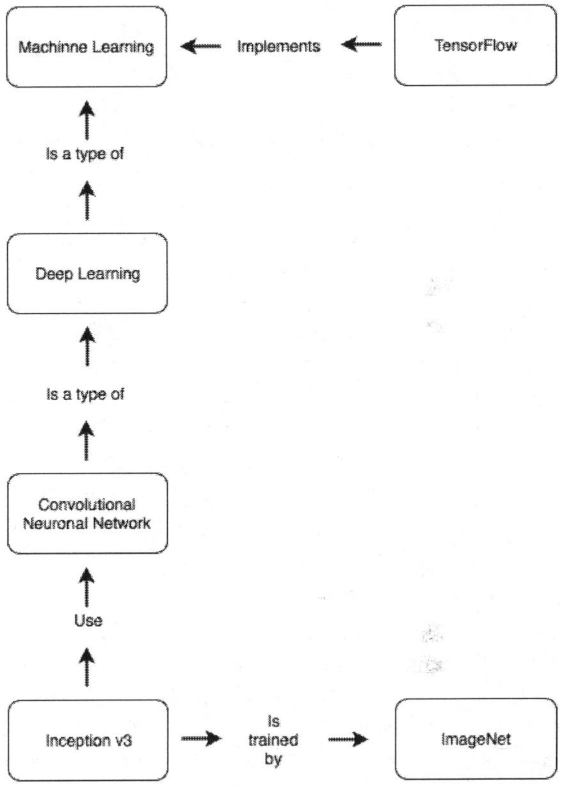

Fig. 1. Conceptual framework.

A. Machine Learning

Machine learning emerged in the 60's as an idea of artificial intelligence but it was until the 80's that it gained importance [19]. Machine learning refers to the practice of training computers through algorithms and mathematical formulas giving the computer the ability to learn and remember from historical data and thus suggest a possible future scenario [20].

The goal of machine learning is to create a model that allows to solve a task. In machine learning, it is desirable that the model is trained using a large amount of data. Through operations and algorithms, the model learns from this data and is able to make predictions. As a result, large companies such as Amazon, Baidu, Google, IBM, Microsoft, and others, use this tool for their business.

There are two types of machine learning approaches: supervised learning and unsupervised learning. On one hand, supervised learning is about training a model from a set of input data with the expected outputs. On the other hand, in unsupervised learning, training is performed with a set of unlabeled input data [21]. This research work is focused on supervised learning.

B. Deep Learning

Deep learning, or better known as deep neural networks, is a branch of artificial intelligence. It emulates the learning approach that human beings use to obtain certain types of knowledge [22]. Deep learning became popular recently when the media headlines showed that Google's AlphaGo beat the world champion of Go, a complex game with thousands of possible combinations [23].

Deep learning allows the processing of computational models composed of multiple layers to learn representations of data with different levels of abstraction. These methods have dramatically improved techniques in image and audio recognition [24].

Deep learning carries out the automatic learning process by means of using an artificial neural network that is composed of a number of hierarchical levels. At the first layer of the hierarchy, the network learns something simple and then sends that information to the next layer. On the second layer, for example, edges are combined by constructing simple shapes, such as a diagonal line or a right angle. In the third layer, the simple forms of the previous layer are combined and more complex objects are obtained like ovals or rectangles. In the next layer, ovals and rectangles could be combined, giving shape to figures in the image [23].

C. Convolutional Neural Networks

Convolutional neural networks are a category of artificial neural networks that have proven to be very efficient in areas such as image recognition, classification, and speech recognition [25]. Convolutional neuronal networks use several identical copies of the same neuron [26]. LeNet was one of the first convolutional neuronal networks that helped drive the field of deep learning since 1990 [27].

CNNs have four main operations [28]: 1) convolution, 2) non-linearity (Relu), 3) pooling or sub-sampling, and 4) classification. These operations act on images that can be represented as a matrix with pixel values [29]. These four operations are explained below:

- *Convolution:* Convolution is a continuous nonlinear function that transforms an input signal into a new output signal. The main purpose of the convolution in the case of the convolutional neuronal network is to extract features from the input image [30]. For example, in Figure IV-C a 5x5 image whose values are only 0s and 1s is considered. Another 3x3 matrix is the filter or kernel. The filter slides over the original matrix from the first pixel, and for each position the multiplication and sum of the elements between the two matrices is calculated. The result is placed in a new matrix. .
  By modifying the filter values, different maps of the same input image are obtained. Figure 3 shows the effects of convolution when applying different filters to an image. Through these filters it is possible to perform operations

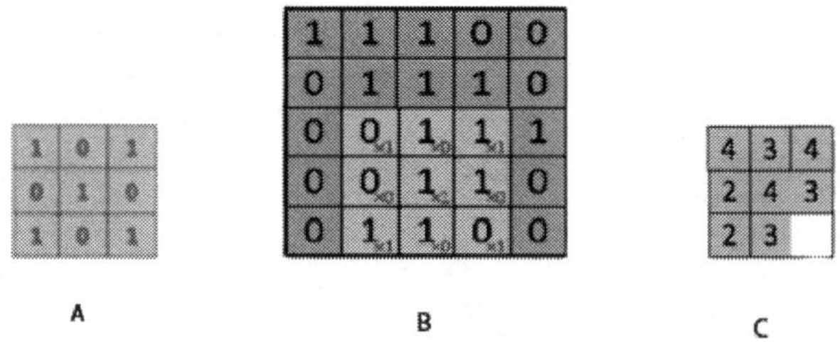

Fig. 2. Filter or kernel (A). Matrix of the image (B). Convolved feature (C) [28].

such as edge detection, sharpness, and blurring. In these operations, the values of the filter matrix are combined before the convolution. This means that different filters can detect different features of an image, for example, edges, curves, lines, etc. [28].

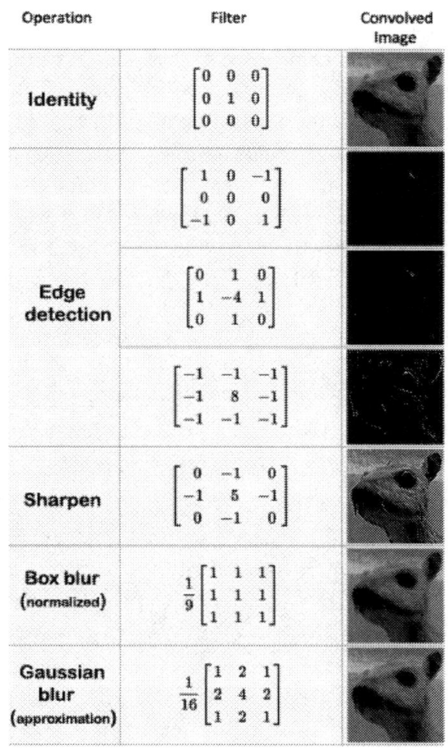

Fig. 3. Different filters [28].

- *Non-linearity (Relu):* Non-linearity is an operation that is applied to each pixel and replaces all negative values of pixels to zeros. The objective of Relu is to introduce non-linearity in the convolution since most of the data that the artificial neuronal network wishes to learn is non-linear [31]. The Relu operation can be seen in Figure 4.
- *Grouping or sub-sampling:* Grouping reduces the dimension of each feature map while retaining the most important information. The grouping can be of different types: maximum value, average value, sum, etc. These functions allow to detect objects inside the image no matter where they are [32]. For example, in the case of max pooling, the largest element of the map features is taken. Figure 5 shows an example with the max pooling

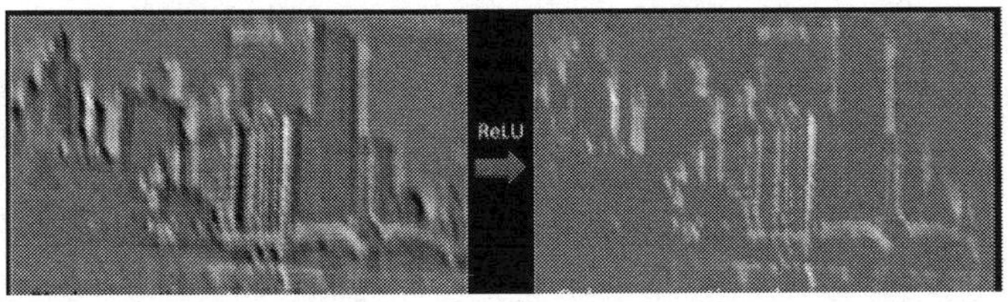

Fig. 4. Operation Relu [28].

operation in a function map [33].

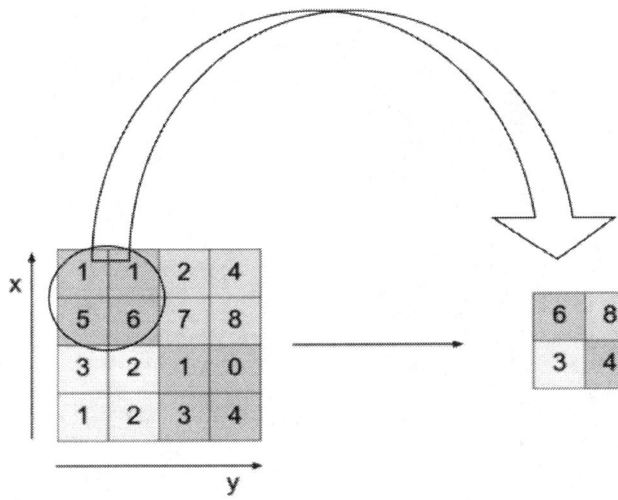

Fig. 5. Max Pooling [28].

- *Fully Connected Layer:* As a whole, the stages of convolution, Relu, and grouping or sub-sampling stages extract useful features, introduce non-linearity in the network, and reduce the dimensions of features to make them smaller and more manageable. Finally, the output of the grouping or sub-sampling layer acts as an input layer to the Fully Connected layer [32]. The objective of this layer is to use the features obtained in previous layers for the classification of the input image [28].

D. TensorFLow

TensorFlow is used in a large number of applications or tools that we use today, such as Google's speech recognition [34]. The TensorFlow API was launched as an open source package in November 2015. TensorFlow uses numerical calculations using data flow graphs. The nodes of the graph represent mathematical operations, while the tensors of the graph handle multidimensional data matrixes to achieve communication between nodes [10], [35]. The value of the tensor can be calculated using Session.run when the graph is executed [36].

E. ImageNet

ImageNet is an image bank organized according to the hierarchy of WordNet. It is a free and accessible resource for researchers and educators around the world [37].

F. Inception v3

Inception-v3 is trained for the ImageNet Large Visual Recognition Challenge using the data from 2012. This is a standard task in computer vision, where models try to classify images into 1,000 classes.
[11].

V. RESULTS

This section presents the methodology that was used in this research work and the results obtained.s

A. Methodology

The activities that were carried out in each of the stages of this research work are described as follows.

1) Preparation of the training environment: In order to train the classification model, 25 pictures of the fundus of the eye were taken from people who have a confirmed diagnosis of glaucoma. Also, 19 pictures of the fundus of the eye were taken from patients who do not show symptoms of glaucoma. These pictures were taken in a period of 3 months at the Instituto de la Visión. All the pictures used in the experiments are available online[4].

To take the pictures of the fundus of the eye of patients with glaucoma, the following procedure was performed:

1) An ophthalmologist confirms that a patient has a clinical diagnosis of glaucoma. To this end, tomographic and campimetria diagnoses were carried out previously.
2) The patient is informed of the importance of taking the picture of his or her optic nerve.
3) The patient signs a medical consent in which he or she accepts that a picture of the fundus of his or her eyes will be taken for research. At this point, the patient is informed about the procedure and future use of the pictures.
4) To take a picture of the fundus of the eye, the pupil of the patient is dilated with phenylephrine eye drops.
5) With the pupil dilated, the picture is taken with the VISUCAM NM / FA machine.

The pictures of the fundus of the eye of patients who do not have a diagnosis of glaucoma were also taken with the VISUCAM NM / FA machine. This machine already had in storage several pictures of healthy patients. As a result, the aforementioned steps did not have to be taken.

Figure V-A1 shows two pictures of the fundus of the eyes of two different patients. On one hand, Section A of this figure shows a picture of the fundus of the eye of a patient with glaucoma. On the other hand, section B shows a picture of the fundus of the eye of a healthy patient. With respect to nerve fibers, the eye at the left is deteriorated.

[4]https://goo.gl/ufjRqP

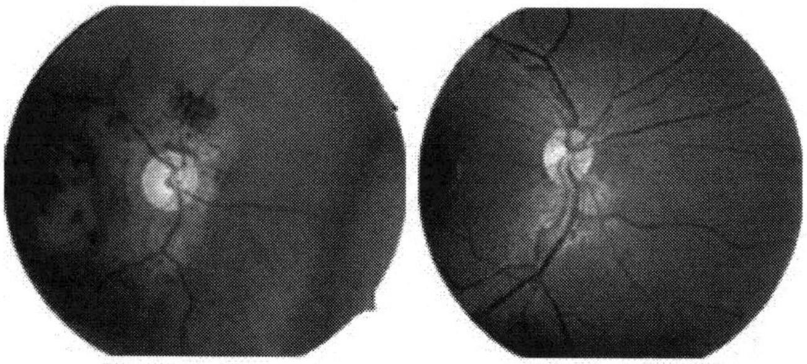

Fig. 6. Pictures of the fundus of the eye: A) with glaucoma and B) without glaucoma.

2) Re-training the Inception v3 convolutional neuronal network : This step consists of re-training the Inception v3 convolutional neuronal network. To this end, a MacBook Air computer with MacOS high Sierra V. 10.13.3 operating system was used. This machine has a 1.6 GHz Intel Core i5 processor and 8 GB 1600 MHz DDR3 of RAM memory. Also, TensorFlow version 1.5.0 was installed and executed. Specifically, the following tools were installed and the following downloads were made:

1) Python version 2.7 was installed from a terminal with the following instruction: "sudo pip install python".
2) TensorFlow was installed through the terminal with the following instruction: "pip install tensorflow".
3) The code label_image.py was downloaded. This code uses the Inception model to classify images that are passed to the model from the command line[5].
4) The code retrain.py was downloaded. This code allows to adapt the pretrained Inception network for other classification problems. A detailed overview of this script can be found online[6].

The command line used to retrained the Inception v3 model is the folloiwng:

sudo python retrain.py --bottleneck_dir /tf_glaucoma/bottlenecks --model_dir /tf_glaucoma/inception --output_graph /tf_glaucoma/retrained_graph.pb --output_labels /tf_glaucoma/retrained_labels.txt --image_dir ~/DataSet/glaucoma

This instruction indicates the script that carries out the retraining (retrain.py) on the Inception model. Also, it indicates the output graph and the labels that are used for training, glaucoma and no glaucoma. The path where the pictures are found is the following: ~/DataSet/glaucoma. In this path, there are two directories. One with the pictures of the fundus of the eye of patients with glaucoma and another with pictures of healthy patients.

From the 44 pictures taken at the Instituto de la Visión, 6 were separated for testing. Specifically, 3 pictures were separated from the 19 pictures without glaucoma and 3 pictures were separated from the 25 pictures with glaucoma. The retraining was done in 8 minutes.

[5]https://goo.gl/hDYKnG
[6]https://goo.gl/b7EcBe

B. Presentation of the Results

The results are shown in Tables V-B and V-B. Table V-B shows the results obtained by entering the 3 pictures of the fundus of the eye with glaucoma to the computer. Each image shows a percentage of accuracy. The evaluations of the three pictures shown to the computer were correctly labeled with an average accuracy of 99%. Although these results are promising, we believe that a better predictive model could be generated by retraining the algorithm using more fundus images.

Table 1. Evaluation of pictures of the fundus of the eye with glaucoma.

Evaluations	No glaucoma	Glaucoma
1 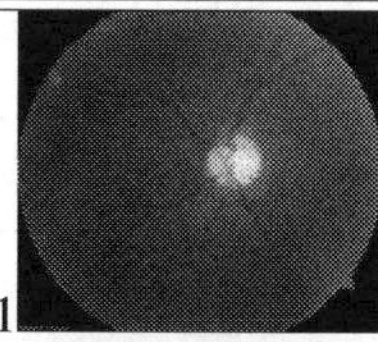	0.00246	0..99754
2 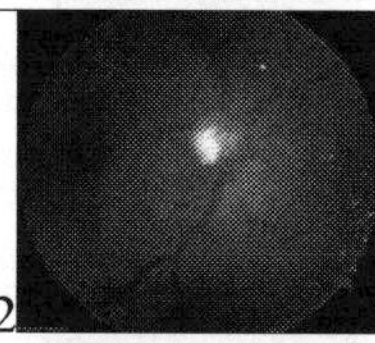	0.00011	0.99989
3 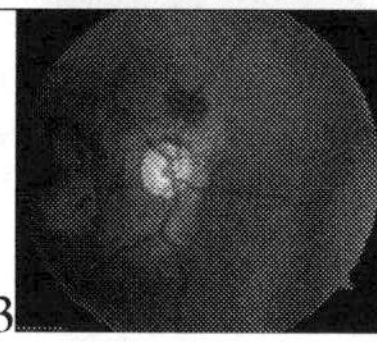	0.00869	0.99624
Average	0.00375	0.99624

Table V-B shows the results of the three pictures of the fundus of the eye that do not have glaucoma. In these cases, the classification model has an average accuracy of 99%.

Table 2. Evaluation of pictures of the fundus of the eye without glaucoma.

Evaluations	No glaucoma	Glaucoma
1 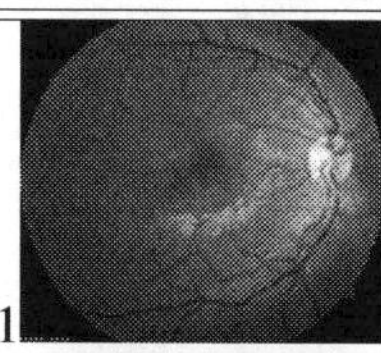	0.99762	0.00238
2 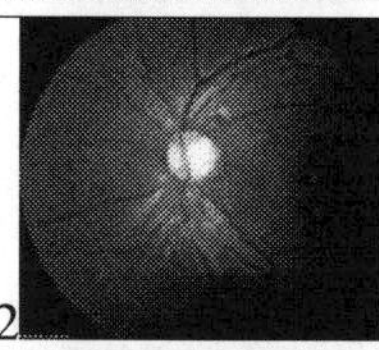	0.99444	0.00556
3 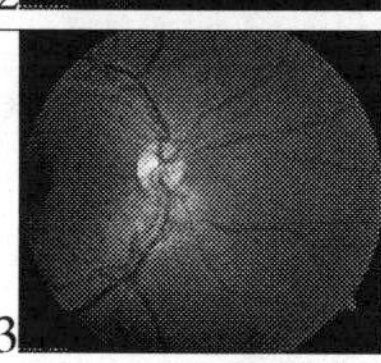	0.9948	0.00052
Average	0.99718	0.00846

VI. Conclusion and Future Work

This research work was conducted to prove that convolutional neural networks implemented in TensorFlow can be used for the early automatic detection of glaucoma. To this end, the Inception v3 model was extended with 44 photographs taken at the Instituto de la Visión at Universidad de Montemorelos, Mexico. An evaluation of the classification was carried out with 6 pictures. As a result, the trained model obtained in average a 99% accuracy for classifying glaucoma and no glaucoma.

As future work, although the results in this research work were promising, the sample of pictures of the fundus of the eye of healthy and sick patients will be extended in order to improve the classification. Likewise, it is expected to extend the predictive model so that it does not only detect glaucoma, but also to assess stages of its severity. Also, we expect to extend the model for the early detection of other diseases such as retinal pathology.

References

[1] S. Pamela, "Diagnostic tools for glaucoma detection and management," November 1, 2015. [Online]. Available: https://www.ncbi.nlm.nih.gov/pmc/articles/PMC2643302/

[2] W. Havener, "Importance of early detection of glaucoma," January 16, 2018. [Online]. Available: https://jamanetwork.com/journals/jama/article-abstract/302280?redirect=true

[3] D. Calkins, "Glaucoma," Tech. Rep. 88-207450, 2016. [Online]. Available: https://www.glaucoma.org/GRF_Understanding_Glaucoma_ES.pdf

[4] The National Institutes of Health, "Results–Ocular Hypertension Treatment Study (OHTS)," n.d. [Online]. Available: https://nei.nih.gov/glaucomaeyedrops/ohts_backg

[5] K. Boyd, "What is glaucoma," August 08, 2017. [Online]. Available: https://www.aao.org/salud-ocular/enfermedades/que-es-la-glaucoma

[6] C. Traverso, "Glaucoma the importance of early detection and early treatment," *European Ophthalmic Review*, vol. 13, no. 4, pp. 13–14, 2011. [Online]. Available: http://www.touchophthalmology.com/articles/glaucoma-importance-early-detection-and-early-treatment

[7] Q. Ha, "Number of people with glaucoma worldwide," *The British Journal of Ophthalmology*, vol. 80, no. 5, pp. 389–393, May 1996. [Online]. Available: https://www.ncbi.nlm.nih.gov/pubmed/8695555

[8] C. Zeiss, "Visucam 524 fundus imaging," 2016. [Online]. Available: https://www.zeiss.com/meditec/us/products/ophthalmology-optometry/retina/diagnostics/fundus-imaging/visucam-fundus-imaging.html

[9] C. Shallue, "Inception V3 model," 2018. [Online]. Available: https://www.kaggle.com/google-brain/inception-v3

[10] Google, "TensorFlow," January 27, 2018. [Online]. Available: https://www.tensorflow.org/

[11] C. Szegedy, V. Vanhoucke, S. Ioffe, J. Shlens, and Z. Wojna, "Rethinking the inception architecture for computer vision," *CoRR*, vol. abs/1512.00567, 2015. [Online]. Available: http://arxiv.org/abs/1512.00567

[12] E. Oh, "Artificial neural network approach for differentiating open-angle glaucoma from glaucoma suspect without a visual field test," vol. 26, March 14 de 2016.

[13] M. Goldbaum, "Comparison of machine learning and traditional classifiers in glaucoma diagnosis," *Transactions on Biomedical Engineering*, vol. 49, no. 9, 2002.

[14] H. Ling, "Development and comparison of automated classifiers for glaucoma diagnosis using stratus optical coherence tomography," *Investigative ophthalmology & visual science*, vol. 46, no. 11, pp. 4121–4129, 2005.

[15] O. Sheeba, *Glaucoma Detection Using Artificial Neural Network*, IACSIT, Ed. IACSIT, April 2014, vol. 6, no. 2.

[16] D. Abhishek, "Automated glaucoma detection using support vector machine classification method," *International Journal of Innovative Research in Computer and Communication Engineering*, vol. 3, no. 1, 2015.

[17] P. Sahithya Sri, P. Chitra, and K. Mahalakshmi, "A survey based on glaucoma detection," *Imperial Journal of Interdisciplinary Research (IJIR)*, vol. 6, pp. 1605–1611, 2015.

[18] H. Eckerson, "Deep learning past, present, and future," may 2017. [Online]. Available: https://www.kdnuggets.com/2017/05/deep-learning-big-deal.html

[19] C. Robert, *Machine learning, a probabilistic perspective*. Taylor & Francis, 2014.

[20] G. Wiederhold, J. McCarthy, and E. Feigenbaum, "Arthur Samuel pioneer in machine learning," *Communications of the ACM*, vol. 33, no. 11, pp. 137–139, 1990.

[21] R. Salas, "Redes neuronales artificiales," *Universidad de Valparaiso. Departamento de Computación*, vol. 1, 2004.

[22] I. Goodfellow, Y. Bengio, A. Courville, and Y. Bengio, *Deep learning*. MIT press Cambridge, 2016, vol. 1.

[23] C. Moreno, "Qué es deep learning y para qué sirve?" 2018. [Online]. Available: https://www.indracompany.com/es/blogneo/deep-learning-sirve

[24] Y. LeCun, Y. Bengio, and G. Hinton, "Deep learning," *Nature*, vol. 521, no. 7553, p. 436, 2015.

[25] A.-H. Ossama, "Applying convolutional neural networks concepts to hybrid NN-HMM model for speech recognition," in *Acoustics, Speech and Signal Processing (ICASSP), 2012 IEEE International Conference on*. IEEE, 2012, pp. 4277–4280.

[26] C. Olah, "Conv nets a modular perspective," p. 1, July 8, 2014. [Online]. Available: https://colah.github.io/posts/2014-07-Conv-Nets-Modular/

[27] E. Culurciello, "Neural network architectures," Mar. 2017. [Online]. Available: https://towardsdatascience.com/neural-network-architectures-156e5bad51ba

[28] U. Ujjwalkarn, "An intuitive explanation of convolutional neural networks," August 11, 2016. [Online]. Available: https://ujjwalkarn.me/2016/08/11/intuitive-explanation-convnets/

[29] A. Geitgey, "Deep learning and convolutional neural networks," Jun 13, 2016. [Online]. Available: https://medium.com/@ageitgey/machine-learning

[30] P. Méndez and J. Ibarra, "Implementación de una red neuronal de convolución para el reconocimiento de poses en imágenes de rostros," *ACI Avances en Ciencias e Ingenierías*, vol. 6, no. 2, 2014.

[31] R. Fergus, "Neural networks," MLSS 2015. [Online]. Available: http://mlss.tuebingen.mpg.de/2015/slides/fergus/Fergus_1.pdf

[32] K. Alex and Sutskever, "Imagenet classification with deep convolutional neural networks," in *Advances in neural information processing systems*, 2012, pp. 1097–1105.

[33] J. Jhonson, "Convolutional neural networks for visual recognition," 2017. [Online]. Available: http://cs231n.github.io/convolutional-networks/

[34] S. Pichai, "TensorFlow smarter machine learning, for everyone," Nov. 2015. [Online]. Available: https://googleblog.blogspot.mx/2015/11/tensorflow-smarter-machine-learning-for.html

[35] M. Abadi, A. Agarwal, P. Barham, E. Brevdo, Z. Chen, and C. Citro, et al., "TensorFlow large scale machine learning on heterogeneous distributed systems," Google, Tech. Rep., Nov. 2015. [Online]. Available: http://download.tensorflow.org/paper/whitepaper2015.pdf

[36] C. Fredrik, "tf.tensor," January 27, 2018. [Online]. Available: https://www.tensorflow.org/api_docs/python/tf/Tensor

[37] O. Russakovsky, "ImageNet," 2016. [Online]. Available: http://www.image-net.org/about-overview

A novel approach for classification of Cancer subtypes using Differentially Expressed Genes from RNA-Seq

Uday R[1] and Anu Mary Chacko[2]
[1] [2]Department of Computer Science and Engineering, National Institute of Technology, Calicut, Kerala, India

Abstract—*Detection of cancer subtypes is a very complex task since there are not many ways of measuring gene expressions accurately. RNA-Seq is an emerging technology for analyzing gene expression content by directly sequencing the mRNA molecules in a sample. In this paper, we propose a gene-expression-based cancer subtype classification pipeline for identifying potential gene markers and use the same to classify between normal and cancerous samples. The proposed approach was applied to two datasets, taken from The Cancer Genome Atlas (TCGA) and its performance was evaluated using two validation schemes called holdout and 10-fold validation. Using it, we are able to identify the minimum number of significant genes required to effectively classify samples with an average accuracy of 95%.*

Keywords: RNA-Seq, Differentially Expressed Genes (DEGs), microarray, Support Vector Machine (SVM), DESeq2, Dimensionality Reduction

1. Introduction

Cancer is a heterogeneous disease, that is, each cancer may have a number of subtypes. Identifying cancer subtype is of great importance in cancer diagnosis and drug discovery. Accurate prediction of cancer subtypes can help in providing better treatment and toxicity minimization for the patients [1]. Occurrence of cancer alters genetic expression of a group of cells or collectively known as a tissue and there are not many techniques for measuring genetic expression of cells. The advent of RNA-Seq technology has made it possible to study different gene transcripts that are significantly affected by cancer [2].

During the last decade, classification was done using microarray-based gene expression. Of late, the technology for quantifying gene expression has changed from microarray to RNA-Seq. The output of RNA-Seq has a number of advantages over the output of microarrays such as providing less noisy data, detecting novel transcripts and not requiring pre-arranged transcripts. Presently, it is also the best suited technique for discovery based experiments. RNA-Seq is used for gene-expression-based classification to identify significant genes, distinguish biological samples and predict the outcomes from large scale gene expression data [3]. One of the challenges while working with RNA-Seq data is to identify a subset of significant or differentially expressed genes which can be used to train a classifier to classify between different classes.

A gene is considered to be differentially expressed if a statistically significant difference is observed in read counts between two experimental conditions. The pattern of differential gene expression is approximated using statistical distributions. Differentially Expressed Genes are usually selected by an expression change threshold and a score cutoff [4]. This set of genes are called Differentially Expressed Genes (DEGs). Computationally speaking, this set of DEGs can be used to effectively classify between conditions. This is further used to build and train a classification model to classify between normal and cancerous samples.

2. Related work

The concept of RNA sequencing is fairly new and it overcomes the drawbacks encountered while dealing with microarray data. Some of the most recent work done using RNA-Seq data is mentioned below.

Gargi Mukherjee et al. [5] developed a protocol using mRNA-Seq data to identify patients likely to have early recurrence of their disease. The authors identified genes that are responsible for prediction of recurrence, based on Kaplan-Meier recurrence free survival and Generalized Matrix Learning Vector Quantization (GMLVQ).

Gokmen Zararsiz et al. [3] conducted a simulation study to examine the effect of several parameters such as number of genes, overdispersion, number of classes, sample size, transformation method and differential-expression rate on model performances using two mRNA datasets. The authors concluded that a power transformed PLDA may be a good choice for a count-based classifier.

Juliana Costa-Silva et al. [6] conducted a review of methods for the identification of differentially expressed genes (DEGs). The authors evaluated six mapping methods and nine main methods for the DEGs identification and the integration of these methods. The results showed that DEG analysis are barely affected mapping methods.

Zhilong Jia et al. [7] proposed an approach that makes use of discriminant non-negative matrix factorization (DNMF) for RNA-seq data. Differential expression analysis using DNMF-based gene ranking method was applied on four RNA-seq datasets. The Area under the Curve analysis of the entire experiment demonstrated that DNMF-based gene ranking method outperformed other popular methods. The authors concluded that DNMF is computationally efficient by substantially outperforming all other benchmarked methods.

In terms of computation, the challenge of identifying Differentially Expressed Genes (DEGs) from RNA-Seq data and using them to construct a classification model is a type of Dimensionality Reduction problem. Hence, we chose to explore this area for the purpose of classifying cancer subtypes. We aim to achieve maximum overall accuracy of the classifier by using minimum number of DEGs to effectively classify between samples that belongs to different classes.

3. Proposed approach

Gene is a genetic marker that can be used to identify individuals. When an individual is affected with cancer, a set of protein-coding genes belonging to that individual are altered. Cancer subtype classification is a type of supervised machine learning problem where we construct a classification model based on set of genes which are significantly altered on occurrence of a specific type of cancer. The proposed approach primarily focuses on the method of obtaining Differentially Expressed Genes (DEGs) and the number of genes to be considered for the purpose of classification.

3.1 Datasets

The following datasets were downloaded from The Cancer Genome Atlas (TCGA) Data Coordinating Center.

Renal cell cancer (RCC) dataset contains 1,020 samples and their corresponding 20,530 known human RNA transcript counts. Samples are separated into three distinct subclasses. Out of 1,020 samples, 91 samples belong to kidney chromophobe carcinoma (KICH) samples, 323 samples belong to kidney renal clear cell (KIRC) and 606 samples belong to kidney renal papillary cell (KIRP).

Lung cancer dataset contains read counts of 20,531 transcripts belonging to 1,128 samples. Samples are separated into two distinct subclasses. 576 out of 1,128 samples, correspond to lung adenocarcinoma (LUAD) and the remaining 552 samples correspond to lung squamous cell with carcinoma (LUSC).

3.2 Pipeline architecture

Objective : To create a pipeline for classification of cancer subtypes for RNA-Seq data. It consists of two modules :

Module-1 : Gene selection

Input : 25 sample pairs of gene-level transcription estimates before and after treatment for each cancer subtype.

Output : A set of significant genes which are responsible to effectively classify between normal and cancerous samples for each cancer subtype.

Process : 25 sample pairs corresponding to each cancer subtype, is fed into differential expression analysis tool one at a time, and a set of significantly altered genes of the inputted cancer subtype is obtained. Genes whose adjusted p-value is less than 0.05 are selected as DEGs.

Module-2 : Cancer subtype classification

Input : Significant gene-level transcription estimate of 1000 samples belonging to different subtypes.

Output : Overall accuracy of the classifier.

Process : Building a classification model involves training the model and testing it using appropriate validation techniques. We use Holdout and 10-fold cross validation to do the same. A model is built using all of the DEGs resulting in Module-1 and its overall classification accuracy is checked. A gene that is differentially expressed for one subtype may also be differentially expressed for another subtype. Next, we eliminate such common DEGs as follows :

Suppose x is the resulting set of DEGs for subtype A, similarly y and z for subtype B and C, then

$$\begin{aligned} x &= x - ((x \cap y) \cup (x \cap z)) \\ y &= y - ((y \cap x) \cup (y \cap z)) \\ z &= z - ((z \cap x) \cup (z \cap y)) \end{aligned} \tag{1}$$

Now, we have a unique set genes for each subtype. Let the union of these genes be called set S.

$$S = x \cup y \cup z \tag{2}$$

A classification model is built using S genes and validated. The general block diagram of the proposed pipeline is shown in Figure 1.

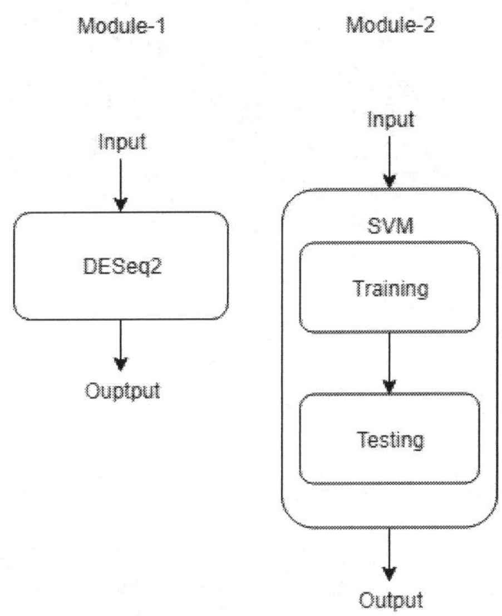

Fig. 1: Proposed pipeline

3.3 Tools used

DESeq2 on Rstudio [8] is used for differential expression analysis in Module-1. Other popular differential expression analysis tools were initially developed to analyze only microarray data. Also, Deseq2 uses Negative Binomial distribution which is best suited for modelling gene counts.

Support Vector Machine (SVM) on Matlab R2015a is used for the purpose of classification in Module-2 because of its strong mathematical background and learning capability.

4. Results

Module-1

When a particular gene is altered, it can either be above or below a certain normal. When an altered gene is above normal, it is called an Up-regulated gene and otherwise it is called a Down-regulated gene. Total number of DEGs obtained and the number of up and down regulated genes among them for each cancer subtype is shown in Table 1 and 2.

Cancer sub-types	# of Up regulated	# of Down regulated	Total # of genes
KICH	2079	391	2470
KIRP	1369	286	1655
KIRC	1017	393	1410

Table 1: Number of DEGs for RCC dataset

Cancer sub-types	# of Up regulated	# of Down regulated	Total # of genes
LUAD	609	477	1086
LUSC	1442	1136	2578

Table 2: Number of DEGs for Lung cancer dataset

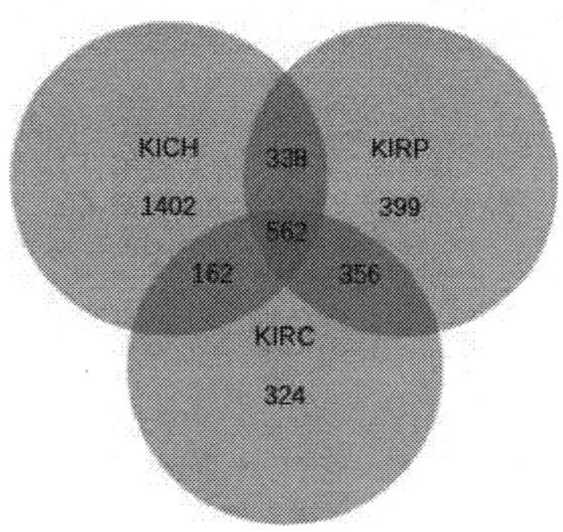

Fig. 2: DEGs overlap for RCC dataset

Result of DESeq2 for RCC dataset : 2470 out of 20530 genes are significant to classify between KICH and normal samples with maximum accuracy. Similarly, 1655 for KIRP and 1410 for KIRC. Out of which, 562 DEGs are common for all 3 RCC subtypes, 900 DEGs are common for KICH and KIRP, 918 DEGs are common for KIRP and KIRC and 730 DEGs common for KIRC and KICH.

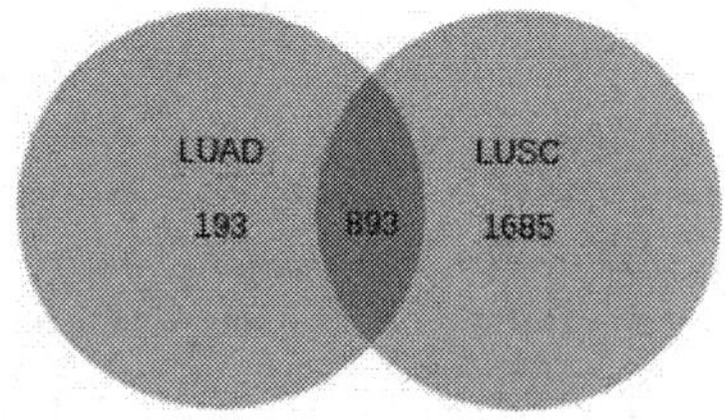

Fig. 3: DEGs overlap for Lung cancer dataset

Result of DESeq2 for Lung cancer dataset : 1086 out of 20530 genes are differentially expressed for LUAD and 2578 for LUSC. Out of which, 893 DEGs are common for both.

Data preparation : Among 1020 samples present in RCC dataset, we eliminated 10 samples each from KIRP and KIRC to obtain a total of 1000 samples. Now, we have 126 normal samples, 524 KIRC samples, 284 KIRP samples and 66 KICH samples. Among 1128 samples present in Lung cancer dataset, we eliminated 76 samples from LUAD and 52 samples from LUSC to obtain a total of 1000 samples. Out of which 97, 448 and 455 belongs to normal, LUAD and LUSC, respectively.

Module-2

Total number of unique DEGs for datasets with and without overlap of common DEGs between cancer subtypes is as shown in the table below.

Cancer dataset	with overlap	without overlap
RCC	3549	2125
Lung	2771	1878

Table 3: Number of DEGs for model building

Holdout validation with 70% of data for training and the remaining 30% for testing is performed to check the overall accuracy of the classifier. Along with this, 10-fold cross validation is also used to evaluate the performance of the classification model. The results of Holdout and 10-fold cross validation for classifiers built using DEGs with and without overlap is shown in Table 4 and 5.

(Overall accuracy in %)		
Validation methods	RCC dataset	Lung dataset
Holdout	95.8	94.7
10-fold cv	95	95.6

Table 4: Result of classifiers built using DEGs with overlap

(Overall accuracy in %)		
Validation methods	RCC dataset	Lung dataset
Holdout	96.3	95.6
10-fold cv	95.3	95.8

Table 5: Result of classifiers built using DEGs without overlap

There is rise in overall accuracy of classifiers in spite of reducing 1,424 DEGs for RCC and 893 DEGs for Lung cancer dataset.

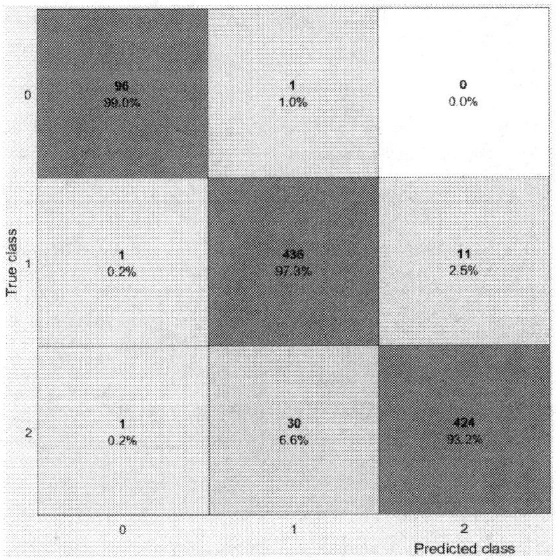

Fig. 4: 10-fold cross validation confusion matrix for Lung cancer dataset with overlap

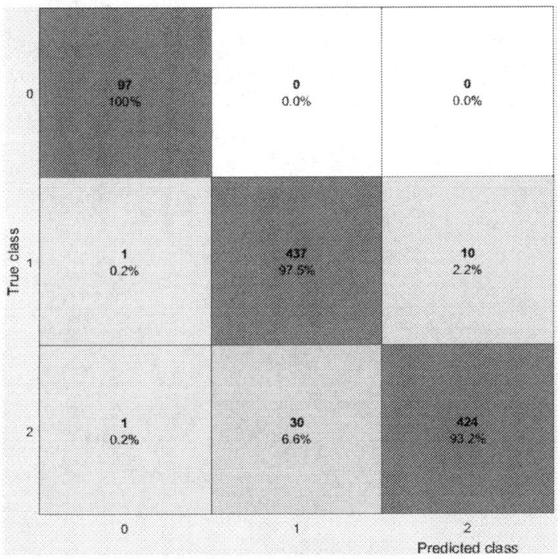

Fig. 5: 10-fold cross validation confusion matrix for Lung cancer dataset without overlap

Class-0 corresponds to normal samples, Class-1 corresponds to LUAD samples and Class-2 corresponds to LUSC samples.

5. Conclusion and Future scope

Cancer is a heterogeneous disease consisting of many different subtypes. The importance of classifying cancer patients into their respective subgroups has led many research teams, to study the application of machine learning (ML) methods. In this work, we propose a pipeline for identifying differentially expressed genes (DEGs) and use the same to classify between normal and cancer subtypes. When a DEG is common for two or more cancer subtypes, it hinders with the performance of the classifier. Hence, in our approach we have eliminated common DEGs that exists between cancer subtypes and our results show improvement in accuracy of the classifier. Also, this framework is applicable to all heterogeneous diseases provided the data is available in Level 3 TCGA format.

In our case, we have looked at disease classification as a computational problem. Whether the selected set of DEGs suggest the underlying biological mechanism(s) responsible for occurrence of a particular cancer is something that only a domain expert can confirm. Statistically, they are significant. As a future extension, the DEGs identified can be verified with the help of a domain expert to understand if there is any deviation. Another extension of this work can be, use of other parameter(s) along with DEGs to further improve accuracy of the classifier.

References

[1] Gopika Rani GU and J Jesu Vedha Nayahi. "Review of Cancer Subtypes Prediction: Progress and Challenges." In: (2013).

[2] Ujjwal Maulik, Anirban Mukhopadhyay, and Debasis Chakraborty. "Gene-expression-based cancer subtypes prediction through feature selection and transductive SVM." In: *IEEE transactions on biomedical engineering* 60.4 (2013), pp. 1111–1117.

[3] Gökmen Zararsız et al. "A comprehensive simulation study on classification of RNA-Seq data." In: *PloS one* 12.8 (2017), e0182507.

[4] Anjum Arfa et al. "Identification of differentially expressed genes in rna-seq data of arabidopsis thaliana: A compound distribution approach." In: *Journal of Computational Biology* 23.4 (2016), pp. 239–247.

[5] Gargi Mukherjee et al. "Predicting recurrence in clear cell Renal Cell Carcinoma: analysis of TCGA data using outlier analysis and generalized matrix LVQ." In: *Evolutionary Computation (CEC), 2016 IEEE Congress on*. IEEE. 2016, pp. 656–661.

[6] Juliana Costa-Silva, Douglas Domingues, and Fabricio Martins Lopes. "RNA-Seq differential expression analysis: An extended review and a software tool." In: *PloS one* 12.12 (2017), e0190152.

[7] Zhilong Jia et al. "Gene ranking of RNA-seq data via discriminant non-negative matrix factorization." In: *PloS one* 10.9 (2015), e0137782.

[8] Michael I Love, Wolfgang Huber, and Simon Anders. "Moderated estimation of fold change and dispersion for RNA-seq data with DESeq2." In: *Genome biology* 15.12 (2014), p. 550.

Improving Diagnosis in Health Care Systems

Luckeciano Melo, Victor Ulisses Pugliese, Daniela America da Silva, Fabiana Rocha, Rodrigo Monteiro de Barros Santana, Gildarcio Sousa Goncalves, Luiz Alberto Vieira Dias, Adilson Marques da Cunha, Paulo Marcelo Tasinaffo,
Brazilian Aeronautics Institute of Technology, São José dos Campos, São Paulo, Brazil

Abstract - *Uniting the learning process of new and emerging technologies together with application projects for society is something that has been done lately in the Brazilian Aeronautics Institute of Technology (Instituto Tecnológico da Aeronáutica - ITA). An Interdisciplinary Problem-Based Learning (IPBL) with almost 30 undergraduate and graduate students from 3 different courses has been used, during 17 academic weeks in the 1st Semester of 2017. On these courses, students have modeled and developed a Computer System applied to a health system, for the management of epidemic crises, with the aim of assisting government authorities and private sectors for managing and making appropriate decisions. Differently from other existing products from universities, research centers, governmental agencies, and other public and/or private companies, this product was developed, using the agile Scrum method and its best practices, along with Big Data, Internet of Things (IoT), and other emerging Information Technologies (ITs) from the market.*

Keywords: health system; big data; predictive models; Internet of Things (IoT); agile methods; problem-based learning.

1 Introduction

This academic project was conducted by the Brazilian Aeronautics Institute of Technology (Instituto Tecnológico de Aeronáutica - ITA), using Interdisciplinary Problem-Based Learning (IPBL) for the integration of the graduate courses of CE-240 Database Systems Project, CE-245 Information Technologies, and CE-229 Software Testing, applying the Scrum agile method and its best practices [1] [2].

The project was named, in Portuguese, Solucoes Tecnologicas Aplicaveis a Midias e Produtos em Saude (STAMPS) and, in English, Technological Solutions Applicable for Health Care (TSA4HC). It was driven by the ITA to generate bioengineering expertise, as a natural continuation of previous projects, considering the development of a Computer System based on Big Data, Internet of Things (IoT), and other emerging technologies using the agile Scrum method for system development and verifying software quality, reliability, safety, and testability.

In addition, some aspects of certification standards were taken into account as the International Classification of Diseases (ICD-10) standard [4] and also the Health Level 7 (HL7) standard [3].

To develop a computer system for providing crises management in a period of just 17 academic weeks, a TSA4HC Academic Project Prototype was developed and divided into the following 4 application subsystem components with high cohesion and low coupling characteristics: PATIENTS, PHYSICIANS, HOSPITALS, and SUPPLIERS.

The development of each group of subsystem was distributed in 4 student teams from those 3 courses previously mentioned. They have taken responsibility for defining requirements, functionalities and verifying quality, reliability, safety, and testability.

An integration strategy between groups of subsystem was designed and implemented on top of the 4 subsystems and named the STAMPSNet. It was modeled as an intelligent system architecture component to define the macro integration strategy between the teams. This STAMPSNet, shown in Figure 1, was created to involve the main step events processed and sent by subsystems, according to the following fases: Detection, Screening, Treatment, and Response.

A general backlog of the TSA4HC Academic Project Prototype was created for all teams, prioritizing User Stories (USs) for better system integration, to be developed and achieved during 3 planned sprints.

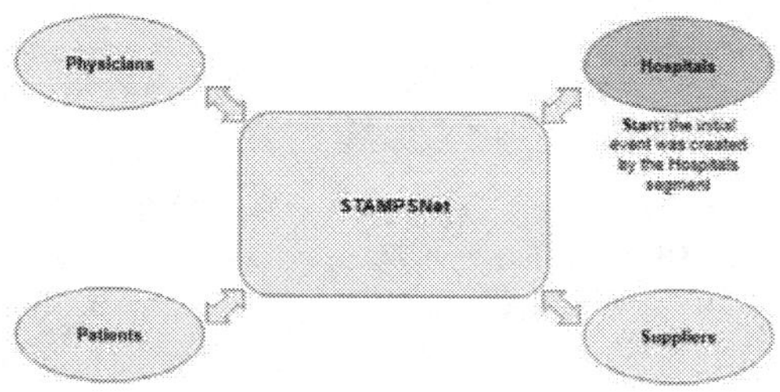

Figure 1. The Proposed STAMPSNet

2 The Interdisciplinarity

2.1 The Graduate Courses

This TSA4HC Academic Project, as previously mentioned, has involved the following three graduate courses:

- CE-240 Database Systems Project, tackling the main techniques for the development of database systems;
- CE-245 Information Technologies, tackling the main Information Technologies (ITs) used in the process of developing computer systems; and

- CE-229 Software Testing, tackling the main foundations used for software testing.

2.2 The Scrum Agile Method and Its Best Practices

According to Jeff Sutherland [1], Scrum is an iterative and incremental framework for projects, products, or applications development. The Scrum structures the development in cycles of work, also defined as sprints. Sprints usually take place one after the other and have fixed duration, typically from 2 to 4 weeks. Each sprint must end on a specific date, whether the work has been completed or not. It is never extended and must be also time-boxed. At the beginning of each sprint, a Sprint Planning Meeting must take place.

Teams' Product Owners (POs), teams' Scrum Masters (SMs), and Teams' Developers (TDs) must periodically review the Product Backlog and discuss goals and context of items. Each Scrum team must select items from the Product Backlog and commit to complete development of them by the end of the sprint, starting at the top priority items of the Product Backlog.

Each selected item from the Product Backlog must be designed and then broken down into a set of individual tasks. The Scrum roles within Scrum teams are typically defined as shown in Table 1.

TABLE 1 - THE SCRUM ROLES

Role	Description
Product Owners (POs)	represent Stakeholders, by defining the Vision artifact, product requirements, and team goals, in order to deliver something of value to be delivered at the end of the sprint [6] [7];
Team Developers (TDs)	are the self-organized and self-managed members of the team responsible for product development and delivery [8];
Stakeholders	represent customers or anyone that have interest, is involved or affected by the outcomes of the product; and
Scrum Masters (SMs)	are responsible for assisting the team in the process execution, in order to maximize efficiency and achieve the goal of a sprint [6].

After the adoption of the Scrum method for this TSA4HC Academic Project Prototype, professors involved with TDs must take the role of Stakeholders. Then, one student from each team, usually the most experienced or the most skilled one in the process, must be chosen and assigned by all its TDs to perform the SM role.

During this TSA4HC Academic Project Prototype development, all students must participate as TDs. At this time, both CE-240 and CE-245 students were assigned for modeling, programming, and evaluating the compliance with the ICD-10 and HL7 standards; and the CE-229 students were assigned for defining and executing acceptance testings and their oracles. Table 2 presents the main Scrum roles used in this TSA4HC Academic Project Prototype.

TABLE 2 - THE STAMPS ACADEMIC PROJECT ROLES

Roles	Who was responsible for
Product Owners (POs)	CE-229 Students
Team Developers (TDs)	Students from all 3 graduate courses
Stakeholders	Professors
Scrum Masters (SMs)	1 student from each Development Team (DT)

2.3 Applying Global Standards

Table 3 shows the global standards applied in the TSA4HC Academic Project Prototype development.

TABLE 3 - The Global STANDARDS

Standards	Details
The ICD-10 Standard	The International Classification of Diseases (ICD-10) was designed as a health care classification system, providing a system of diagnostic codes for classifying diseases, including nuanced classifications of a wide variety of signs, symptoms, abnormal findings, complaints, social circumstances, and external causes of injury or disease. The ICD-10 data was loaded in the MongoDB, a NoSQL database in English, and it was used to map symptoms and to suggest potential diagnosis of PATIENTS from the TSA4HC Academic Project.
The HL7 Standard	The Health Level 7 International Standard (HL7) was designed for providing a comprehensive framework and related standards for the exchange, integration, sharing, and retrieval of electronic health information that supports clinical practice, management, delivery, and evaluation of health services [3]. In the TSA4HC Academic Project Prototype, it was used Level 4 of the HL7 that defines standards for Data Exchange.

2.4 The Architecture Overview

The TSA4HC Academic Project Prototype application was developed in a cloud system and had each of its subsystems hosted in the Heroku Platform as a Service. It has allowed source-code in Phyton, Java, or PHP programming language.

It also has used: MySQL, for the Relational Database; MongoDB, for the best of relational using innovations from NoSQL; JSON, for the data-interchange format; Apache Kafka, as a messaging system; Django, as a Phyton Web Framework for rapid development; and Github, as a development platform to review code, manage the project, and remotely build the software working collaboratively with developers and testers.

At the end, results were integrated through a common data bus to operate according to the definition of the STAMPSNet architecture.

2.5 The Testing Methods

The TSA4HC Academic Project Prototype was implemented by using the Acceptance Test Driven Development (ATDD) technique, having requirements turned into very specific test cases and being prepared since the first week of the first Sprint.

The development was done, by taking into account test cases specifications. The product was validated against those tests cases every week of each Sprint, through an iterative development process, where requirements have evolved through collaborations between TDs, SMs, POs, and Stakeholders.

Teams have to be self-organized to determine issues to be tested in advance, differently from conventional methods when testing used to be performed only after implementations. In the TSA4HC Project scenario, testings were performed during all its implementation.

3 The TSA4HC Academic Project Prototype

Designed to host application systems by using cloud-computing resources, the Heroku is a cloud service platform, which provides support for various programming languages. Some of its benefits are: abstraction of services configuration; support for various programming languages; practicality in application management - continuous deployments; and freedom for testing cloud applications [10][11].

Within the PHYSICIANS subsystem, it was also implemented some digital component key features of the TSA4HC Project to help PHYSICIANS in consultations and/or visits per PATIENTS, allowing benefits such as identifying symptoms, diagnosis, and number of visits, according to geo-locations.

The TD assigned for developing this subsystem was responsible for delivering 10 USs within the 3 sprints of 4 weeks each. At the end of the 2nd Sprint, the TD of PHYSICIANS have integrated its developed application subsystem with other related TDs through a STAMPSNet intelligent system, running on top of this TSA4HC Academic Project Prototype application subsystem.

4 The Intelligent Diagnosis System

This intelligent system developed within the STAMPSNet was initially divided into two main parts. The first part has focused on the automatized diagnosis of PATIENTS. It plays an important part for treating data coming from the Web. The second part of this intelligent system focuses on epidemics' tracking, by using information inferred from the first part and also from the diagnosis of some real doctors.

4.1 The Diagnosis System

The diagnosis system had the purpose of inferring the state of potential PATIENTS through their symptoms arriving in the STAMPSNet. In a first version of this diagnosis system, developed during the second Sprint, the STAMPSNet has used the Jaccard Index as a similarity metric.

At that time, this model has shown to be very limited for the needs of the STAMPSNet. Although more general for diagnosing, every kind of disease from the ICD-10 database, using the Jaccard Index was limited, mainly because it considered all symptoms as statistically likely in the diagnosis also being limited only to binary symptoms.

Furthermore, this model has increased its dissimilarities, when adding additional symptoms of PATIENTS, which can be also be a problem for PATIENTS with multiples diseases. Hence, the TD of PHYSICIANS proposed a new diagnosis model, based in a weighted similarity index. Figure 2 shows the whole proposed subsystem for PATIENTS diagnosis.

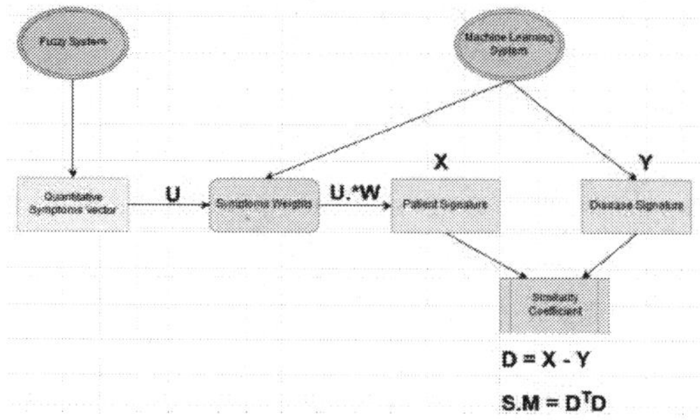

Figure. 2. The Proposed Diagnosis Subsystem

On this subsystem, the fuzzy part corresponds to convert binary symptoms (a person may have a symptom or not) into a quantitative measure of each symptom, because it is known that a symptom can be more intense in some diseases if compared to others. For example, a headache is worse in an Ebola PATIENT than in a Flu PATIENT.

$$U = u_1 u_2 .. u_n \quad (1)$$

As shown in Equation (1), the output of the fuzzy system is a quantitative symptoms vector, composed by all PATIENTS symptoms and each dimension is a (0,1) value based.

The next part of the system is composed by a Machine Learning (ML) system, which purpose is to optimize the parameters of symptom weights' vector to represent the disease signature. The symptom weights' vector, as shown in Equation (2), is a vector of parameters, for a specific disease, in a way that each element corresponds to a symptom of the disease:

$$\theta = \theta_1 \theta_2 .. \theta_n \quad (2)$$

The value of these positive parameters follows two rules:

1. The value of the parameter is related to how much that symptom defines the disease. For example, fever has little influence in the Ebola diagnosis - several diseases present this symptom. On the other hand, joint pain is a symptom that better defines this disease, because it is a more specific symptom; and

2. The sum of the squares of all parameters is an unit, as shown in Equation (3). This constraint normalizes and calibrates the final similarity coefficient, in a way that the most non-similar pair (PATIENT signature/ disease signature) results in an unit.

$$\theta^T \theta = \theta_1 \theta_2 .. \theta_n \theta_1 \theta_2 .. \theta_n = 1 \quad (3)$$

ISBN: 1-60132-479-0, CSREA Press ©

On the other hand, the disease signature is a vector which represents the value of symptoms for a specific disease. The greater the similarity between this vector and the PATIENT signature vector, the greater the probability of the PATIENT having the specified disease.

The Machine Learning (ML) system receives PATIENTS records as training data. These records have symptoms as parameters, specified in the same way as the quantitative symptoms vector. At this time, two models are trained: the first outputs the symptoms weight vector with the more appropriated influence of each symptom; and the second outputs the signature of a specific disease.

Finally, the PATIENT has a signature as a result of an element-wise multiplication between the quantitative symptoms vector and the symptoms weights vector, as shown in Equation (4). This vector is compared with the disease signature, by using the similarity metric presented in Figure 3.

$$X = U.^{*}\,\theta = u_1\theta_1 u_2\theta_2 .. u_n\theta_n \quad (4)$$

As shown in Equation (5), each signature corresponds to a point in an N-Dimensional space of symptoms. The similarity is calculated by the euclidean distance between the representation of the patient symptoms and the disease representation.

Firstly, vectors are subtracted. Then, the similarity metric is the length of the resultant vector.

$$D = X - Y = x_1 x_2 .. x_n - y_1 y_2 .. y_n \quad (5)$$

As shown in Equations (6) and (7), in terms of percentage, the calibrated score can be presented as:

$$Similarity(\%) = (1 - S.M) * 100\% \quad (6)$$

$$S.M = \langle D, D \rangle = d_1 d_2 .. d_n\, d_1 d_2 .. d_n \quad (7)$$

This system was implemented in the STAMPSNet, with some simplifications. First of all, in its implementation, it was used one-hot encoding in symptoms, mocking up the fuzzy system, due to the fact that teams don't have specialized knowledge about medical diagnosis.

Furthermore, the ML system was mock up due to the lack of patients' records - there is no public dataset available due to privacy reasons.

As shown in Equation (8), in this simplified model, the value of similarity is given by:

$$Similarity(\%) = \overline{u_1 u_2 .. u_n}\theta^2{}_1\theta^2{}_2 .. \theta^2{}_n * 100\% \quad (8)$$

As the parameters chosen are based on statistical inferences of how the symptom determines the disease, it is possible to simplify the last Equation (9) as a simple linear model:

$$Similarity(\%) = u'_1 u'_2 .. u'_n\, \theta'_1\theta'_2 .. \theta'_n * 100\% \quad (9)$$

As shown in Equation (9), this is the final mathematical model implemented in the STAMPSNet. Due to the calibrated score of similarity, this value is analogue to a probability coefficient: if a patient with all symptoms is 100\% likely to have the disease, for example. Then, the main results and test cases of this model are further analyzed, as presented later on Section 6 The Main Agile Testing and Results.

4.2 The Disease Occurrence Calculation

A predictive model was implemented to identify possible alerts to be sent to the system based on the level of a disease. The Disease Occurrence Calculation was based on the following 6 levels of disease, as per definition of the US Department of Health and Human Services, Centers for Disease Control, and Prevention [12][13], as shown in Table 4. There are some recent examples of those level of diseases as shown in Table 5.

In the STAMPSNet, through diagnoses of medical consultations, bio-statistical calculations of Maximum Expected Occurence will be done to measure the spread of a disease, and it really comes down to how many people are infected with a disease. There are 3 type of alerts related to the level of a disease, as shown in Table 6. Any suspected case must be immediately notified to the health authorities of the city, state, and health surveillance.

TABLE 4 - THE DISEASE OCCURRENCE CALCULATION

Disease	Details
Endemic	refers to the constant presence and/or usual prevalence of a disease or infectious agent in a population within a geographic area
Hyper-endemic	refers to persistent high levels of disease occurrence;
Epidemic Occasionally	is when the amount of disease in a community rises above the expected and this level refers to an increase, often sudden, in the number of cases of a disease above what it is normally expected in a population area;
Outbreak	carries the same definition of epidemic, but is often used for a more limited geographic area;
Cluster	refers to an aggregation of cases grouped in place and time that are suspected to be greater than the number expected, even though the expected number may not be known; and
Pandemic	refers to an epidemic that has spread over several countries or continents, usually affecting a large number of people.

TABLE 5 - LEVEL OF DISEASES EXAMPLE

Disease	Where
Endemic	Malaria is a constant worry in parts of Africa;
Epidemic	Ebola started in West Africa, as an outbreak, but it has evolved into an epidemic and more than 28,600 people were infected with Ebola during the 2014-15 outbreak in West Africa and around 11,300 people died [15]; and
Pandemic	H1N1 pandemic has occurred between 2009-2010, when the H1N1 virus that caused that pandemic is now a regular human flu virus and continues to circulate seasonally worldwide [14].

TABLE 6 - THE ALERT LEVELS

Alert	Type	Details
Green	Normal	When no occurrences are registered for a disease. For example, in case of an Ebola Epidemic Risk, if no occurrence has been logged in the last 42 days, then the STAMPSNet sends a Safe Area message to all subsystems;
Yellow	Outbreak Risk	When the PHYSICIANS subsystem listens and checks match of PATIENTS' messages. If a PATIENT diagnosis matches more than 80\% of Ebola symptoms, then it counts +1 occurrence. If occurrences are more than 4 cases, then the STAMPSNet sends an Outbreak Risk message to all subsystem; and
Red	Epidemic Risk	When the PHYSICIANS subsystem listens for confirmed Ebola medical diagnoses and checks social media incidents with suspected Ebola. If the sum of medical diagnoses and social media incidence, both with Ebola, are more than 4 occurrences, then the STAMPSNet sends a Critical Alert for Epidemic Risk message to all segments.

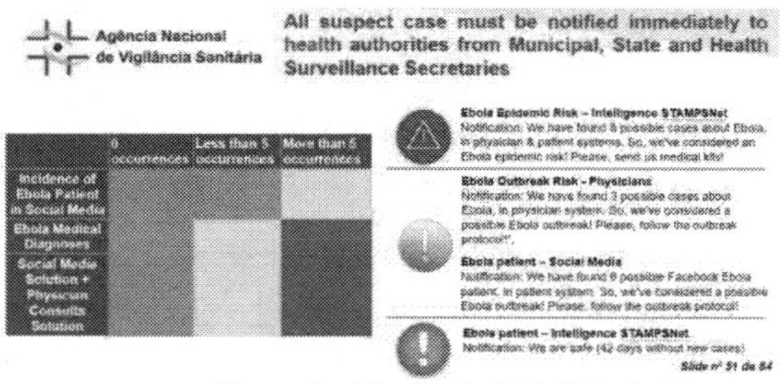

Figure. 3. The Ebola Risk Calculation

5 The Proof of Concept Presentation as an Assigned Mission

This TSA4HC Academic Project Prototype was inspired on the needs of public and/or private organizations involved in crises management tackling health events (e.g. epidemics), needing to manage data and information for decision making. At the end of 17 academic weeks, a simulated Proof of Concept (PoC) was applied to an assigned mission to verify the efficiency of using the TSA4HC Academic Project Prototype in a fictitious epidemics of EBOLA. Table 7 shows some details of this PoC.

TABLE 7 - The Proof of Concept Applied to an Assigned Mission

Phases	Details
Detection Phase	During a national holiday, a person (eventual PATIENT) goes awry and faints in the middle of a Shopping. The security team at a Local Care Office or near HOSPITAL receives this PATIENT, where a PHYSICIAN analyses symptoms such as very high fever, tremors, vomiting with blood, red eyes, and mental confusion. The event is detected by the STAMPSNet and the PATIENT 1 is identified by the system. On this Detection Phase, the STAMPSNet receives information from the PATIENTS subsystem informing potential EBOLA events collected from social midia. It also receives information from the PHYSICIANS subsystem informing potential PATIENTS consultations/visits having EBOLA symptoms.
Screening Phase	Considering also reports of the PATIENT about his severe joint pains and his recent work in an area affected by the EBOLA epidemic, a medical team reports that everything indicates that this PATIENT is infected by the EBOLA virus. From there on, this PATIENT can be considered as the first PATIENT to start an epidemic in a region, if it is readily identified. As a result, this PATIENT 1 will be registered in the PHYSICIANS subsystem and any new consultations/visits indicating an EBOLA infection will be also registered in the PHYSICIANS subsystem.
Treatment Phase	A set of epidemiological events are managed in such way that: - Those who have had contact with Ebola's infected PATIENT 1 are promptly identified and/or cared for;and - At this point in time, it was assumed that the population/society has an available computational tool like this TSA4HC Academic Project Prototype capable of providing appropriate records, management, and controls since the emergence could evolve into an epidemic;
Response Phase	A set of epidemiological events are managed in such way that: - The HOSPITAL subsystem must have the computational means to collaborate in the process of managing large flows of efficient patient care, by using appropriate technologies and efficient screening methods; - The involved HOSPITALS subsystem and the SUPPLIERS subsystem is able to provide needed medicines and devices and also have appropriate tools to participate in an inventory management process of devices and medicines.

On the Treatment Phase, in order to identify an EBOLA infection, the PHYSICIANS subsystem uses Jaccard index measuring similarity for the two sets of ICD-10 data and Patient Symptoms, with a range from 0\% to 100\%, also weighted by potential symptoms. In this Ebola case study, some symptoms are fever, headache, muscle pain and chills. Later, a person may experience internal bleeding, resulting in vomiting or coughing blood.

On the Screening Phase of consultations/visits by PHYSICIANS subsystem and also based on information shared with the PATIENTS subsystem related to feeds coming from social midia, the PHYSICIANS subsystem may also identify when to send an epidemics alert based upon statistical methods. And, if more than 4 occurrences indicating an EBOLA case do occur, then a YELLOW preventive alert may be sent to the STAMPSNet, informing all subsystems PATIENTS, PHYSICIANS, HOSPITALS, and SUPPLIERS, that there is an ATTENTION STATE, preventively preparing it for an EBOLA epidemics. If occurrences do evolve to above 5 Ebola cases, for example, then a CRITICAL STATE reactive alert may be sent to the STAMPSNet, informing all subsystems PATIENTS, PHYSICIANS, HOSPITALS, and SUPPLIERS to properly react to an EBOLA epidemics.

On the Response Phase, the alert message from the Treatment Phase is sent to the STAMPSNet, and processed by the HOSPITALS subsystem in the Response Phase. At this time, the HOSPITALS subsystem may identify the number of rooms available, and may start medical treatments.

Also in the Response Phase, the HOSPITALS subsystem may send an alert to the STAMPSNet requesting the SUPPLIERS subsystem to provide medicines, materials, and/or devices, in order to properly manage crises. This notification may be also sent to authorities such as city hall, red cross, army, among others.

After the crises situation is under control, the alert may be closed. The first EBOLA symptoms may appear from 2 days to 3 weeks after infections. And the end of an Ebola outbreak can only be officially declared after the end of 42 days without any new confirmed cases. Figure 4 presents an example of an Ebola diagnosis.

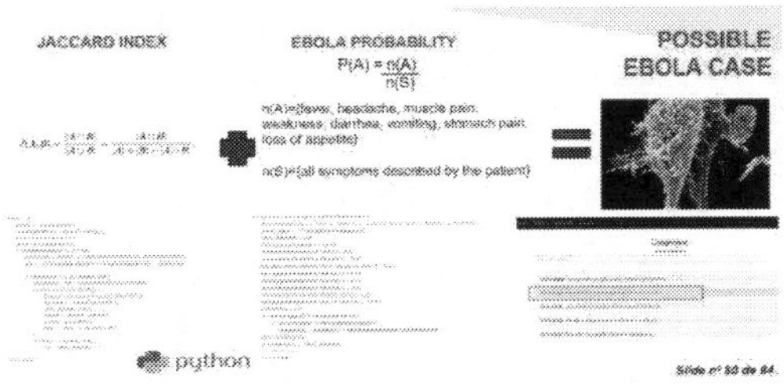

Fig 4. An example of Ebola Diagnosis

6 The Main Agile Testing and Results

The TSA4HC Academic Project Prototype was developed by using the Acceptance Test Driven Development (ATDD) technique, in order to guide the development-oriented test, as it should be written before implementing the system itself. The ATDD cycle has the following steps: (i) add a test; (ii) run and observe; (iii) write the code; (iv) run the automated tests; and (v) re-factor the code [16].

Some specific Test Cases were developed to guarantee proper results based upon User Stories requirements. As the product has been verified against those tests cases, the iterative and incremental Scrum agile method was applied in the development process. Then, requirements have evolved through collaborations among TDs, POs, and Stakeholders and the self-organized Scrum Teams have determined issues to be addressed in advance. This happened, differently from conventional methods where tests are usually performed only after implementation.

The following main Test Cases were used to test the Intelligent Diagnosis System: the Disease and Symptom's List; and the Diagnosis Matches.

6.1 The Disease and Symptom's List Test Case

The first main Test Case was expecting a tool for supporting the PHYSICIANS subsystem, during the process of identifying and/or certifying possibles diseases in his patients, based on inputted symptoms.

Using the ICD-10 standard as a database, a list of registered diseases was shown based upon the information provided.

Figure 5 shows one example of the Disease List utilization.

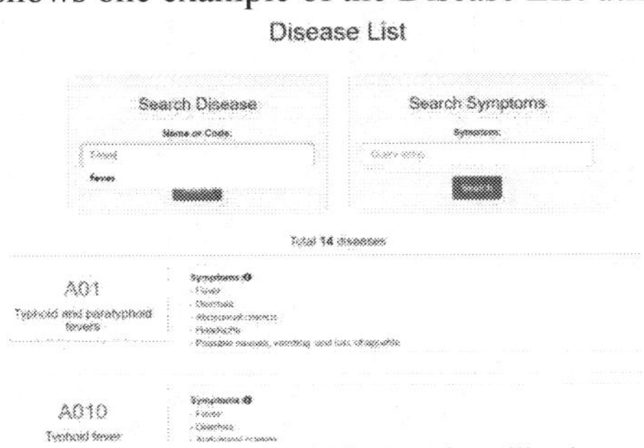

Figure 5. An example of Disease List utilization

6.2 The Diagnosis Matches Test Case

The second main Test Case implemented was expecting also a tool for supporting the PHYSICIANS subsystem. But, to support the PHYSICIANS subsystem for predicting probable diseases based on different symptoms from the PATIENTS subsystem, based on similarity percentages from each possible disease, refer to Figure 6.

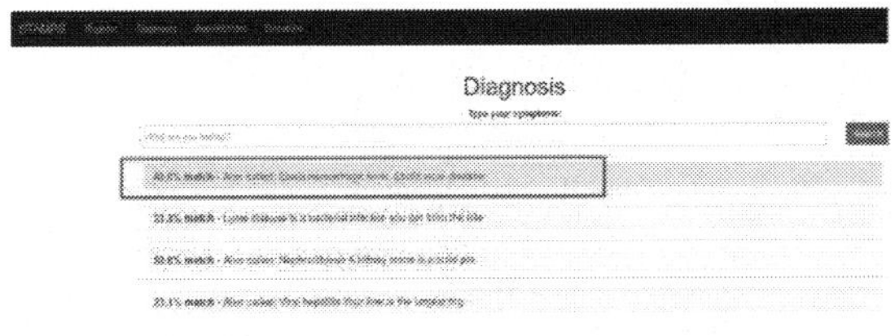

Figure 6. Using Jaccard Index to Match Potential Diagnosis

7 Conclusions

This paper described the development and implementation of an academic interdisciplinary project using the Scrum agile method and its best practices. In order to do so, an Academic Project Prototype named Technological Solutions Applicable for Health Care (TSA4HC) was developed as a Proof of Concept (PoC), by using cloud-computing resources. It has described the development and application of the TSA4HC, as an Integrated Problem-Based Learning (IPBL) project, using Big Data, Internet of Things (IoT), and other emerging technologies for governmental organization and private sector.

The purpose of this system was to aggregate data and integrate actors such as Patients, Hospitals, Physicians, and Health Suppliers within a decision making process related to crisis management involving epidemics' events of a health systems. To fulfill these requirements, the TSA4HC Academic Project Prototype was developed by students from 3 different courses taught at the Brazilian Aeronautics Institute of Technology (Instituto Tecnologico de Aeronautica – ITA), on the 1st semester of 2017.

7.1 Specific Conclusions

The use of interdisciplinarity on 3 Computer Science courses has worked as expected, since the students got to know how to work in teams to successfully develop a complex Information Technology (IT) and Real-Time Embedded System. A cloud computing environment was extensively used by students, in order to allow collaborative work at distance, by using hangout meetings, personal sites, and an official project website.

The Scrum method was adapted to the reality of the Brazilian Aeronautics Institute of Technology (ITA) academic interdisciplinary environment, helping all the 4 Scrum Teams of almost 30 students to deliver value to Stakeholders, at the end of each 3 Sprints of 4 weeks each, and also at the end of the TSA4HC Project.

The application of Acceptance Test Driven Development (ATDD) within the project was closely related to the adopted interdisciplinary approach, since acceptance tests were specified and created by students from the CE-229 Software Testing course, while the software was implemented by students from the CE-240 Database Systems Project and CE-245 Information Technologies (ITs) courses. The results of this TSA4HC Academic Project Prototype were successful, as reported on Sections III, IV, V and VI.

At the end, students have successfully completed and presented the TSA4HC Academic Project Prototype in their final examination, as a Proof of Concept (PoC) to professors, entrepreneurs, and also to some invited guests from industry and academia.

7.2 General Conclusions

According to the authors, the academic development of a critical intelligent system is a rewarding experience, which can be used in different graduate and undergraduate courses. The use of interdisciplinarity, cloud-computing, Machine Learning (ML) and agile methods appears to be a new interesting and motivational way of achieving academic goals, in just one semester of 17 weeks, and can be also extended to other courses and knowledge domains.

7.3 Recommendations

The authors recommend the assigned mission be proposed and clearly defined at early stages of any academic project. In this TSA4HC Project, its requirements specification took a few weeks to be defined. For future projects, it is recommended the mission be defined right since the first academic week. It is also recommended the integration of different layers be done also as early as possible, using for example ANSYS / Esterel SCADE tools, allowing different teams to work on communication protocols, layouts refinements, and testing, also on the early stages of the project.

Finally, the authors also recommend the use of automated testing tools and procedures to accelerate the development process, while increasing the quality of the product. The automation testing tools with Phyton could be used for automation, since it does provide some testing automation, but there was no time for the students to take the full advantage of it in this project.

7.4 Future Work

It is suggested that the process used in this TSA4HC Academic Project Prototype can be extended to other embedded systems projects, as for example in the health domain, within the area of using wearables to collect and track personal health conditions. As future work, it is suggested to continue the implementation of a fuzzy system to quantify symptoms, and also implement a Machine Learning (ML) algorithm to extract information about disease symptoms. It is also suggested to extend cooperation with industry, in order to obtain academic projects selection aligned with up-to-date market needs.

8 Acknowledgement

The authors would like to thank: 1) The Brazilian Aeronautics Institute of Technology (Instituto Tecnologico de Aeronautica - ITA); 2) The Casimiro Montenegro Filho Foundation (Fundacao Casimiro Montenegro Filho - FCMF); 3) The Software Engineering Research Group (Grupo de Pesquisa em Engenharia de Software - GPES) do ITA; and 4) The Brazilian Ecossistema enterprise, for their infrastructure, data set, assistance, advice, and financial support for this work, during the development of this Technological Solutions Applicable for Health Care (TSA4HC) Academic Project Prototype.

9 References

[1] Sutherland J., 2010, SCRUM Handbook, Scrum Training Institute Press.

[2] Cohen D., et. al., 2004, An Introduction to Agile Methods, Fraunhofer Center for ExperimentalSoftware Engineering, ADVANCES IN COMPUTERS, VOL. 62.

[3] HL7, 2017, Health Level Seven International, http://www.hl7.org/documentcenter/public/training/IntroToHL7/player.html

[4] ICD, 2017, International Classification of Diseases, http://www.who.int/classifications/icd/en/

[5] WHO, 2017, World Health Organization, http://www.who.int/about/en/

[6] Cohn M., 2010, Succeeding with agile: Software development using Scrum, 1st Edition, Pearson Education, Inc.

[7] Leandog, 2012, Agile Discussion Guide, Version 3.1, Cleaveland, Ohio.

[8] Larman, C, 2004, Agile and iterative development: a manager's guide, Addison-Wesley Professional

[9] S Niwattanakul, J Singthongchai, E Naenudorn, 2013, Using of Jaccard Coefficient for Keywords Similarity, Proceedings of the International MultiConference of Engineers and Computer Scientists 2013 Vol I, IMECS 2013, March 13 - 15, 2013, Hong Kong

[10] Freeman, E.; Bates, B.; Sierra, K.; Robson, E. Head, 2004, First Design Patterns: A Brain-Friendly Guide, O'Reilly Media, Inc

[11] Holovaty, A, Kaplan-Moss, J, 2017, The DJango Book, Available: https://djangobook.com/ in August, 06th 2017.

[12] CDC, 2017, Center For Disease Control and Prevention, Available: https://www.cdc.gov/ in August, 13th 2017, US Department of Health and Human Services

[13] CDC, 2017, Center For Disease Control and Prevention, Principles of Epidemiology in Public Health Practice, Third Edition, An Introduction to Applied Epidemiology and Biostatistics, Available: https://www.cdc.gov/ophss/csels/dsepd/ss1978/lesson1/section11.html in August, 13th 2017, US Department of Health and Human Services

[14] CDC, 2017, Center For Disease Control and Prevention, The 2009 H1N1 Pandemic: Summary Highlights, April 2009-April 2010, Available: https://www.cdc.gov/h1n1flu/cdcresponse.htm in August, 13th 2017, US Department of Health and Human Services

[15] BBC, 2017, Ebola 'super-spreaders' cause most cases, Available: http://www.bbc.com/news/health-38955871 in August, 13th 2017, US Department of Health and Human Services

[16] JORGENSEN, P. C. "Software Testing – A Craftsman's Approach". 4th Edition. Boca Raton, FL: CRC Press, 2014

[17] KMeansHan, Longfei; Luo, Senlin; Wang, Huaiqing; Pan, Limin; Ma, Xincheng; Zhang, Tiemei, 2017, An Intelligible Risk Stratification Model based on Pairwise and Size Constrained, JBHI Medical Informatics Volume 21 Issue 5, available http://ieeexplore.ieee.org/document/7762039/

[18] Hoogendoorn, Mark; Berger, Thomas; Schulz, Ava; Stolz, Timo; Szolovits, Peter, 2017, Predicting Social Anxiety Treatment Outcome based on Therapeutic Email Conversations, JBHI Public Health Informatics Volume 21 Issue 5 available http://ieeexplore.ieee.org/document/7546552/

[19] Yoon, Jinsung; Davtyan, Camelia; van der Schaar, Mihaela, 2017, Discovery and Clinical Decision Support for Personalized Healthcare, JBHI Medical Informatics Volume 21 Issue 4 available http://ieeexplore.ieee.org/document/7482682

SESSION

POSTER PAPERS

Chair(s)

TBA

ISBN: 1-60132-479-0, CSREA Press ©

A Study on the Improvement of Cognitive Function by Analog-based Board Game and Four Sensory Stimulus Digital Convergence

Jeong-Won Kang[1], **and Ki Young Lee**[2]
[1,2] Department of Information and Telecommunication Engineering
Incheon National University Incheon, Korea
[1]jwkang0107@inu.ac.kr

Abstract - *The scope of this study is to use the functional play equipment as a medium which can improve depression and senile dementia that may be caused by the decline of the cognitive ability and strengthen ties between generations, and to obtain empirical results data on cognitive function improvement especially by "digital function convergence that can stimulate four senses in an analog-based board game"*

Keywords: Analog Board Game, Four Sensory Stimulus, Digital Convergence, Cognitive Function

1 Introduction

As the elderly population increases, social problems are increasing due to the declining cognitive ability of the elderly. Most of the elderly mental diseases, including dementia or elderly depression are caused by the decline of the cognitive ability, and the physical and mental suffering of family members is serious. For the elderly, as well as for disabled persons without normal cognitive development, or for children whose brain development is ongoing, training is required to improve their cognitive ability.

However, training to improve the cognitive ability can maximize the effect of training when voluntary and active participation of participants is presupposed. Most cognitive ability training programs have had problems that it was difficult to derive participants' active participation and hard to get enough effect of the training because they have been approached from a medical perspective.

In this study, we are focused on procedure that naturally allows participants to require repeated training by encouraging the participants' interest based on the play-based perspective game rather than the medical treatment perspective. And we develop the mobility-oriented games that cannot be implemented in static games such as TVs, smart phones, and traditional games. Throughout this study, the effect of the elderly cognitive ability improvement by the collaborative game will be evaluated.

Practical authentication method for game chips used by players for fair game operation is also devised.

2 Related Works

Depression is a major symptom shown in 40-50% of the demented elderly with the overall decline of the cognitive function. The experimental result of the integration program for prevention of dementia stimulating the five senses showed that depression was reduced significantly [1]. It has been proved that the intervention in the elderly with suspected dementia in the early stage is effective when integrated. In addition, it provides an important implication for the improvement of their cognitive function in the future in that the elderly can maintain their interest and keep participating when based on the play therapy approach [2]. Recently, selling books, computer programs and games to enhance "brain health" or keep the brain young has exploded in recent years, showing the public's aspiration to maintain their brain and cognitive ability with age. However, there is only empirical evidence that supports or refutes these claims [3].

It is important to maintain the cognitive function rather than prevent dementia for aging brain health, and it is recommended that continuous cognitive stimulus and exposure, addition of new cognitive challenge, cognitive improvement activities, and stimulus through social interaction in order to maintain or improve the cognitive function [4]. Multiple sensory stimuli (light, color, sound, music, etc.) to the cognitive function, depression, anxiety and quality of life of the elderly with dementia improve communication and social interactions with the effect of reducing anxiety and depression [5].

3 Improvement of Cognitive Ability Through Usability Evaluation

The purpose of this paper is to find out the effect of cognitive function improvement through a digital, analog convergence board game that can stimulate four senses (sight, hearing, touch, perception) for elderly people aged 60 or older. Four hypotheses are developed for this study:

1) A four-sensory stimulus digital convergence board game will be more effective in improving the cognitive function of the subjects than a single analog board game.

2) Simple operations and dynamic game rules will be more effective in improving the cognitive function of the subjects than simple game rules of identifying friend or foe.
3) A collaborative 2:2 (doubles) game will be more effective in improving the cognitive function of the subjects than a 1:1 (singles) game.
4) The cognitive function improvement effects of the subjects will be great in the order of 1) < 2) < 3).

Details of measurement methods and test specifications are summarized in Table 1 below.

TABLE 1. DEFINITIONS OF MEASUREMENT METHODS AND TEST SEPCIFICATION

Attributes	Description
Test pecification	Measured by the number of people who have showed the improvement of the cognitive ability compared to the number of participants (sample) through MMSE-k, qualitative assessment
Usability evaluation method	A type of cognitive interview, focusing on how effectively respondents use the system to accomplish their goals and derives objective results data on the cognitive ability before and after the game through the usability evaluation for 40 ~ 50 elderly people.
Measure-ment method 1	A smart board game is used to measure the improvement rate by a questionnaire for orientation, memory, attention and calculation function, language function, visual composition ability changed before and after the game
Measure-ment method 2	Games are divided into the analog only board game group and analog, digital convergence game group to measure the results and compare evaluation
Measure-ment method 3	Measurement and evalaution comparison by separating game rule applied to two groups; one is with operations game, another is in the form of identification of friend or foe
Measure-ment method 4	Measurement and evalaution comparison after sequentially performing the singles game and the collaborative doubles game
Measure-ment method 5	Phased classification and comparison of the results of the cognitive improvement of all the subjects who participated in the usability evaluation

The existing digital form of cognitive enhancement game is characterized by the way that the game is played by the elderly alone participating in the game and by the help of the medical person for treatment. In this study, we are to use a "Analog Board Game and digital function convergence to stimulate four senses" type board game to reduce the participants' repulsion and induce interest, naturally allowing participants to require brain stimulation repetition training and analyze the effects of cognitive function improvement and draw up a utilization plan with collaborative games that enable social bonds and in a way that includes a simple operation function.

4 Conclusion

The loneliness, depression, and dementia symptoms due to aging cannot be expected to be solved fundamentally by improving the temporal cognitive function by a simple game program. Therefore, this study may be of significance for presenting objective indicators to secure the possibility of reducing the loneliness / alienation of the elderly in daily life by improving the cognitive ability with task performance by cooperation, natural whole body exercise as well as sense training to improve the cognitive ability, especially analog board games and four sensory stimulus digital convergence board games in which concurrent participation is possible without distinction of sex or age.

5 References

[1] Lee Yun Mi and Park Nam Hee, "The Effects of Dementia Prevention Program on Cognition, Depression, Self-esteem and Quality of life in the Elderly with Mild Cognitive Disorder," Korean Journal of Adult Nursing, Vol. 19, No. 5, pp. 104~114, 2007.

[2] Hye Won Shin, and Soon Dool Chung, "Program Development and Evaluation of Integrative Play Therapy for Elder People with Suspected Early Dementia", Korean Association for the Psychological Rehabilitation of Children, The Journal of Play Therapy, Vol.19, No.3, 2015.

[3] Tiffany F Hughes, MPH. "Promotion of Cognitive Health Through Cognitive Activity in the Aging Population", US National Library of Medicine, National Institutes of Health, PMC2850280. Aging Health. Vol.6, No.1, pp.111–121, 2010.

[4] Asenath La Rue, "Healthy Brain Aging: Role of Cognitive Reserve, Cognitive Stimulation, and Cognitive Exercises" Clin Geriatr Med. Vol.26, No.1, pp.99-111, 2010.

[5] Amir Vazini Taher, Maryam Khalil Ahmadi, and Faraz Pak Zamir, "Effects of multi-sensory stimulation on cognition function, depression, anxiety and quality of life in elderly persons with dementia", International Journal of Sport Studies. Vol.5, No.3, pp.355-360, 2015.

Combining Advanced Machine Learning with Situation Awareness for Big Data Health Informatics Applications

Kenny C. Gross
Oralce Physical Sciences Research Center
Oracle Corporatio
kenny.gross@oracle.com

Dieter Gawlick
Oracle Database Group
Oracle Corporation
dieter.gawlick@oracle.com

POSTER ABSTRACT

Situation Awareness (SA) is arguably the best method to extract the highest value for data; Oracle's KIDS (Knowledge Intensive Data-management Services) is one model for achieving SA. A significant challenge for achieving SA with Big Data applications in Life Sciences and Healthcare IoT applications is to efficiently discover anomalies in real-time, even if the new anomalies have not previously been encountered. The Multivariate State Estimation Technique (MSET) is an advanced prognostic pattern recognition method that was originally developed in the 1990's for high-sensitivity prognostic applications in complex safety-critical industries by discovering anomalies with the provably lowest-possible false positives/negatives, and with low resource consumption. Although MSET is mature and well proven for prognostic applications across many IoT industries, MSET more recently has found compelling value-add for SA enablement, because MSET solves issues that confuse humans in the loop, and confound the best conventional machine-learning (ML) algorithmics: issues that include disambiguation between faulty sensor values versus anomalies in the monitored sensed parameters, faulty timestamps (from instrumentation clock missmatch issues), extraction of high-accuracy information content from low-resolution transducers, and optimal "imputation" (not interpolation) of missing values in multivariate time series. This poster presentation focuses on the combination of MSET (for anomaly discovery, and for auditable certification of the *absence* of anomalies) and Situation

ISBN: 1-60132-479-0, CSREA Press ©

Awareness to achieve a compelling value proposition for Big Data life sciences and healthcare applications, as well as for newly emerging dense-sensor Internet-of-Things (IoT) applications and human-in-the-loop supervisory-control applications.

MSET Informatics: Automated Training/Tuning/Optimization Process

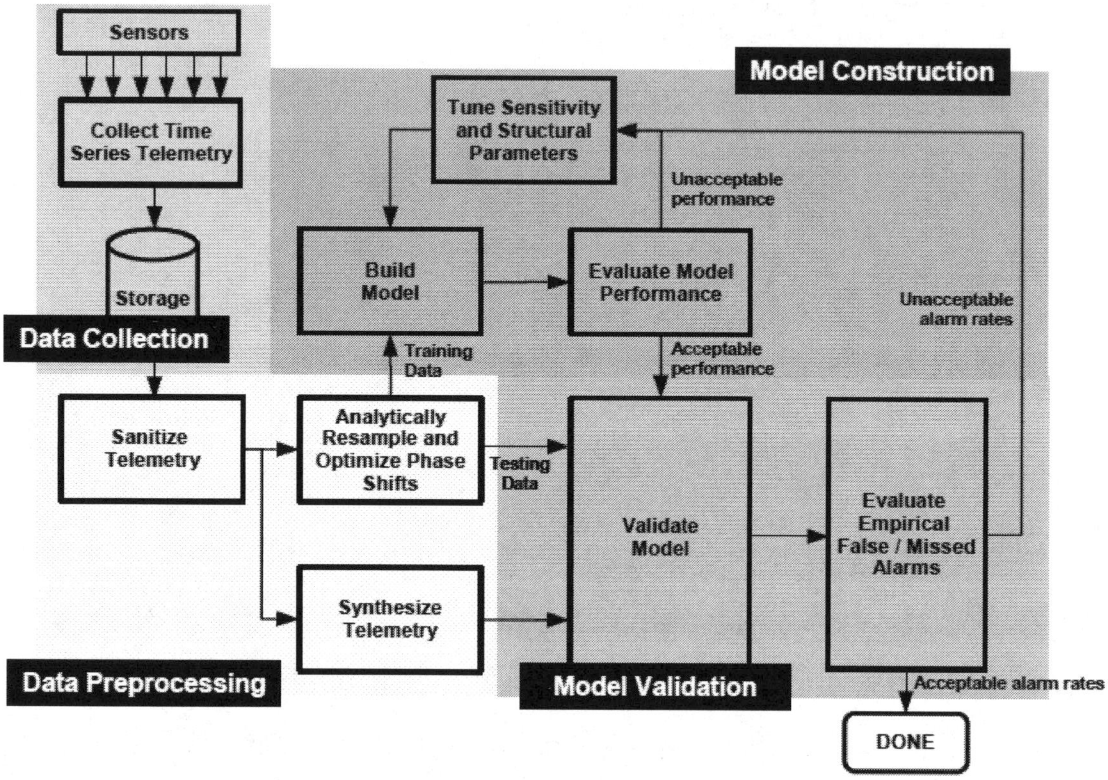

Process/Data Flow for Health-Informatics Use Cases

Multi level processing

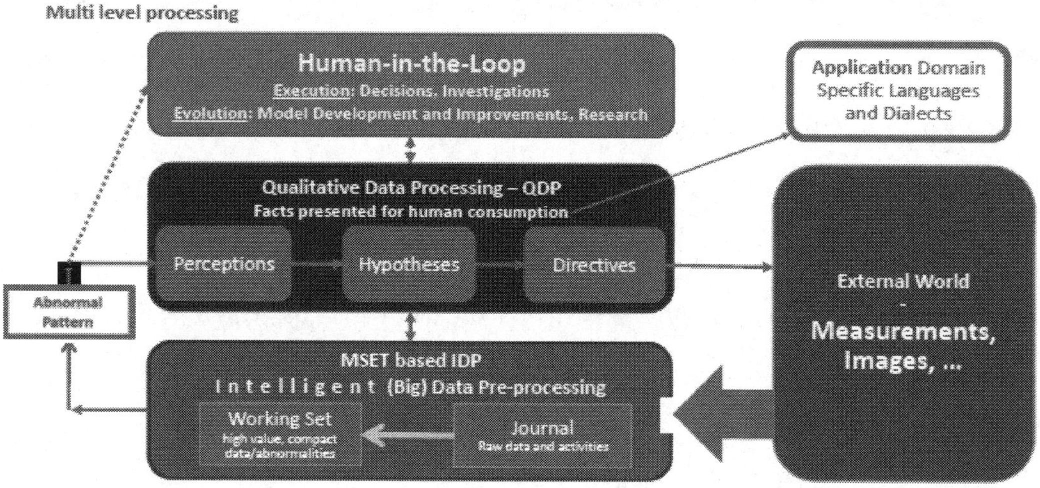

Feature Extraction and Data Validation Analysis for Clustering Physical Stability of Trainee

Sang-Ho Hwang[1], Sanghun Yun[1], Sang-Ho Lee[1], *Won-Seok Kang[1]
[1]Wellness Convergence Research Center, DGIST, Daegu, Republic of Korea

Abstract - *In this paper, we propose two feature extraction methods for clustering the physical stability of trainees. The proposed methods extract features by processing data such as sleep, rest, and activity intensity collected from wearable devices. In the experiment, we performed k-means to show the efficiency of the proposed feature modeling. The prediction strength score method was conducted in validation experiment. The score generated was 0.95, when the number of clusters was k=3 which means "stable", "normal" and "unstable" status.*

Keywords: Unsupervised learning, Clustering, Validation, Wearable device, Physical stability

1 Introduction

The physical stability of trainees is very important for safety in the fields such as chemical plants, nuclear power plants and aviation maintenance. However, these industrial sites' managers do not consider the physical stability of trainees, or assess it by self-diagnosis of trainees.

To solve this problem in the industrial sites, there have been many studies to classify physical stability of trainees or workers [1, 2]. However, these studies used questionnaires to classify physical stability or only measured one feature modelling method such as activity based on Heart Rate Reserve (*HRR*) [2].

In this paper, we propose a new feature modelling method to perform better classification accuracy than the previous approach. We used the retained physical data such as sleep, activity, heart rate and so on to test the feature-modellings using *k*-means to show the efficiency. We used the prediction strength score method in validating the clustered results. The proposed method utilizes only the data of specific period of the entire data, taken exception to the personal life patterns.

2 Feature extraction

In a broad sense, the physical stability includes physical fitness, health, and fatigue excluding mental factors. It is difficult to understand causality for fatigue, because it has appeared in multiple relationships with the physical, psychological, pathological or environmental [3]. In this paper, the definition of fatigue is limited to the state of sleep and activity, called physical stability.

The raw data collected through wearable devices consist of sleep status enumerated in integer value (0, 1, 2, 3), heart rate enumerated in integer value (0 ~ 220), the step count. Each data is measured per one minute for 7 months. The resting heart rate of the whole heart rate is collected in awaken status.

Our final application target is to make an assessment method of trainees to handle complex industrial devices. The retained data are not real data generated in the trainees. We guess that the normal physical stability data is equal to any person. We suppose that the subject of the retained data is trainees. The data of the trainee's condition assessment is used from AM. 1 to AM. 5 for sleep status and from AM. 10 to PM. 2 for activity status. We selected the period's data sets to classify and validate the proposed feature modelling. Table 1 and Table 2 are the proposed feature modelling method adopted in our assessment system to classify a physical status for complex industrial trainees.

Table 1 shows the first proposed model consisted of two features and used in classifying and validating the accuracy of deciding the trainee's physical status.

R is the one dataset consisted of sleep and activity periods ($R \in \{1,2,\ldots,d\}$, d = total number of datasets). S_{i_R} means the sleep status in *i* period (unit 1 minute) of the *R* dataset and the *S* has four statuses: active(0), sleeping(1), sleepless(2), and awake(3). $Steps_{i\_R}$ is the count of steps in *i* period of the R dataset. $f1$ means the total time that the trainee was assumed to have taken a deep sleep. $f2$ means the amount of activity of the trainee based on the count of steps.

Table 2 shows the second proposed model consisted of four features. Instead of the *Step* features in the first model, we adopted the new feature : *HRR* in purpose of measuring activity intensity of trainees [2]. Equation 1 shows *HRR* to measure the activity intensity.

$$HRR_{i\_R} = \frac{HR_{i\_R} - HR_{rest}}{HR_{\max} - HR_{rest}} \tag{1}$$

where, HR_{i_R} is the heart rate in *i* period of *R* dataset and HR_{rest} is the resting heart rate. HR_{max} is the maximum heart rate, estimated by the Tanaka formula [4]. In table 2, HRR_i is the activity intensity in *i* period. $f'1$ and $f'2$ mean the total time of sleep and non-sleep status from AM. 1 to AM. 5, respectively. $f'3$ means the total number of times of work

Table 1. Proposed model 1 : two features modelling for physical stability

Formula
$f1_R = \sum_{i=1}^{240} S_{i\_R} == sleeping\ ?\ 1\ :\ 0\ (i \leftarrow i + 1\text{min})$
$f2_R = \sum_{i=241}^{480} INT(Steps_{i\_R})$

$S = \{active, sleeping, sleepless, awake\}$

* Corresponding author : Won-seok Kang (wskang@dgist.ac.kr)

Table 2. Proposed model 2 : four features modelling for physical stability

Formula
$f'1_R = \sum_{i=1}^{240} S_{i\_R} == sleeping?\ 1\ :\ 0\ (i \leftarrow i+1\text{min})$
$f'2_R = \sum_{i=1}^{240} (S_{i\_R} == active\ or\ S_i == awake)\ ?\ 1\ :\ 0$
$f'3_R = \sum_{i=241}^{480} HRR_{i\_R} \leq 0.0\ ?\ 1\ :\ 0$
$f'4_R = \sum_{i=241}^{480} HRR_{i\_R} > 0.5\ ?\ 1\ :\ 0$

activities assumed to take a rest or have a sedentary lifestyle. *f'*4 means the total number of times of work activities where the percentage of activity intensity is more than 50%. These activities are assumed to perform an excessive workload and trainees who have continued these activities need to take an adequate rest.

In the experiment, data were collected from 290 (265/25, male/female) workers at four worksites (Hanwa, LG Display, LG Innotek, and KCC). We used the Fitbit Charge HR, a wristband type wearable health device. We collected 44,400 raw data from March 2016 to September 2016. There are 40,103 male data sets and 4,337 female data sets. The data may have missing values for reasons, such as low power, environment, and so on. We excluded raw data with missing values within the sleep and activity periods to improve the accuracy of clustering. Among the retained raw data, we only used 4,068 raw data with no missing value. We used K-means algorithm to cluster the physical stability status of trainees, and used Prediction strength to measure clustering validation [5]. We compared the proposed feature modelling methods with *HRR*-model. *HRR*-model used two features, a total time of work activities with a moderate workload (0-30% *HRR*), and a total time of work activities with an excessive workload (over 40% *HRR*) during the same period using our feature modelling method [2].

Figure 1 shows a result of the prediction strength score

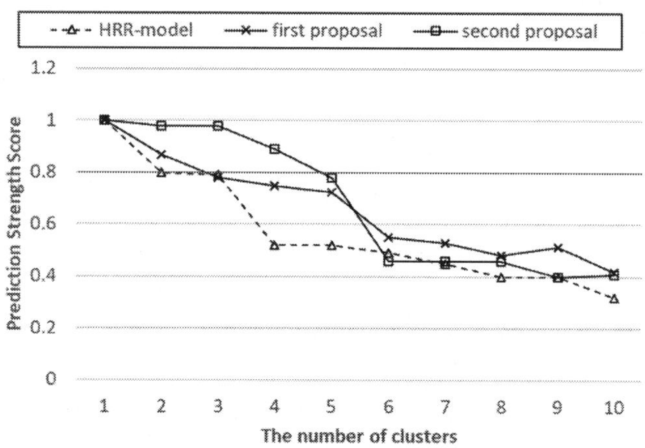

Figure 1. Prediction strength scores according to the incremental cluster *k*-value

according to the incremental cluster *k*-value. When the cluster *k*-value is from 1 to 3, The second proposed feature modeling method have the best validation degrees because all of the prediction strength score is greater than 0.8. Therefore, unlike the other models, the proposed second model is suitable for generating three clusters for the assessment of trainees' the physical stability. The first feature modeling method also has a better validation score than the previous *HRR*-model.

To show the classification accuracy, we generated the learning and test data set for ANN(Artificial Neural Network)-based classification evaluation with *k-value=3* and each proposed feature modeling. All data set of each cluster are labeled by "stable", "normal" and "unstable". ANN layer structure is 800-800 architecture. We confirmed that the tested accuracies were about 98% and 99%, respectively.

3 Conclusions

In this paper, we proposed two feature modeling methods to make a learning and a test set to be used in classification algorithms in order to decide a complex industrial trainee's physical status. Our proposed feature modeling methods show better performance than the previous feature modeling in classification approach within the limit of sleep, rest, and activity intensity data which is collected by wristband type wearable devices such as commercial model : Fibit and Xiaomi's band.

4 Acknowledgment

This work was supported by the Technology Innovation Program (10077260) funded by the Ministry of Trade, Industry & Energy (MOTIE, Korea) and DGIST R&D Program of the Ministry of Education, Science and Technology of Korea (18-IT-02). All collected data was used after receiving permission of Institutional Review Board (IRB) approval (no. DGIST-160303-HR-012-01) from DGIST.

5 References

[1] Zahra Maman, Sedighi, et al. "A data-driven approach to modeling physical fatigue in the workplace using wearable sensors." Applied ergonomics Vol. 65, pp. 515-529, 2017.

[2] Sungjoo Hwang, and SangHyun Lee. "Wristband-type wearable health devices to measure construction workers' physical demands." Automation in Construction Vol. 83 pp. 330-340, 2017.

[3] Chen, Martin K. "The epidemiology of self-perceived fatigue among adults," Preventive medicine, Vol. 15, No. 1, pp. 74-81, 1986.

[4] Tanaka, Hirofumi, Kevin D. Monahan, and Douglas R. Seals. "Age-predicted maximal heart rate revisited," Journal of the American College of Cardiology, Vol. 37, No. 1, pp. 153-156, 2001.

[5] Tibshirani, Robert, and Guenther Walther. "Cluster validation by prediction strength," Journal of Computational and Graphical Statistics, Vol. 14, No. 3, pp. 511-528, 2005.

SESSION

LATE BREAKING PAPERS

Chair(s)

TBA

ISBN: 1-60132-479-0, CSREA Press ©

Dynamic Consent in Cybersecurity for Health

Arianna Schuler Scott[1], Michael Goldsmith[1], Harriet Teare[2], Sadie Creese[1] & Jane Kaye[2]
[1]Department of Computer Science, University of Oxford, Oxford, UK
[2]Centre for Health, Law and Emerging Technologies, University of Oxford, UK

Abstract *- Patient care is becoming individualized, moving away from traditional models of medical care. As part of this migration, healthcare services are becoming reliant on data being hosted and decisions being made online. As an institution, the National Health Service (NHS) is grounded in principles of individual welfare like informed consent and duty of care but a patient-centred approach cannot put the responsibility for data protection directly onto patients because those who control and process information are better placed to leverage the appropriate risk controls. This paper explores whether moving healthcare decisions online helps or hinders, presenting a framework for dynamic consent (consent withdrawal, two way engagement and long term thinking) as a way to mitigate cybersecurity risk. Consent decisions must lie with the data subject but those with oversight and expertise must be responsible for wider implementation of these controls and communicating them via institutional policy.*

Keywords: dynamic consent, cybersecurity, data-protection, digital health, cyber-risk.

1 Introduction

Moving information online has become standard practice because it is cheaper, more accessible and introduces resilience: where data may have been lost or deleted there is now a way to retrieve what was lost. 'Healthcare data' (the terms information and data are used interchangeably) as a term had widened – what was once confidential records collected in a clinical practice has expanded due to an increase in the number of data sources and general demand for information sharing: in the UK, provision of care for individuals lies with the National Health Service but data needs to be shared across organisations (like Public Health England for example whose remit is the wellbeing of the national population). Strength lies in this migration of data online but there must be safeguards in place to protect patients. Responsibilities are mandated by legislation like the Data Protection Act 2018 (DPA18) and General Data Protection Regulation (GDPR) and risk lies in ignoring these. This paper argues that data protection makes the case for the importance of security when dealing with patient information.

A system is needed that allows oversight for decision-makers and control for individuals, emphasising the protection of data and mitigation of harm and facilitating a two way conversation that benefits both sides. Consent is problematic in that despite agreed principles and regulatory mechanisms, variance lies in implementation. Problems include a lack of understanding from others (Kumar, 2013), consent being treated as a one-off decision (Wiles et al, 2005) even though people change their minds and information sharing agreements that are ill thought through. Data sharing enables collaboration; innovation allows external parties to develop tools, analyses and treatments to help healthcare providers deliver more effective treatment but risk lies in the abuse of these relationships. To mitigate this risk, policy-making will need to balance power dynamics between individuals and those who control how personal information is used.

The Data Protection Act defines a data subject as an individual who is the subject of personal data, data controllers as determining how and why information is processed and data processors as analysing data on behalf of the controller (Data Protection Act, 2018). Cybersecurity presents multi-stakeholder problems and to approach them, stakeholders need common metrics. Inflexible legislation stifles innovation and constricts new technology, with national policy being pressured rather than facilitated by change. Recent efforts towards protecting individual rights in the General Data Protection Regulation (GDPR) and new Data Protection Act (DPA) mean that regulatory requirements must be translated into technical ones but the intangibility of data makes it difficult to conceptualise harms mitigated by data protection controls. High profile data breaches in sectors like retail (Target), telecommunications (TalkTalk) and social media (Facebook) demonstrate public awareness and opinion but highlight a lack of outlets for public debate. Responsible use and protection of data provides individual liberties, evidence of accountability in a court of law and the freedom to exist in a democratic society. By understanding and communicating risk, institutions can begin to identify and mitigate threats. Comparing a record of how an individual wants their data to be used to how it actually is being used identifies conflict, providing a starting point from which to audit, address and respond to those conflicts in real time.

Dynamic consent rests on revocation, engagement and persistence over time. Consent withdrawal, the changing of consent preferences and two-way communication 'between patient and... provider' (Kaye et al., 2015) put control in the hands of individuals. Moderation of consent decisions, the opportunity for people to feed back into the process and auditing of consent choices present a richer data exchange (Williams et al., 2015). Dynamic consent suits large-scale data-sharing and can be built into new systems, but its implementation in existing ones will mean assessing current practice, re-drawing working relationships and amending existing policies (Budin-Ljøsne et al, 2017). Dynamic consent is a privacy control, a trust-building instrument (Kanellopoulou, 2009). Hospitals have a duty of care towards patients which makes confidentiality non-negotiable and trust relies on confidentiality (Caldicott, 2013). Healthcare as a sector depends on trust between patient and practitioner to provide effective diagnoses and treatments, with trust lending legitimacy to practice (Aitken et al., 2016).

1.1 Cybersecurity risks in healthcare

In this position paper we consider the risks that exist around patient data. Information security literature uses 'CIA' tried to conceptualise risk. Patient data needs to be kept *confidential* (accessed only by authorized parties), with *integrity* (only authorized changes may be made) and *available* when necessary. The scale, complexity and heterogeneity of users render the maintenance and enforcement of risk controls a challenge.

Medical devices: pacemakers, insulin pumps and cochlear implants are examples of devices that cannot be easily taken out for maintenance. Wireless communication is becoming prevalent and maintaining the confidentiality of data collected by these sensors mitigates the unauthorised collection of personal data or control of the device (Loukas, 2015).

Access control: hospitals are busy environments, where many users need to access health records for many reasons. There are simple ways to make sure certain people see certain information about a patient but if these rules are not thought through in their design and information is withheld (through no fault of the practitioner) then delivery of care may be affected.

Information sharing agreements: Institutional inattention towards data protection presents a problem for healthcare practitioners in that innovation invites risk, so when involving external partners the information to be shared and the use for which it is being shared is paramount. Industry partners will prioritise earning potential over patient confidentiality, for example.

1.2 Institutional responsibility

As hospitals have a duty of care to patients, data controllers now legally have a duty of care to their data subjects. Users can be ill-informed, incompetent or apathetic to security concerns so responsibility for data-protection cannot lie solely with them. Data controllers must take responsibility for this as they have oversight and capacity to do so. Institutional policy (specific rules) and procedure (specific actions implementing policy) need to be in place to assess whether these responsibilities are being met.

Leaders and decision makers need to be engaged with overarching objectives for healthcare as this directs practice. Both governance and technical solutions must follow the same principles of data-protection: consent, autonomy and privacy, but dialogue between technical and non-technical stakeholders is expensive. Time and budget constraints mean that technical interpretation is often left to software developers, while policy-makers are often accused of being 'left behind' by technology. This divide causes a lack of understanding about what needs to be done to ensure data-protection, and how. The GDPR introduces controls to prioritise the privacy and autonomy of individuals, like compulsory data-breach notifications and named 'data-protection officers' (European Parliament, 2016).

2 Background

2.1 Digital health

Digital health is an implementation of technology-enabled, personalised healthcare which makes use of physical hardware and intangible software to support care providers in diagnosing and treating individuals. Personal trackers like FitBits and mobile devices are one kind of physical technology and in-clinic machines enabling diagnoses are another. Software ranges from applications on a mobile device to social media, from MyFitnessPal to Twitter. Some physical devices have multiple software tools running on them, like a mobile phone used to access a food planner and glucose calculator for someone with diabetes, while others run a single piece of software for a specific use, such as Magnetic Resonance Imaging (MRI) machines.

The digitalisation of healthcare eases administration, lowers budget requirements and allows for provision of care beyond the clinic. Confidence introduced by Internet access and self-diagnosis, alongside perceptions of a lax and underfunded health service in the UK (Martin et al, 2017) has increased the demand for a patient-centred service with more transparency around care and treatment. Reviews of the National Health Service (NHS) over time demonstrate this change; 'Caldicott Guardians' were originally appointed to ensure patient confidentiality (Caldicott & Britain, 1997) and a later review emphasised this duty of care towards data by using people, process and technology to secure information sharing behaviour.

2.2 Moving data online

Decisions about who can access information and under what circumstances are changing due to these processes and databases moving online. An online system could encourage shared decision-making between patients and healthcare providers, but there must be an understanding of associated security implications. Without access controls in place, storing data online presents a higher risk of exposure. Sensors collecting biological information, like Fitbits and other Internet-connected devices communicate to external servers. Vulnerabilities lie in these connections as well as the machine itself.

The Internet makes data-sharing in health services easier, replacing paper records with specific digital access which can be granted for diagnosis and treatment. Centralising access to patient records provides oversight, allowing wider use across a network of clinical and research bodies. The risk this exposes patients to must be discussed and an adaptive threat response developed.

2.3 Data protection

Patient-identifiable information (P-II) was defined in a review of the National Health Service (NHS) as 'items of information… [enabling a] person's identity to be established by one means or another' (Caldicott & Britain, 1997). Protecting data should limit its misuse. The Data Protection Act of 1998 (Act, 1998) dictates that processing personal information must be lawful and specific. Data must be relevant, accurate and kept for no longer than necessary. The European General Data Protection Regulation (GDPR) builds on these principles, giving guidelines for consent and emphasising privacy-by-design early on in development. All organisations owning, maintaining or developing systems that process personal data have a legal responsibility to put data-protection principles into practice.

The Caldicott principles of data use established specific information use on a need-to-know basis and Caldicott Guardians were installed in hospitals to oversee the implementation of these principles. Governance describes the management of data-handling, ensuring confidentiality and sharing information to support patient care, defined in a later report as a tool for establishing lawful data protection practices. (Caldicott, 2013).

2.4 Cybersecurity

Significant privacy concerns around specific healthcare responses like genomics or precision medicine but these lie outside the scope of this paper. As a position paper we address cybersecurity challenges for general digital health. There exist many ways to assess and mitigate cybersecurity risk and understanding data protection principles allows us to conceptualise where these problems lie and mitigate them early on e.g. taking a safety-first approach to data protection like Data Minimisation rather than relying on a complete understanding of the risk landscape (Nurse, Creese & De Roure, 2017).

Technical systems are built on qualitative (functional) and quantitative (non-functional) requirements and security often blurs the boundary between the two. Functional requirements have an expected input and output (a user enters their name; their name is then displayed back to them). Non-functional requirements can be subjective (saving a new name should take no longer than 0.2 seconds). Cybersecurity takes human behaviour into account which in a hospital includes a computer being left logged on or sensitive records being left lying on a desk. Cybersecurity considerations include data protection, physical and psychological harm as well as reputational and cultural harm:

Physical: Physical impact. A denial of service attack overloads a machine to stop all functions. A machine providing life support needs to be secured.

Psychological: Emotional or cognitive impact. Manipulative scare tactics are used by ransomware developers who lock a machine until a user pays for its release.

Reputational: Impacts relationships. Supply chain attacks target a large company's infrastructure via a smaller service provider who is usually less protected. Other companies may avoid working with them in the future.

Cultural: Disruption of stability. If a cyber-attack caused a loss of patient records, **mass** withdrawal from public health services could cost years of development.

Current legislation seeks consent for specific data to be shared, allowing revocation to ensure that data sharing is driven by the needs of healthcare providers and their patients. A blanket approach to consent is nearer current practice however, with indiscriminate hovering up of data.

2.5 Dynamic consent

Consent is an underlying principle in the medical field but implementation problems mean that questions around what it means to be 'informed' and whether there is a 'genuine consent' are often revisited. A dynamic framework for consent allows an individual to have a say in what they share and what is shared about them. Three things are involved: allowing consent withdrawal (revocation of data access), a two way conversation (engagement between data subject and controller) and an awareness of data's persistence (that it is kept over time). Our focus lies with the responsibilities residing with data controllers.

Revocation of access allows data subjects a level of control over who sees their information, but is not often exercised (Whitley, Kanellopoulou & Kaye, 2012). There are several corner-cases to consider, such as many subjects revoking access at the same time. If a hospital experienced a data breach, an ineffective public relations response may cause a loss of trust and group revocation. This could delay or prevent care.

Data persists over time so the consent process should cater to that. Dynamic consent maps consent preferences to an individual, allowing information control over a period of time. Different healthcare providers may require access to an up-to-date patient record. The way that institutions share data and the way data flows are designed, built and maintained is important because if doctors cannot are accessing out of data information they cannot provide optimal medical care.

The more comfortable a person is, the more likely they are to disclose information (Whitley, 2009). By engaging with data subjects' attention, a controller can make them feel more at ease and scope out effective information delivery mechanisms (Abawajy, 2014). A dynamic framework for consent is one way to put into practice legislation like GDPR, the Data Protection Act and the e-Privacy Act. Neglecting the principles underlying legislation and finding workarounds risks considerable financial penalty.

3 Discussion

3.1 Revocation

Revocation works to establish a relationship between data controller (in this case a scientist or researcher) and subject (participant or patient). The right to revoke access is enshrined in the General Data Protection Regulation and Data Protection Act. Being able to change how others use personal data (Pearson & Casassa-Mont, 2011) gives individuals control over their own information. Dive & Newson (2018) describe autonomy as deliberate, informed and free from external and internal influences like extortion and addiction. Patients need to be able to make their own decisions as well as trust experts inform those decisions. Trust is essential in the delivery of successful diagnoses and treatments (Meyer & Ward, 2008) and revocation helps build trust (Agrafiotis et al., 2009).

Informing individuals about revocation options may present the illusion of choice. Technology designed to enable revocation could constrain healthcare delivery if that functionality is not supported and this degrades trust (Anders, 1996). Risk lies in not knowing what expected behaviour looks like and the potential for de-anonymisation of records. It is impossible to predict every eventuality when designing new systems or when adding to existing ones, the complexity of interconnected technologies increase in complexity as they scale, which can cause problems (Leonard-Barton, 1988). We need discussion around corner-cases, like someone revoking consent as the controller is processing that data (Agrafiotis et al., 2010).

3.2 Engagement

Dynamic consent relies on a communication framework termed 'Engagement 2.0' by Teare et al (2015), based on principles of active participation, autonomy, knowledge and consent. The authors recommend interaction with research participants as a way to gather feedback to improve practice as well as collect data, as evidenced by the RUDY project, a study platform changing the delivery of clinical care (Javaid et al., 2016). Patients want to actively engage and feel that their choices are respected (Hammami et al, 2014). The RuDY project consults a patient forum for feedback and works this into their practice.

Engagement shapes discourse across healthcare, research and the public sector. Researchers focus on societal trends rather than individual impact (Mitchell et al., 2017), but one of the largest vulnerabilities in cybersecurity is caused by a general lack of user education and awareness. Security needs to be everybody's problem (Adams & Makramalla, 2015). Hospitals are notorious for their insecure behaviour – in 2016 the NHS and DeepMind, a subsidiary of Alphabet, announced development of an early-warning system for kidney disease. The hospital had provided confidential patient records including those of patients who do not suffer from kidney disease (Powles & Hodson, 2017). DeepMind published press releases and engaged with the academic community whereas the hospital was held up as an example of poor data practice by the Information Commissioner's Office (ICO, 2018). Hospitals do not have the resources to hire media and public-relations professionals on a day-to-day basis, relying rather on governance and best practice.

3.3 Persistence

Data is kept over time. This persistence, while employees change, new policies are put into practice and emerging technologies develop means that consent decisions and preferences over time should be recorded. Consistency in practice is important – for researchers this may mean treating every participant in exactly the same way to mitigate changes in personnel. A similar principle exists for clinicians – patients expect a consistent level of care regardless of who they are being treated by. As data is stored over time, planning for the long term mitigates a short-sighted approach to risk.

Changing how organisations handle data balances management oversight with the autonomy of teams making those changes (Sirkin, Keenan & Jackson, 2005). Emerging cyber-threats, such as the 'WannaCry' software that held a number of NHS computers to ransom, are not always targeted at hospitals; but due to a lack of investment in security, the impact can be much wider that necessary (O'Dowd, 2017). With a significant lack of expertise and low prioritisation of security in the healthcare sector, the question arises – are we institutionally prepared to roll out consistent security changes?

4 Conclusion

With individual rights such as the right to be informed about data breaches, the right to revoke consent and the right to be forgotten enshrined in recent legislation alongside guidance as to who holds responsibility for the protection of data and mitigation of any related risk, direction must come from decision-makers as to how to invest in and prioritise cybersecurity in healthcare. A dynamic framework for consent grounded in the concepts of effective engagement, granular revocation and persistence over time addresses risk by respecting the autonomy of individuals and empowering them to take control of their own decisions. Informed consent does not mean overloading data subjects with procedural decisions. The responsibility for policy design and decisions around the storage, sharing and access of data lies with decision-makers in an institutional framework with regular feedback mechanisms.

Identifying and mitigating risk is central tenet of cybersecurity. Categorising types of risk like denials of service, employee negligence and data theft, and potential harms such as blackmail, targeting and interruption to provision of care, provides a framework around which to make decisions. Dynamic consent translates directly into cybersecurity requirements: revocation of data provides a level of oversight and control, an active dialogue fosters a better understanding of data use and long term thinking models security risks over time. Understanding and communicating risk helps identify and mitigate threats ahead of time. This paper argues that a dynamic framework for consent provides data minimization which can be used as evidence of good governance and best practice. Comparing a record of how an individual wants their data to be used against how data is actually being used identifies possible conflict, providing a starting point from which to audit, address and respond to those conflicts in real time.

5 References

[1] Abawajy, J. "User preference of cyber security awareness delivery methods"; Behaviour & Information Technology, 33(3), 237 – 248, 2014.

[2] "Data Protection Act"; Online, retrieved from http://www.legislation.gov.uk/ukpga/1998/29/contents [Accessed 20 April, 2018], 1998.

[3] Adams, M. and Makramalla, M. "Cybersecurity skills training: an attacker-centric gamified approach"; Technology Innovation Management Review, 5(1), 2015.

[4] Agrafiotis, I., Creese, S., Goldsmith, M., & Papanikolaou, N. "Reaching for informed revocation: Shutting off the tap on personal data"; IFIP PrimeLife International Summer School on Privacy and Identity Management for Life, 246-258, Sept 2009.

[5] Aitken, M., Cunningham-Burley, S., & Pagliari, C. "Moving from trust to trustworthiness: Experiences of public engagement in the Scottish Health Informatics Programme"; Science and Public Policy, 43(5), 713-723, 2016.

[6] Budin-Ljøsne, I. et al. "Dynamic Consent: A Potential Solution to Some of the Challenges of Modern Biomedical Research"; BMC Medical Ethics 4, 18(1), 2017.

[7] Caldicott, D. F., & Britain, G. "Report on the review of patient-identifiable information (pii)"; London: Department of Health, 1997.

[8] Caldicott, F. "Information: To share or not to share"; Information Governance Review, 2013.

[9] Anders, G. "Health against wealth: HMOs and the breakdown of medical trust"; Houghton Mifflin Harcourt, 1996.

[10] "Data Protection Act 2018"; Online, retrieved from https://www.gov.uk/government/ collections/data-protection-act-2018.

[11] Dive, L. L., & Newson, A. J. "Reconceptualizing Autonomy for Bioethics", 2018.

[12] European Parliament. "Regulation (EU) 2016/679 of the European Parliament and of the Council of 27 April 2016 on the protection of natural persons with regard to the processing of personal data and on the free movement of such data, and repealing Directive 95/46/EC (General Data Protection Regulation)"; Official Journal of the European Union, Vol. L119, pp. 1-88, 2016.

[13] Hammami, M. M., Al-Gaai, E. A., Al-Jawarneh, Y., Amer, H., Hammami, M. B., Eissa, A., & Al Qadire, M. "Patients' perceived purpose of clinical informed consent: Mill's individual autonomy model is preferred"; BMC medical ethics, 15(1), 2, 2014.

[14] Javaid, M. K., Forestier-Zhang, L., Watts, L., Turner, A., Ponte, C., Teare, H.. & Barrett, J. "The RUDY Study Platform–a novel approach to patient driven research in rare musculoskeletal diseases"; Orphanet journal of rare diseases, 11(1), 150, 2016.

[15] Kanellopoulou, N. "Legal philosophical dimensions of privacy"; EnCoRe Project Briefing Paper, 2009.

[16] Kaye, J., Whitley, E. A., Lund, D., Morrison, M., Teare, H., & Melham, K. "Dynamic consent: a patient interface for twenty-first century research networks"; European Journal of Human Genetics, 23(2), 141, 2015.

[17] Kumar, N. K. "Informed consent: Past and present."; Perspectives in clinical research, 4(1), 21, 2013.

[18] Kun, L. "Editorial DeepMind"; Health and Technology, 8, 1 – 10, 2018.

[19] Leonard-Barton, D. "Implementation as mutual adaptation of technology and organization"; Research policy, 17(5), 251-267, 1988.

[20] Loukas, G. "Cyber-physical attacks: A growing invisible threat"; Butterworth-Heinemann, 2015.

[21] Martin, G., Martin, P., Hankin, C., Darzi, A., & Kinross, J. "Cybersecurity and healthcare: how safe are we?"; BMJ, 358, j3179, 2017.

[22] Meyer, S. B., & Ward, P. R. "Do your patients trust you?: a sociological understanding of the implications of patient mistrust in healthcare professionals."; Australasian Medical Journal (Online), (1), 1, 2008.

[23] Mitchell, C., Ploem, C., Chico, V., Ormondroyd, E., Hall, A., Wallace, S. & Taylor, J. C. "Exploring the potential duty of care in clinical genomics under UK law"; Medical law international, 17(3), 158-182, 2017.

[24] Mont, M. C., Pearson, S., Creese, S., Goldsmith, M., & Papanikolaou, N. "A conceptual model for privacy policies with consent and revocation requirements"; IFIP PrimeLife International Summer School on Privacy and Identity Management for Life, 258-270, Aug 2010.

[25] Nurse, J. R., Creese, S., & De Roure, D. "Security risk assessment in Internet of Things systems"; IT Professional, 19(5), 20-26, 2017.

[26] O'Dowd, A. "Major global cyber-attack hits NHS and delays treatment"; BMJ: British Medical Journal (Online), 357, 2017.

[27] Pearson, S., & Casassa-Mont, M. "Sticky policies: An approach for managing privacy across multiple parties"; Computer, 44(9), 60-68, 2011.

[28] Powles, J., & Hodson, H. "Google DeepMind and healthcare in an age of algorithms"; Health and technology, 7(4), 351-367, 2017.

[29] Information Commissioner's Office. "Royal Free - Google DeepMind trial failed to comply with data protection law"; Online, retrieved from https://ico.org.uk/about-the-ico/news-and-events/news-and-blogs/2017/07/royal-free-google-deepmind-trial-failed-to-comply-with-data-protection-law [Accessed 18 March, 2018], 2017.

[30] Sirkin, H. L., Keenan, P. & Jackson, A. "The hard side of change management"; Harvard business review, 83(10), 108, 2005.

[31] Teare, H. J., Morrison, M., Whitley, E. A. & Kaye, J. "Towards 'Engagement 2.0': Insights from a study of dynamic consent with biobank participants"; Digital Health, 1, 2015.

[32] Whitley, E. A., Kanellopoulou, N. & Kaye, J. "Consent and research governance in biobanks: evidence from focus groups with medical researchers"; Public Health Genomics, 15(5), 232-242, 2012.

[33] Whitley, E. A. "Informational privacy, consent and the "control" of personal data"; Information security technical report, 14(3), 154-159, 2009.

[34] Wiles, R., Heath, S., Crow, G., & Charles, V. "Informed consent in social research: A literature review"; NCRM Methods Review Papers NCRM, 1, 2005.

[35] Williams, H., Spencer, K., Sanders, C., Lund, D., Whitley, E. A., Kaye, J. & Dixon, W. G. "Dynamic consent: a possible solution to improve patient confidence and trust in how electronic patient records are used in medical research"; JMIR medical informatics, 3(1), 2015.

Applying Deep Learning Methods for Short Text Analysis in Disease Control

Ekpe Okorafor[1] and Ezema Abraham[2]
[1,2]Department of Computer Science, African University of Science and Technology, Abuja, Nigeria

Abstract – *The recurrence of infectious disease outbreaks has intensified in developing countries. Coupled with the limitation of traditional disease control strategies, other approaches have been explored for disease control – with social media at the forefront. Data from this source are short, noisy, and informal in representation thus, conventional natural language processing (NLP) methods are not well adapted for their structure. Hence, a deep learning approach for character-level language modeling was explored to classify disease-related tweets, and an adaptive prediction model for outbreak monitoring was developed – Ebola virus disease (EVD) as a use case. Our system showed comparable classification performance on EVD-related tweets. Also, our predictive model showed correlation with official reported cases with an early warning of fourteen days.*

Keywords: Disease control, Deep learning, Short text analysis.

1. Introduction

The explosion of data in recent times has marked a new age for the human society. Social media platforms such as Facebook, LinkedIn and Twitter offer a place for people to share information in real time. Also, in 2016, Africa alone aggregated a total of 120 million Facebook users each month, and the statistics for other social media platforms have shown similar growth [1], [2]. In the space of a decade, the increasing Twitter coverage has transformed into improved acceptance by disparate users in expanded locations, and has cut across projects like event surveillance, masses' perception evaluation, and information extraction thus, its recommendation in disease control strategies. Disease control interventions aim to reduce disease spread, lethality, and incidence to a practicable extent [3]. Strategies could be for disease prevention which involves disease event surveillance, preparedness, and rapid response or eradication that involves isolation, treatment, and rehabilitation of infectious people. It is worth noting that a good disease control strategy involves both prevention and eradication activities and their execution tend to overlap at various stages of the intervention process.

Africa has been plagued with epidemic disease outbreaks from years preceding the 15th century. These occurrences tend to retard the growth of the human population in the region, and the development expectations [4]. Recorded cases show a trend of outbreak recurrence in previously affected nations and migration to neighboring countries [4], [5]. Alas, the recurrence rate and its associated mortality, question the level of preparedness, surveillance efficacy and control efforts in place. Hence, over the years, web and social media monitoring have been explored to mitigate disease propagation due to its advantage in timely and geo-spatial detection of disease outbreaks [6].

Notwithstanding the potential of social media in disease control, it is characterized by a number of complexities that have caused a rather slow adoption in present day disease control strategies. This work aims to make contributions in addressing a number of these conditions by applying deep learning methods in text analytics. Unlike formal documents, social media data follow the short text standard (limited to 500 characters), are unstructured, sparse, informal (do not follow the syntax and semantics of the target language) and are fused with native languages – which is peculiar to Africa. As a result, traditional natural language processing (NLP) techniques are not well adapted to their noise level.

NLP tasks have to do with text understanding by machine programs, they span across sentiment analysis, machine translation, question type classification, part of speech (POS) tagging, named entity recognition, and topic categorization. Predictive models based on neural networks made groundbreaking progress in language modeling to capture the distributional similarity of words leveraging word embedding [7]–[10]. Subsequent works have built on this baseline to show the efficacy of deep learning approaches in complex NLP tasks. Language modeling is central in text processing; count-based language models adopt statistical co-occurrence of words but take less precedence to Neural language models (NLMs) due to their associated sparsity and large dimension. However, NLMs require immense preprocessing and vocabulary consideration, which make them very large. They give poor embeddings for infrequent words and do not capture words with inflections; as a result, affecting their consideration for social media data processing.

The character-level paradigm for language modeling has shown outstanding result in NLP tasks; it requires less feature engineering, preprocessing, seamless adaptation in morphologically rich languages, reliable cross-domain classification, and applications in various NLP tasks [11]–[13]. The convolutional neural network (CNN) model design used in this work for short text analysis stemmed from [11] based on the results achieved and the suitability of the methods to the aforementioned informality associated with social media data. In a stride to achieve early outbreak detection to forestall infectious disease transmission, the subsequent parts of this write up document a framework which monitors the Twitter platform for Ebola-related tweets, uses character-level CNN for topic categorization and leverages its outcome as indicators in an adaptive prediction algorithm for detecting Ebola outbreak. These approaches are incorporated as our Deep Learning for Disease Control (DeepLDC) Framework.

2. The Deep Learning for Disease Control (DeepLDC) Approach

As represented in Fig. 1, DeepLDC involves the following:

i. Twitter data streaming.
ii. Extraction of relevant fields from the unstructured data.
iii. Short text classification using character-level CNN.
iv. Disease outbreak monitoring and outbreak prediction.

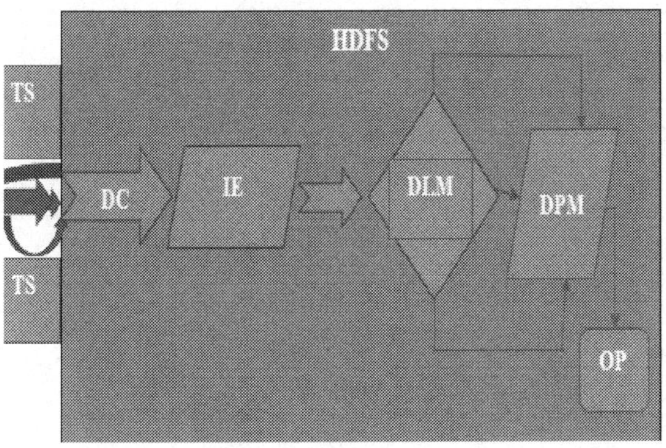

Figure 1. The DeepLDC architecture.
TS stands for twitter stream; DC is the data channel; IE for information extraction; DLM is the deep learning model; DPM is disease prediction model; OP is the output prediction; and HDFS stands for Hadoop file system.

2.1 Data Collection and Processing

Data is a major requirement when designing any model; in the course of this work, data had to be sourced, annotated, and aggregated from scratch. Twitter was selected as our target social media platform because of its wide coverage likewise its provision for streaming and search requests. We also thought it appropriate that for precision, our dataset be solely composed of Ebola-related historic data. We collected a total of 1,320 tweets during previous outbreaks in Liberia, Nigeria, Sierra Leone, and the United States of America; spanning from March 2014 to March 2016. To improve search results, Ebola-related keywords and search operators were utilized; also, the geo-code of target locations was used to improve the search radius results.

2.1.1 Data Annotation

Tweets were manually labelled into the following classes:

1. Outbreak related tweets: contained tweets about spread in a particular area, deaths, new cases confirmed or suspected, reports of illness, flu or fever, new outbreaks, description of disease and its effects.
2. Prevention, control, and management tweets: they were tweets about control efforts, possible cure, end of viral spread, and prevention techniques.
3. Not directly related tweets: were tweets about Ebola workshops, seminars, research papers, study, and Ebola jokes.

2.1.2 Character-Level Text Processing

A predefined dimension of *n* equal to 70 comprising all the 26 letters in English language, all the numbers, punctuations and newline make up the character field. The character field is listed as follows:
a, b, c, d, e, f, g, h, i, j, k, l, m, n, o, p, q, r, s, t, u, v, w, x, y, z, 0, 1, 2, 3, 4, 5, 6, 7, 8, 9, !, “,”, #, $, %, &, (,), *, +, ‘,’, -, ., /, :, ;, <, =, >, ?, @, [, , ,], ^, _, {, |, }, ~, /n,\.

1-of-n encoding was used to represent the input text characters and the input sequence was transformed into vectors of size n with length *w* equal to 148. Thus, only characters within our predefined input span of 148 characters; which is the maximum length of an input sentence were considered. These sequences of characters make up the input frames to our model.

2.2 Deep Learning Model Design

The generated text sequences from 2.1.2, were dynamically set at the input of a CNN model which computes a ‘1–D’ convolution and outputs three probability scores of the classifications enumerated in 2.1.1. Given an input function $i(x) \in [1, w] \to \mathbb{R}$ and a discrete kernel function $f(x) \in [1, m] \to \mathbb{R}$, the Convolution $h(y) \in [1, \lfloor((w-m)+2p)/s\rfloor + 1] \to \mathbb{R}$ between $i(x)$ and $f(x)$ is given as

$$h(y) = \sum_{x=1}^{k} f(x).i(y.s - x + c) \quad (1)$$

Where p is the padding, s is the number of strides, and c = m -s + 1 is an offset constant.

2.2.1 Model Architecture

In an effort to adapt our CNN architecture to the twitter data standard (short text), we used the following settings across layers:

i. clipped the input length to 148 characters.
ii. [Convolutional Layer – rectified linear unit] *2 →[max-pooling]*3 → [Fully connected Layer – rectified linear unit] *2→[Fully connected Layer –softmax]→score of 3
iii. used a 5-layer architecture from (ii) above.

We used non-overlapping max-pooling for down sampling after convolution, padding of zero in all the layers, and the rectified linear unit (relu) activation function because of its non-saturating characteristic for better training performance [14].

2.2.2 Model Specifications

A stride size of '1' was used in the convolution layers. From Table 1, our final output value was '3' because of the task we had at hand – this value varies depending on the expected output. We applied 256 filters per convolutional layer to generate 256 feature maps. From Fig. 2, after flattening the 256 feature maps, (17 * 256) parameters form the input to the fully connected layers.

Table 1. Deep learning model specifications

Convolutional Layer	Number of Filters	Kernel Length	Pool
1	256	7	N/A
2	256	7	2,2,2

Fully connected layer	Output units
3	1024
4	1024
5	3

2.3 Disease Outbreak Monitoring

The tweets classification defined in 2.1.1 is leveraged as an indicator for our disease monitoring approach. Our system detects any abnormal increase in outbreak-related tweets in the form of spikes from Twitter stream. This serves as the event-trigger of our system.

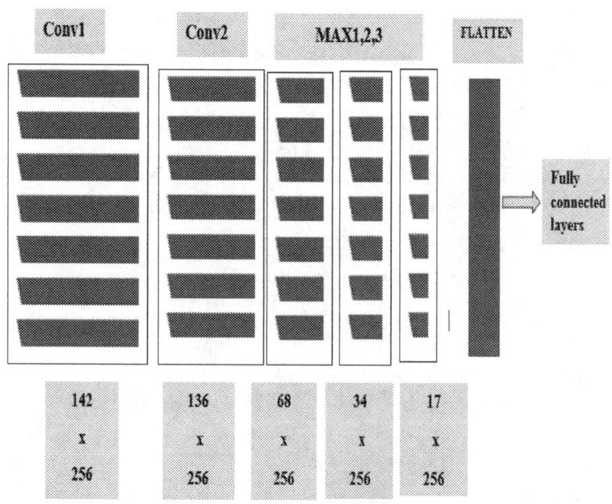

Figure 2. Representing the convolutional neural network block structure

It is worth noting that an increase in disease outbreak event chatter does not necessarily translate to an outbreak therefore, a related spike in the prevention, control, and management related tweets are also evaluated to make decisions on possible outbreak points using outlier detection concepts.

Our system uses the concept of an additive sliding window across previous tweet counts to compare an aggregated signal level against new stream entries. The sliding window comparison to a new stream takes the form of a measure of the momentum of the incoming tweets. This measure serves the function of monitoring the rise in level of new tweet counts as compared to the old momentum; forming two momentum graphs.

At any point where the new count level exceeds the aggregated momentum, an outbreak is possible; we refer to this point as a cross-boundary. We carry out a support test at this point to confirm an outbreak as a form of cross-validation by comparing against the momentum of the prevention, control, and management related tweets. An opposite behavior: count level less than the aggregate momentum; confirms a new disease outbreak in our system. This decision in the confirmatory test is based on the observed trend in collected data that in event of a new outbreak, less data about the other two classes are generated and in cases where there is an even or relative count across all classes, conversations tend to be on general viewpoints, lack firsthand outbreak content and do not indicate panic. The twitter streaming API gives search results for the past seven days; this stream of data can be used for periodical disease event surveillance. Also, for a disease control approach to be timely and preemptive, the monitoring period has to be short enough to capture events of outbreak cases. The method we propose is adaptive and considers the effect of recent readings in evaluation.

2.3.1 Outbreak Prediction Algorithm

$T_{OC} \leftarrow$ $Tweets_{OutbreakCount}$

$T_{WO} \leftarrow$ Outbreak window

$T_{PC} \leftarrow$ $Tweets_{PreventionCount}$

$T_{WP} \leftarrow$ Prevention window

At time t: $T_{woi} = \sum_{j=t-1}^{t-n} T_{ocj}$ (2)

$T_{wpi} = \sum_{j=t-1}^{t-n} T_{pcj}$ (3)

while: T_{oc} *!=0*

If: $T_{oc} \geq T_{woi}$

Output: "Detected case of possible new disease Outbreak (--cross-boundary--)"

If: $T_{pc} < T_{wpi}$

Output: "Confirmed case of a possible new outbreak"

end

Else:

Output: "Cross-validation test indicates no new outbreak"

end

end

end

where:

$i = \{1,2,3,4, \ldots, X \mid i \in \mathbb{N}^+\}$

$j = \{1,2,3,4, \ldots, Y \mid j \in \mathbb{N}^+\}$

$n = \{1; 2; 3; 4; \ldots; Z \mid n \in \mathbb{N}^+\}$

3. Results

The DeepLDC approach was applied to the Ebola Virus Disease (EVD) condition in West African countries. Its classification performance was evaluated and we checked correlation with official reported cases.

3.1 Topic Categorization on Twitter Data

The task was to classify the Ebola-related tweets we collected, as enumerated in 2.1 into classes as explained in 2.1.1. The training dataset comprised the outbreak related data (labelled *#0*); prevention, control, and management data (labelled *#1*); and not directly related data (labelled *#2*). Each having a uniform number of 350 tweets and the validation dataset comprised of 90 tweets respectively.

The following parameters were set when we trained our CNN model:

i. non-overlapping max pooling was used.
ii. rectified linear unit was implemented to give the network more freedom to adjust weights during training [8], [14].
iii. weights were initialized randomly with values from a Truncated normal distribution defined by mean=0.00 and standard deviation=0.05.
iv. the network was trained using backpropagation [14], [15]; utilized adaptive delta (adadelta) stochastic gradient algorithm for optimization; learning rate was initialized to 1, with a reduction of 0.6 after two non-improving training errors.
v. a drop out of 0.5 was inserted between the fully connected layers for regularization and to check overfitting [15].

Our model obtained a validation accuracy of 63.16% and a training accuracy of 99.61%, which shows some degree of overfitting. As shown is Table 2, we obtained scores of 58%, 57%, and 57% as average precision, recall and f1-score respectively.

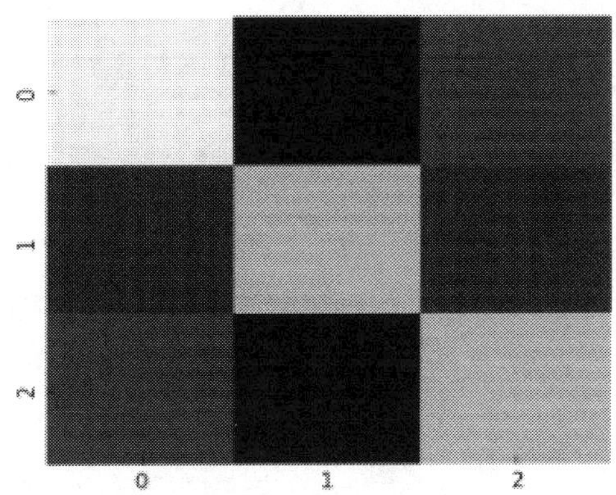

Figure 3. Confusion Matrix from topic categorization

Table 2. Performance evaluation

	Precision	Recall	F1-Score
0	0.56	0.63	0.59
1	0.65	0.54	0.59
2	0.52	0.55	0.54
Average	0.58	0.57	0.57

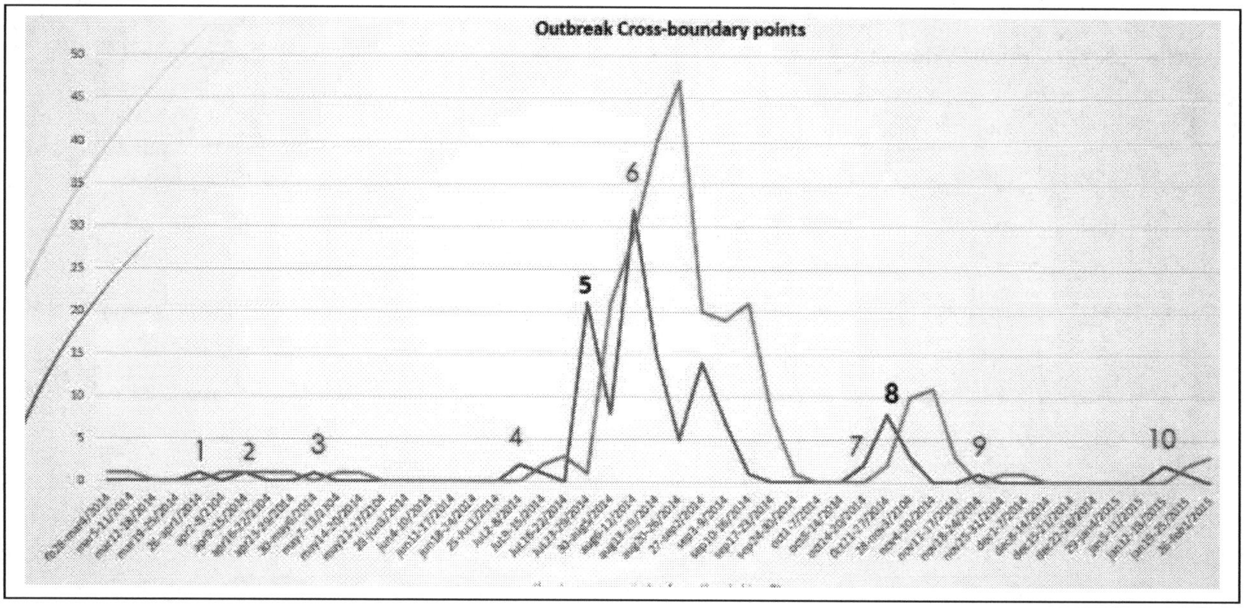

Figure 4. Disease prediction: outbreak-related tweets in Nigeria (February 2014-February 2015).
Red line is the aggregated momentum with window size of (n)=2; Blue line is the incoming tweet count. Points 1,2,3,4,5,6,7,8,9,10 are cross-boundary points.

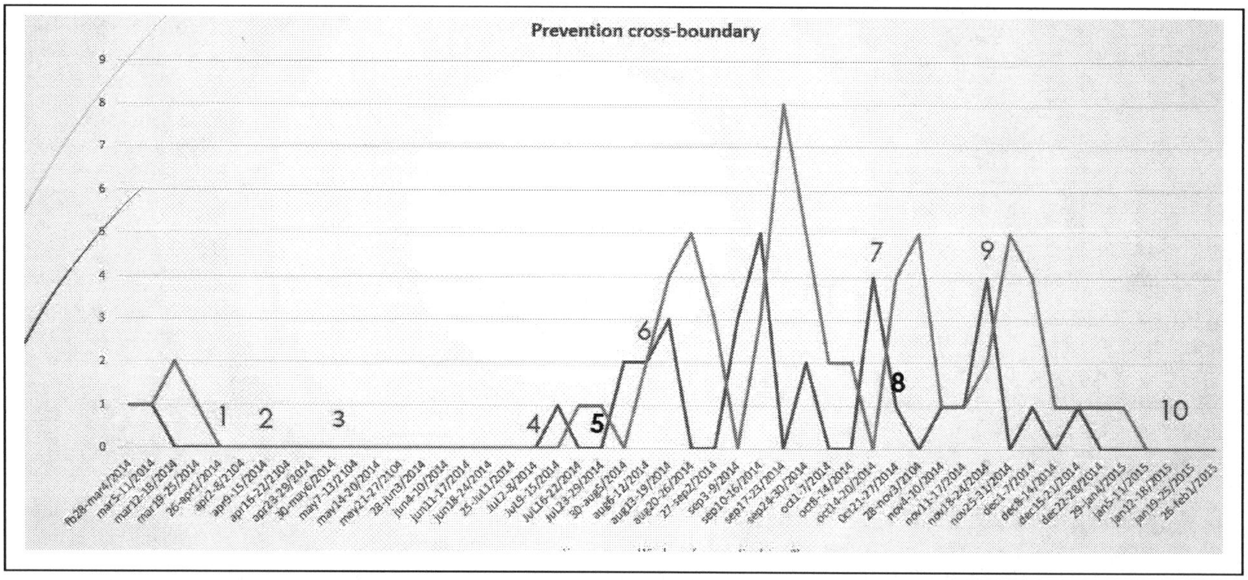

Figure 5. Disease prediction: prevention-related tweets in Nigeria (February 2014-February 2015)
Red line is the aggregated momentum with window size of (n)=2; Blue line is the incoming tweet count. Only points 5 and 8 met cross-validation condition.

3.2 Correlation with Reported Cases

We tested the DeepLDC prediction model from 2.3 on Nigeria during the EVD outbreak period (from February 2014 – February 2015) and obtained the graphs in Fig. 4 and Fig. 5. The data points have a span of seven days – data point 1 equivalent to data collected from the 26th of February to the 4th of March 2014 and data point 49 equivalent to data collected from the 25th of January to the 31st of January 2015. Our model picked out the following points as possible disease outbreak points:

1. Data point 22, labelled point 5 – which corresponds to July 23-29, 2014.
2. Data point 35, labelled point 8 – corresponds to tweets gathered on outbreak in Mali from October 21-27 2014.
3. Other data points did not meet the condition of our confirmatory test.

These points show some consistency with reported cases in Nigeria and its neighboring countries:

i. Nigerian health minister confirms first case of Ebola 6th of August 2014, five new cases being treated. Source: [17].
ii. Ebola strikes at the heart of Nigeria, doctor who treated Sawyer dies 19th of August 2014. Source:[18].

Therefore, it can easily be interpreted from the corresponding date of label 5 in Fig.4 and Fig. 5 that there is a significant difference between our approach detection time and official reports (from July 23rd – 6th of August,2014). Thereby, achieving a 14-day early notification for disease control strategies to commence.

4. Related Works

In an effort to prevent epidemic, early disease detection is necessary for infectious disease control. This can be carried out using a number of disease surveillance mechanisms. Recent works have explored novel mechanisms [6], [19], [20], [21] although, more have been related to social media adaptations.

[20] proposed an approach using emotion classification of health-related incidents to monitor disease outbreaks. Signs of outbreaks can be noticed by detecting a shift in the nature of discuss about a specific disease thus, exploiting the relationship of public mood and socio-economic events. A shift in discuss entails a change in the distribution of emotions around supposedly affected areas immediately after and prior to incidents. Using this approach, the need for text classification into predefined categories of discuss is avoided.

The approach of [21] involved the use of epidemiology models to analyze the underlying mechanisms in disease transmission. Social media data provided information about the exact contact network and mixing within the population which epidemiology models lack. Tweet counts were used as inputs to the compartment model to obtain the underlying contact network. As a result, the work could explore the strengths of these two approaches. However, due to the possibility of misinformation on social media, it may be difficult to establish an accurate measure of the required model parameters that characterize the general population, thereby affecting results.

[22] achieved surveillance by matching tweets that had relevant disease-related keywords with predefined locations of interest for 14 different diseases. Tweets were geo-tagged based on the location mentioned in the post body, from geo-code searches, and from the geolocation provided in the user's profile. Outbreak related topics were identified by unsupervised clustering also. Similarity of documents in the generated time series clusters was performed using the Jaccard coefficient and the result differed for all the diseases at different locations. Results showed high correlation for mumps, Ebola, Botulism and Ehec when compared with ProMED-mail reports.

5. Conclusion and Future Work

This work makes contribution to an emerging field of deep learning for disease control. Character-level approach for topic categorization is implemented on EVD-related tweets from previous periods of outbreaks and we achieved comparable performance with limited dataset. In a similar way, our DeepLDC approach shows merits in checking alert by means of it cross-validation test. Its event triggers are sensitive to both high and low changes in signal level. It implements an adaptive decision process that defeats the need to set a constant threshold value and mitigates spillovers after the trauma of a new outbreak. Despite the work done so far, progressive efforts to improve the classification accuracy of the deep learning model is essential. The present result is envisaged to improve with more data to aid better model generalizations and reduce overfitting. Attempts to locate the exact location of outbreaks in tweets using named-entity-recognition (NER) will greatly improve efforts for swift intervention in cases of outbreak in multiple locations.

References

[1] P.Parke. "How many people use social media in Africa.";Cnn.com,14-Jan.-2013. [Online].Available: http://edition.cnn.com/2016/01/13/africa/africa-social-media-consumption/index.html. [Accessed:10-March-2017]

[2] Fuseware and World Wide Worx, "SA Social media landscape 2016"; pp. 3–6, Feb. 2016.

[3] W. R. Dowdle. "The principles of disease elimination and eradication"; *Bull. World Health Organ.*, vol. 76, no. SUPPL. 2, pp. 22–25, 1998.

[4] S. Kebede, S. Duales, A. Yokouide, and W. Alemu. "Trends of major disease outbreaks in the African region, 2003-2007"; *East Afr J Public Heal.*, vol. 7, no. 1, pp. 20–29,March 2010.

[5] C. A. Spinage and W. House. "*African ecology - benchmark and historical events*". Springer Heidelberg Dordrecht London New York, 2012.

[6] J. Choi, Y. Cho, E. Shim, and H. Woo. "Web-based infectious disease surveillance systems and public health perspectives: a systematic review"; *BMC Public Health*, vol. 16, no. 1, p. 1238, Dec. 2016.

[7] Y.Lecun, L.Bottou, & Yoshua Bengio. "Gradient-based learning applied to document recognition";

PROCEEDING OF THE IEEE,1998,p. 86(11):2278-2324, Nov. 1998.

[8] X. Glorot, A. Bordes, and Y. Bengio. "Deep sparse rectifier neural networks"; *AISTATS '11 Proc. 14th Int. Conf. Artif. Intell. Stat.*, vol. 15, pp. 315–323,April 2011.

[9] T. Mikolov *et al.* "Distributed representations of words and phrases and their compositionality"; *Nips'14*, vol. cs.CL, pp. 3111–3119, Dec. 2013.

[10] T. Mikolov, G. Corrado, K. Chen, and J. Dean. "Efficient estimation of word representations in vector space"; *Proc. Int. Conf. Learn. Represent. (ICLR 2013)*, pp. 1–12, Sept 2013.

[11] X. Zhang and Y. LeCun. "Text understanding from scratch"; *Computer Research Repository ,Vol.abs/1502.01710, pp .1-10, April* 2016. [online].Available: http://arxiv.org/abs/1502.01710.[Accessed:05-July-2017].

[12] Y. Kim, Y. Jernite, D. Sontag, and A. M. Rush. "Character-aware neural language models"; *Proceedings of the Thirtieth AAAI Conference on Artificial Intelligence (AAAI'16)*; pp. 2741-2749, Feb. 2016.

[13] X. Chen, L. Xu, Z. Liu, M. Sun, and H. Luan. "Joint learning of character and word embeddings"; *IJCAI Int. Jt. Conf. Artif. Intell.*, vol. 2015–Janua, no. Ijcai, pp. 1236–1242,July 2015.

[14] A. Krizhevsky, I. Sutskever, and G. E. Hinton. "ImageNet classification with deep convolutional neural networks"; *Adv. Neural Inf. Process. Syst.*, pp. 1–9, Dec. 2012.

[15] M. Andrychowicz *et al.* "Learning to learn by gradient descent "; *Computer Research Repository ,Vol. abs/1606.04474,*pp.1-17,Nov 2016. [online]. Available: http://arxiv.org/abs/1606.04474.[Accessed:25-Aug-2017].

[16] N. Srivastava, G. Hinton, A. Krizhevsky, I. Sutskever, and R. Salakhutdinov. "Dropout: A simple way to prevent neural networks from overfitting"; *J. Mach. Learn. Res.*, vol. 15, pp. 1929–1958,June 2014.

[17] M.Mark. "Ebola outbreak: nurse who treated first victim in Nigeria dies"; The Guardian, 06-Aug-2014.[Online].Available: https://www.theguardian.com/world/2014/aug/06/ebola-outbreak-nurse-nigeria-dies.[Accessed: 05-Oct-2017].

[18] A.Akinremi & S.Balogun. " Ebola strikes at the heart of Nigeria: Ameyo, daughter of Kwaku Adadevoh, grand daughter of Herbert Macaulay dies";ThisdayLive,21-Aug-2014.[Online]. Available: https://web.archive.org/web/20140821181052/http://www.thisdaylive.com/articles/ebola-strikes-at-the-heart-of-nigeria-ameyo-daughter-of-kwaku-adadevoh-great-grand-daughter-of-herbert-macaulay-dies/186843/. [Accessed:05-Oct-2017].

[19] L. Simonsen, J. R. Gog, D. Olson, and C. Viboud. "Infectious disease surveillance in the big data era: Towards faster and locally relevant systems"; *J. Infect. Dis.*, vol. 214, no. Suppl 4, pp. S380–S385, Nov,2016.

[20] B. Ofoghi, M. Mann, and K. Verspoor. "Towards early discovery of salient health threats: a social Media emotion classification technique"; *Pac. Symp. Biocomput.*, vol. 21, pp. 504–515, 2016.

[21] L. Zhao,J.Chen,F.Chen,W.Wang,C. T. Lu , and N. Ramakrishna. "SimNest: Social media nested epidemic simulation via online semi-supervised deep learning"; *Proc. - IEEE Int. Conf. Data Mining, ICDM*, vol. 2016–Janua, no. i, pp. 639–648, Jan 2016.

[22] N. Kanhabua and W. Nejdl. "Understanding the diversity of tweets in the time of outbreaks"; *Proc. 22nd Int. Conf. World Wide Web - WWW '13 Companion*, pp. 1335–1342,May 2013.

Newsvendor Games with Budget Constraint in A Multi-hospital System

Min LUO
[1]School of Science and Engineering,
The Chinese University of Hong Kong, Shenzhen,
Shenzhen, Guangdong, 518172, P.R. China.
[2]School of Management,
University of Science and Technology of China,
P.R. China.
Emai: luomin@cuhk.edu.cn

Xiaoqiang CAI
Shenzhen Research Institute of Big Data,
The Chinese University of Hong Kong, Shenzhen,
Shenzhen, Guangdong, 518172, P.R. China.
Email: xqcai@se.cuhk.edu.hk

Abstract—**In this paper, we study a class of cooperative games among multiple hospitals. The optimization problems with the newsvendor games are formulated as deterministic and stochastic programs respectively. We analyze the cooperative allocation decision using the notion of a core. Start with the elegant result of a deterministic linear programming case where we assume the demand is definite larger than the supply, we prove the nonemptiness of the core and use the duality theory to find an imputation in the core. We further investigate it as a stochastic linear programming problem. The proposed method with strong duality theory is applied to show the nonemptiness of the core and suggests a way to find an element in the core.**

Index Terms—**healthcare; newsvendor games;stochastic; linear programming; duality theory.**

Contact author: Min LUO
Regular Research Paper

1. Introduction

Hospitals and care systems face unparalleled pressures in many countries and regions in the current environment. Growing populations, harsh environmental conditions and scarce medical resources are straining the budgets. In a populous country like China, public hospitals are always overcrowded and the time assigned for each patient is far from enough. On the contrary, private care organizations with higher charges need to advertise to improve the utilization of their capacity. Provision of high quality and affordable health care becomes one of the greatest challenges to the society. To solve these problems, health care systems must become more efficient at delivering care and preventing disease. As we know, waiting is the consequence of a mismatch between the needs for service and the availability of resources to provide that service. This mismatch might be the result of having too little of needed resources, or perhaps the needs themselves are excessive. Also it is likely that the resources and needs have not been adequately synchronized with each other.

We believe it is important to explore the resource allocation problem in the long run, especially when information system makes it possible for cooperation between health care sectors. We should strive for a well-coordinated system that delivers care with great efficiency and quality, at reasonable cost, matching the resources for care to where (and when) they are needed most.

The concept of sharing inventory has been studied a lot in centralized news-vendor model. Which can be conjectured that when demands are uncertain, centralization of capacity can help the hospital reduce resource investment and improve patient satisfaction. In our previous work [Luo and Cai(2016b)], we formulate an inter-hospital collaboration problem and derive solutions when capacities are available over multiple hospitals. To operationalize the sharing of capacity in the integrated system, we need to secure the willingness of the various parties to cooperate with each other, which leads to our current research. Specifically, we investigate, based on the concepts and methodologies of cooperative game and an inter-hospital cooperation problem for elective surgery planning. Based on some preliminary exploration [Luo and Cai(2016a)], we will show, this represents a new research effort and many interesting but challenging questions have to be addressed.

In recent years, several collaborative actions have been reported in various industries including pharmaceutical, fashion, automobile, and post-sales support (see [Anupindi and Bassok(1999)] [Chen and Zhang(2009)] for their motivating examples). The main driver of these collaborative activities is the cost benefit due to economies of scale and risk pooling, which can be achieved in several operations including logistics, purchasing, and inventories. Among them, inventories have a special importance because in many supply chains they constitute a big portion of the overall investment and resources [Anupindi et al.(2001)Anupindi, Bassok, and Zemel].

In a two-party situation, the answer would be easy. Any allocation improving the firms' stand-alone profit will be considered as a winwin case. However, if more firms are involved, they want to know that it is not more advantageous for them to cooperate in a smaller group rather than joining the big group. Existence of such an allocation is crucial for the stability of the cooperation. This problem can be studied using cooperative game theory, which provides, among others, the core as a popular solution concept.

The core is the set of allocations upon which no coalition can improve. Depending on the characteristics of the game, core allocations may exist or may fail to exist, i.e., the core can be empty. Since the lack of related papers in hospital cooperation, we review some of the papers studying inventory cooperation using newsvendor models in combination with the core as solution concept for the allocation problem of anticipated benefits.

The newsvendor model is probably the most celebrated model in inventory literature and it is used extensively to study inventory centralization and cooperation. Newsvendor models are used especially for products with high perishability or short life cycles and they have the ability to capture the basic trade-offs regarding inventory-related decisions.

Inventory cooperation and allocation of benefits has been a subject of inventory literature for a long time. Early papers studied slightly different models and approaches to the problem. [Eppen(1979)] was one of the first to consider the effect of centralization for a multi-location newsboy problem. [Gerchak and Gupta(1991)] proposed different cost allocation rules in centralized inventory systems.

In the last decade, cooperative game theory and the core concept became a main method for studying this problem. This part of the literature is the focus of our review paper. [Hartman et al.(2000)Hartman, Dror, and Shaked] showed that the newsvendor game is balanced, and the core of such a game is nonempty in some interesting cases, such as normally distributed demands.

[Müller et al.(2002)Müller, Scarsini, and Shaked] [Slikker et al.(2001)Slikker, Fransoo, and Wouters] showed that any finite newsvendor game is balanced whenever the random demand vectors has finite mean. [Slikker et al.(2005)Slikker, Fransoo, and Wouters] proved balancedness for games with transshipment costs. [Özen et al.(2008)Özen, Fransoo, Norde, and Slikker] dealt with balancedness for games with several warehouses. [Chen and Zhang(2009)] developed a stochastic programming duality approach to find a core element of these games.

For a review of inventory centralization games of deterministic and stochastic models, see [Fiestras-Janeiro et al.(2011)Fiestras-Janeiro, García-Jurado, Meca, and Mosquera]. For a comprehensive review of game theoretical models of supply chain management, see [Nagarajan and Sošić(2008)].

The paper is organized as follows. In Section 2, we introduce some basic concepts in newsvendor games. In Section 3, the basic game are presented. Section 4 deals with the deterministic situation. Section 5 developed a stochastic programming duality approach and find a core element when the hospital faces random demand.

2. Preliminaries

We first give a brief introduction to cooperative game. We refer to [Peleg and Sudhölter(2007)] for an extended treatment of this subject. In the setting of this paper, the hospitals are planning jointly in order to reach a overall service level and achieve the maximum revenue.

These hospitals are referred as *players*, denoted with a finite set $N = \{1, 2, ..., n\}$. A function $v : 2^N \to \mathbb{R}$, is called *characteristic function*. A subset $S \subseteq N$ is called a *coalition* and $v(S)$ is the the maximum revenue the coalition S can achieve by itself. The set N is often called the *grand coalition*. Given a coalition S, the subgame $\langle S, v_S\rangle$ is the game with grand coalition S and characteristic function v_S such that $v_S(T) = v(T)$ for $T \subseteq S$.

The *allocation* is represented as a vector $x \in \mathbb{R}_\mathbb{N}$ such that $\sum_{i\in N} x_i = v(N)$. Such a vector is a possible way to split the worth of the grand coalition among all players efficiently, that is, without any leftover.

$$core(\langle N, v\rangle) :=$$
$$\{x \in \mathbb{R}_\mathbb{N} : \sum_{i\in S} x_i \geqslant v(S)\ for\ all\ s \subset N, and \sum_{i\in N} x_i = v(N)\} \tag{1}$$

If an allocation is not in the core, then it is not stable, because there exists a coalition S such that $\sum_{i\in S} x_i < v(S)$. This coalition will therefore have an incentive to deviate and achieve $v(S)$by itself rather than join the grand coalition and obtain only $\sum_{i\in S} x_i$.

An allocation $x \in \mathbb{R}^\mathbb{N}$ with the property that $x_i \geq v(\{i\}), \forall i \in N$ is called *individually rational*. x is called *efficient* if $\sum_{i=1}^n x_i = v(N)$.

Call e^i the ith vector of the canonical basis of $\mathbb{R}^\mathbb{N}$ and define $e^S := \sum_{i\in S} e^i$. A map $\gamma : 2^N \to [0, 1]$ is called balanced if

$$\sum_{S\in 2^N\setminus\{\emptyset\}} \gamma(S)e^S = e^N.$$

A game $\langle N, v\rangle$ is called *balanced* if for every balanced map γ, we have

$$\sum_{S\in 2^N} \gamma(S)v(S) = v(N). \tag{2}$$

A game $\langle N, v\rangle$ is called *totally balanced* if it is balanced and each of its subgames is balanced as well. The above condition considers the situations where the players can form subcoalitions (i.e., every balanced map represents a situation where each player i forms coalition S with $i \in S\gamma(S)$ fraction of his time), and checks whether the players, if they organized themselves via these subcoalitions with corresponding weights, can do better than the grand coalition.

3. The Basic Model

We formulate a basic model allows hospitals who could use OR time locally as well as at some other hospitals. The revenues included net profit for lending the room, service fee of surgery team, as well as the costs, are assumed linear and the parameters could vary across the hospitals. Each hospital is faced with her own stochastic demand, which may be correlated with other hospitals. Naturally, we think the decisions can be made at two stages according the realization time of demand. In this complicated situation, one hospital gets the right of use of the OR time lot by paying for it before demand is realized. After the demand is realized, she owns the right to determine how the time lot is to be used, by her team or other hospitals. We analyze the cooperative allocation decision using the notion of a core. In general, not every game has a nonempty core. However, games with cores' existence are much more conducive to cooperation. We demonstrate that the core of this game is not empty, and suggest an allocation mechanism to support it.

The hospital has to decide the amount of surgeries will be provided by different types of surgery group and decide the the amount of OR time used in each hospitals accordingly, knowing that no change and replenishment is allowed. Each hospital faces an independent demand D_j for each of his surgery group $j, j \in M_i$ and order the OR time q_j $(\sum_{k\in N} q_{jk} = q_j)$ for them, then the hospital i obtains a profit:

$$\pi_i = \sum_{j\in M_i} r_j min\{D_j, q_j\} - \sum_{j\in M_i}\sum_{k\in N} c_{jk}q_{jk} \quad (3)$$

where r_j is the revenue that the surgery group j obtained for offering the operation and c_{jk} is the cost for using the OR time in another hospital k. Obviously, $r_j > c_{jk}$.

Let $D_i := \sum_{j\in M_i} D_j$ be the aggregate random demand for hospital i. The operator is defined by the expected total profit for the hospitals who order the optimal amount of OR time:

$$\Pi_N(D) = max_q\ E[\sum_{i\in N} \pi_i(D_i, q_i)], \quad (4)$$

All coalitions have the same anonymous profit function and face the same type of maximization problem, and the only difference between them is the random demand that they face.

We seek a so-called balanced distribution $x_1, x_2, ..., x_n$ such that

$$\sum_{i\in N} x_i = \Pi_N, \quad and \quad \sum_{i\in S} x_i \geq \Pi_S \quad \forall S \in N. \quad (5)$$

These (in)equalities completely describe the cooperative game and are referred to as core (in)equalities. In order to ensure that the grand coalition is stable (i.e., no group of hospitals has an incentive to deviate from the grand coalition N and form a smaller coalition S and no one will be better off by acting independently or cooperating with any subset of hospitals), it is imperative to devise a distribution scheme that meets the core inequalities of the game.

4. Deterministic newsvendor game

Before the investigation of the basic model, we first study the special situation where each surgery team has such a high demand that is definitely larger than the total time each surgery group may be allocated. The problem become a deterministic linear programming (LP) problem, and the corresponding cooperative game reduces to an LP game.

Hospital i obtains a profit:

$$\pi_i = \sum_{j\in M_i} r_j \sum_{k\in N} q_{jk} - \sum_{j\in M_i}\sum_{k\in N} c_{jk}q_{jk} \quad (6)$$

The grand coalition wants to maximize their profits:

$$v(N) = max \sum_{i\in N} \pi_i \quad (7)$$

subject to

$$\begin{aligned} &q_{11} + q_{21} + ... + q_{m1} \leq T_1 \\ &q_{12} + q_{22} + ... + q_{m2} \leq T_2 \\ &\vdots \\ &q_{1n} + q_{2n} + ... + q_{mn} \leq T_n \\ &q_{11}, q_{21}, ..., q_{mn} \geqslant 0 \end{aligned} \quad (8)$$

Theorem 1. The deterministic newsvendor game is balanced.

We consider the dual to the linear program:

$$min \sum_{i\in N} T_i p_i \quad (9)$$

subject to

$$\begin{aligned} &p_1 \geqslant r_1 - c_{11}, \\ &p_1 \geqslant r_2 - c_{21}, \\ &\vdots \\ &p_1 \geqslant r_m - c_{m1}; \\ &p_2 \geqslant r_1 - c_{12}, \\ &p_2 \geqslant r_2 - c_{22}, \\ &\vdots \\ &p_2 \geqslant r_m - c_{m2}; \\ &\vdots \\ &p_n \geqslant r_1 - c_{1n}, \\ &p_n \geqslant r_2 - c_{2n}, \\ &\vdots \\ &p_n \geqslant r_m - c_{mn}; \\ &p_1, p_2, ..., p_n \geqslant 0. \end{aligned} \quad (10)$$

Let $(p_1^*, p_2^*, ..., p_n^*)$ be the solution vector with the grand coalition, then of course:

$$v(N) = \sum_{i\in N} T_i p_i^* \quad (11)$$

$$v(N) \leq \sum_{i\in N} T_i p_i^* \quad (12)$$

Now, we define the payoff vector as u:

$$u_i = T_i p_i^* \tag{13}$$

Obviously,

$$v(N) = \sum_{i \in N} u_i \tag{14}$$

$$v(N) \leq \sum_{i \in N} u_i \tag{15}$$

for every $S \subset N$, thus u is an imputation in the core.

Heuristically, the components $(p_1^*, p_2^*, ..., p_n^*)$ can be thought of as unit equilibrium prices for the capacities. Each of the hospitals is paid for his resources according to the price vector p^*, the resulting payments will always give a vector in the core.

5. Stochastic newsvendor game

In this section, we consider a general situation where each surgery group faces a random demand. Our approach is motivated by the work of [Owen(1975)], who used linear programming duality to show the nonemptiness of the core for the (deterministic) linear production game. Owen's approach has become one of the systematic tools in analyzing cooperative games and has found numerous applications, for example, the inventory centralization games. We expect that the stochastic programming duality approach will find more applications in analyzing cooperative games with uncertainty.

$$\pi_i = \sum_{j \in M_i} r_j E[min(D_j, q_j)] - \sum_{j \in M_i} \sum_{k \in N} c_{jk} q_{jk} \tag{16}$$

The grand coalition's profit is

$$\Pi_N = \sum_{i \in N} \pi_i = \sum_{j} r_j E[min(D_j, q_j)] - \sum_{j \in M} \sum_{i \in N} c_{ji} q_{ji} \tag{17}$$

Their objective is:

$$v(N) = max \Pi_N(D_N) \tag{18}$$

subject to

$$\begin{aligned} &\textstyle\sum_{j \in M} q_{ji} \leq T_i \\ &q_{ji} \geqslant 0, i \in N, j \in M \end{aligned} \tag{19}$$

Then, the dual of the about stochastic program can be written as:

$$min \sum_{i \in N} T_i p_i \tag{20}$$

subject to

$$\begin{aligned} &p_1 \geqslant max_j r_j E[\theta(D_j)] - c_{j1}, j \in M \\ &p_2 \geqslant max_j r_j E[\theta(D_j)] - c_{j2}, j \in M \\ &\vdots \\ &p_n \geqslant max_j r_j E[\theta(D_j)] - c_{jn}, j \in M \\ &p_1, p_2, ..., p_n \geqslant 0 \end{aligned} \tag{21}$$

Let $(p_1^*, p_2^*, ..., p_n^*)$ be the solution vector. Then we have,

$$v(N) = \sum_{i \in N} T_i p_i^* \tag{22}$$

and for any S

$$v(S) \leq \sum_{i \in S} T_i p_i^* \tag{23}$$

Now, we define the payoff vector $u = (u_1, u_2, ..., u_n)$ and

$$u_i = T_i p_i^* \tag{24}$$

So we have $\sum_{i \in N} u_i = v(N)$ and $\sum_{i \in S} u_i \geq v(S)$, therefore u is an imputation in the core.

6. Conclusion

In this paper, we study the cooperative games among the hospitals. We analyze the cooperative allocation decision using the notion of a core. In general, not every game has a nonempty core. However, games with cores' existence are much more conducive to cooperation. We demonstrate that the core of this game is not empty, and suggest an allocation mechanism to support it.

Start with the elegant result of a deterministic linear programming case where we assume the demand is definite larger than the supply, we prove the nonemptiness of the core and use the duality theory to find an imputation in the core. We further investigate it as a stochastic linear programming problem motivated by the special case. The proposed method with strong duality theory is applied to show the nonemptiness of the core and suggests a way to find an element in the core.

Another topic may be investigated in the future is the cooperation among surgery groups in the stage of surgical case scheduling. After more and more information is realized on the random variables as time evolves, a coalition of surgery groups may find it better to combine their surgical cases for an optimal integrated rescheduling over the time slots they have been allocated. This will give rise to a cooperative game of the surgery teams. Due to the nature of the problem, this is basically a sequencing game.

Acknowledgment

The authors acknowledge the support of National Natural Science Foundation of China (No. 71531003 and No. 71432004), Research Grants Council of Hong Kong (No. T32-102/14N), and the Leading Talent Program of Guangdong Province (No. 2016LJ06D703)".

References

[Anupindi and Bassok(1999)] Ravi Anupindi and Yehuda Bassok. Centralization of stocks: Retailers vs. manufacturer. *Management Science*, 45(2):178–191, 1999.

[Anupindi et al.(2001)Anupindi, Bassok, and Zemel] Ravi Anupindi, Yehuda Bassok, and Eitan Zemel. A general framework for the study of decentralized distribution systems. *Manufacturing & Service Operations Management*, 3(4):349–368, 2001.

[Chen and Zhang(2009)] Xin Chen and Jiawei Zhang. A stochastic programming duality approach to inventory centralization games. *Operations Research*, 57(4):840–851, 2009.

[Eppen(1979)] Gary D Eppen. Noteeffects of centralization on expected costs in a multi-location newsboy problem. *Management science*, 25 (5):498–501, 1979.

[Fiestras-Janeiro et al.(2011)Fiestras-Janeiro, García-Jurado, Meca, and Mosquera] M Gloria Fiestras-Janeiro, Ignacio García-Jurado, Ana Meca, and Manuel A Mosquera. Cooperative game theory and inventory management. *European Journal of Operational Research*, 210(3): 459–466, 2011.

[Gerchak and Gupta(1991)] Yigal Gerchak and Diwakar Gupta. On apportioning costs to customers in centralized continuous review inventory systems. *Journal of Operations Management*, 10(4):546–551, 1991.

[Hartman et al.(2000)Hartman, Dror, and Shaked] Bruce C Hartman, Moshe Dror, and Moshe Shaked. Cores of inventory centralization games. *Games and Economic Behavior*, 31(1):26–49, 2000.

[Luo and Cai(2016a)] Min Luo and Xiaoqiang Cai. Cooperative games in an integrated system with multiple hospitals. In *Service Systems and Service Management (ICSSSM), 2016 13th International Conference on*, pages 1–4. IEEE, 2016a.

[Luo and Cai(2016b)] Min Luo and Xiaoqiang Cai. Surgical capacity sharing in an integrated hospital system. In *Service Systems and Service Management (ICSSSM), 2016 13th International Conference on*, pages 1–5. IEEE, 2016b.

[Müller et al.(2002)Müller, Scarsini, and Shaked] Alfred Müller, Marco Scarsini, and Moshe Shaked. The newsvendor game has a nonempty core. *Games and Economic Behavior*, 38(1):118–126, 2002.

[Nagarajan and Sošić(2008)] Mahesh Nagarajan and Greys Sošić. Game-theoretic analysis of cooperation among supply chain agents: Review and extensions. *European Journal of Operational Research*, 187(3): 719–745, 2008.

[Owen(1975)] Guillermo Owen. On the core of linear production games. *Mathematical programming*, 9(1):358–370, 1975.

[Özen et al.(2008)Özen, Fransoo, Norde, and Slikker] Ulas Özen, Jan Fransoo, Henk Norde, and Marco Slikker. Cooperation between multiple newsvendors with warehouses. *Manufacturing & Service Operations Management*, 10(2):311–324, 2008.

[Peleg and Sudhölter(2007)] Bezalel Peleg and Peter Sudhölter. *Introduction to the theory of cooperative games*, volume 34. Springer Science & Business Media, 2007.

[Slikker et al.(2001)Slikker, Fransoo, and Wouters] M Slikker, J Fransoo, and M Wouters. Joint ordering in multiple news-vendor situations: a game theoretical approach. *Beta work-ing paper*, 64, 2001.

[Slikker et al.(2005)Slikker, Fransoo, and Wouters] Marco Slikker, Jan Fransoo, and Marc Wouters. Cooperation between multiple newsvendors with transshipments. *European Journal of Operational Research*, 167(2):370–380, 2005.

Research on an Information Sharing System Considering Urgency and Processing Omission Prevention in the Home Care Field

Yuta Sakasai[1], Yuya Totsuka[1], FManabu Kurosawa[1],Jun Sawamoto[2], Hiroshi Yajima[1] Name[1]
[1]School of Science and Technology for Future Life, Tokyo Denki, University, Kitasenjyut, Adaci-Tokyo, Japan
[2]Regional Cooperative Research Center, Iwate Prefecture University, Iwate Prefecture, Japan
{17FMI12,16FMI21}@msdendai.ac.jp, kurosawar@cck.dendai.ac.jp, sawamoto@iwate-pu.ac.jp,
yajima@mail.dendai.ac.jp

Keywords: Home care, Aging society, Information sharing system, Multi-occupation collaboration, Emergency detection .

Abstract: In Japan, rapid aging is a big problem. Particularly, medical care for elderly people at home requires cooperation of workers of multiple job types. However, since these workers take care of many elderly people and deal with enormous information, information sharing on the elderly is not sufficient. In this research, using the proposed method, each worker always obtains important information for individual elderly persons in a timely manner and proposes a method for leading to appropriate medical care for the elderly. It is characterized in that important information is preliminarily set in a strange form for each elderly person, and the relevant information is promptly pushed to the workers. Also, each care worker can follows up the result of elderly care treatment by watching treatment process flow on bulletin board. The effectiveness of the proposed method is verified by experiments..

1 INTRODUCTION

In Japan, rapid aging is a big problem.(Cabinet Office 2016) Particularly, medical care for elderly people at home requires cooperation of workers of multiple job types. However, since these workers have many elderly people and deal with enormous information, information sharing on the elderly among care workers is not sufficient.

In a conventional medical care field, analog information sharing means such as telephone and FAX is mainstream. On the other hand, however, as an office work, the elderly information is also input to the electronic system.

However, cooperation among the workers is not successful at present(Ministry of Health, Labor and Welfare 2016). The results of the interview found the following. Workers are in charge of many elderly people. For this reason, (1) the information managed by the care workers is enormous, (2) Therefore, the worker can not quickly find important information when necessary.

In addition, employees are obliged to record by paper charts or visiting nursing records(Takashi Yoshino 2016). For this reason, information sharing between workers does not proceed.

In this research, we propose an information sharing method that allows workers to obtain necessary information at necessary timing. Specifically, we will establish a "multi-occupational information sharing system" that notifies Push type information with high urgency needed by each worker.

In the proposed system, information items of interest are set for elderly people in charge of each worker. Then, the information sharing system has a PUSH function that presents important information to the care workers.

The worker obtains information of interest in a timely manner when the corresponding information is input. Information input to the information sharing system can be converted into a format that is properly processed and mandatory and can be outputted. At the same time, the medical care

workers informs the issues concerning the elderly to the other medical care participants.
At the time, it is necessary to confirm whether the contents of the issues are sequentially conveyed among related care participants in a timely manner.
In order to realize this function, we develop a visualization tool for checking the transmission status of the issues content to be sent.

With this method, (1) the worker can acquire the information he / she wants in real time, and (2) the input burden on the information sharing system of each business operator is reduced, Also, (3) the worker can check the transmission status of the issues content that he sends to other care worker.

2. PROBLEM OF INFORMATION SHARING IN HOME CARE

In this research, we address the following issues concerning information sharing among workers in medical care at home.

(1) Each worker is responsible for many elderly people. And care workers have to manage huge amounts of information on elderly people. For this reason, it is difficult to quickly extract pertinent information concerning elderly subjects in emergency or the like Home medical care needs are increasing, but the number of home medical care service providing agencies is small. For this reason, the number of elderly people in charge of individual workers is very large. For example, it is clear from the hearing results that the visiting doctor is in charge of more than 100 elderly people. Under these circumstances, the information of elderly people managed by individual care workers is enormous. For this reason, it is difficult to extract necessary information quickly when necessary such as emergency situations.

Because of administrative processing, submission in paper form is often obliged. In this case, input to the information sharing system requires double input operation. In other words, the input burden is large.

(2) Also, in order to share information in real time, it is necessary to communicate data of elderly using an electronic system. However, when a double input operation is required, it is burdensome for a busy care worker, and usage of an information sharing system has not progressed.

Along with the development of the current ICT technology, there are many researches for digitizing care information carried out by care workers. For example, Nakamura and colleagues built a community medical cooperative network system "Miyagi Medical and Welfare Information Network MMWIN" (Miyagi Medical and Welfare Information Network) (Naoki Nakamura 2016). This system connects medical institutions in Miyagi prefecture by a secure network and stores, shares and manages information.

(3) A close cooperation on the physical condition of the elderly is important among medical care workers. However, there is no way for individual care workers to ascertain whether this linkage is being carried out reliably.

However, many of these medical information sharing systems are focusing on information input methods only and are improving input efficiency. There are few studies that consider the support of the information acquiring side.

3. PRPPOSED METHOD

As a premise of the concept proposal, we set the situation where each care worker shall share information using a PC, mobile terminal, or tablet terminal.

3.1 Concept of the Proposed Method

In this research, we propose a information sharing method that allows workers to obtain necessary information at the necessary timing for the necessary amount.

To realize the concept, when sharing information in this proposed system, each worker preliminarily sets conditions (interest conditions) with high

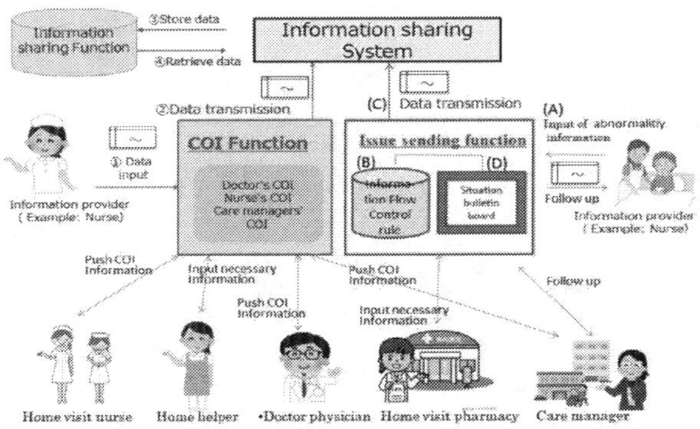

Fig. 1 Whole Image of the Proposed System

interest and urgency for each elderly in charge in the system.

The system detects the important input information (such as contents and notes input by another care worker for a certain elderly) based on this condition, and only when it matches to conditions, the system push notice to care worker.(Fig.1)

The priority notification is displayed on the terminal irrespective of the situation of the worker terminal. With this function, workers can acquire important information in a timely manner to themselves. The reason for setting up the concept is that through interviews with each job type, it was found that information that should be confirmed and frequently handled is confined within a certain range in order for each job type to perform work.

Therefore, (1) information necessary for the worker is set in advance in the information sharing system, and (2) information matching the setting is notified to each worker only when it is input to the system. Through this processing, it is possible to prevent overloading of information of workers.

In addition, the proposed system reduces the time and labor required for input of information sharing contents. Therefore, in this system, electronic key input by keyboard etc. is minimized, specifically, in usage of (1) GUIs such as check boxes and knobs, and (2) voice input for parts where sentences can not be avoided.

3.2 Concern of Interest

For each worker, the condition of interest to the elderly is called "Condition of Interest" (COI) (P.J.Denning 2006) in this study. COI has been defined to pass "necessary information at the necessary timing only the necessary amount". In this research as well, in accordance with this aim, we aim to notify "only the amount that the worker preferentially needs at the timing when the worker needs the information that the worker needs".

3.3 Assumed Worker

In this research, we target four occupations of visiting doctors, visiting nurses, care managers, and nursing care helpers as assumed users of the system. Once the validity of the system is confirmed, it will be extended to physiotherapists, pharmacists, visiting rehabilitation and social workers.

4. INFORMATION SHARING SYSTEM

Information sharing system mainly consists of three function: Information shearing and filtering function, issue sending function and information storing function. Information storing function has been used in usual groupware(Luis Carriço 2009), so we developed Information shearing and filtering function, issue sending function.

4.1 Information shearing and filtering function

The information sharing and filtering function is a function of sharing and filtering information about basic information on patients registered by workers, vital data, meals, medications etc. The main processing of this function is to register, browse, edit, and delete data

The information sharing items to be treated are clarified by interview with care workers. As stated, in this research, before setting information sharing in the proposed system, COI that filter information for each patient in charge of each worker is preset, COI

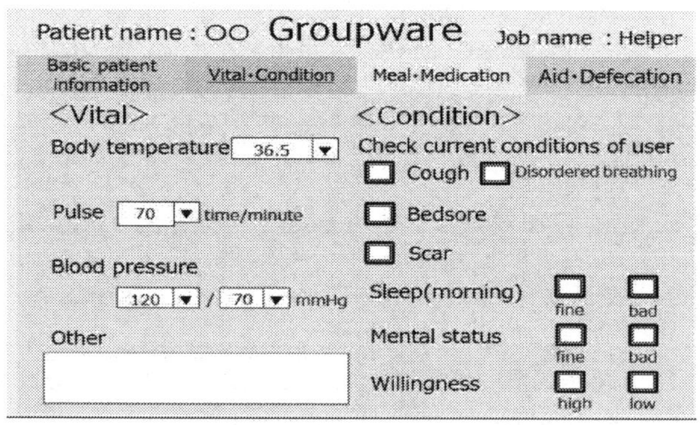

Fig. 2 Information Sharing Items(Vital/State)

items to be set are as follows.

(a) Basic patient information

By registering the basic information of the patient, it is possible to refer to the patient's family composition, medical history, etc. at any time. Basic patient information is patient name, age, profession, main disease name and address etc.

(b)Vital

ISBN: 1-60132-479-0, CSREA Press ©

By inputting patient's temperature, pulse, blood pressure, information is shared. It is the most basic information on patient's life.(FIG.2)

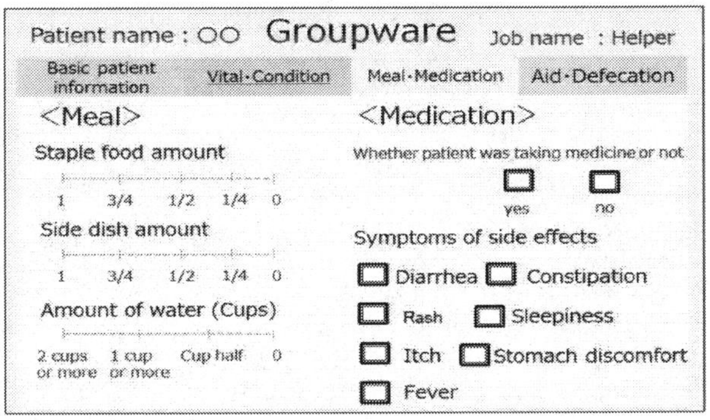

Fig.3 Information Sharing Items(Meal/Medication)

(c) Physical condition of the patient To select from the check box and input about items such as cough, breathing malfunction, scars, sleep, mental state, motivation and so on. Regarding the pressure sores and scratches, an image of affected area is attached when entering. This makes it possible for the viewer to visually confirm changes with time of the scratch. As a result, when the next care worker visits, the care worker can prepares a necessary equipment in advance. (FIG. 2)

(d) meal

The care worker inputs and shares the amount related to the meal when visiting the patient's residence. The items are the staple food amount, the side food amount, and the water content. This information makes it possible to confirm the meal situation of the patient. For example ,The record of meal amount is used as part of the record of visiting nurse. (FIG. 3)

(e) Support

A worker inputs and shares the kind of care work carried out for the elderly with a check box. Many care workers input. Items include bathing assistance, excretion assistance, body cleansing, posture exchanging, dietary assistance, hydration, washing and mouth cleansing. The entry of these items can be used as a record for nursing helper etc.(FIg.4)

(f) Defecation

(g) The worker inputs and shares the amount of excretion of the patient and its state. Shared items are feces quantity, urine quantity, feces / urine condition. . (FIG. 4)

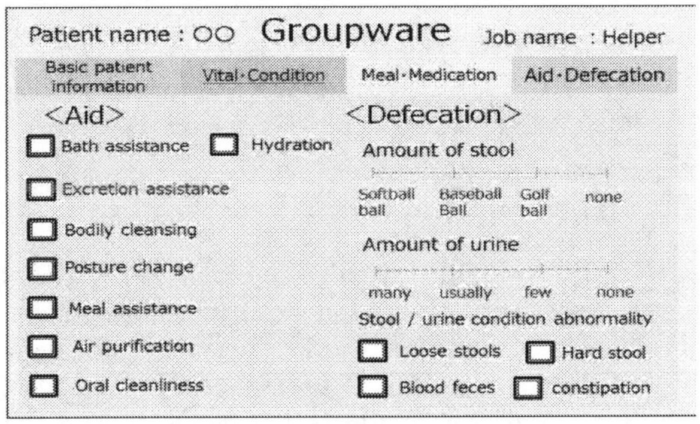

Fig.4 Information Sharing Items(Support/Defecation)

4.2 COI filtering function

In this research, we propose a COI filtering function that takes the following two procedures as a method of input information selection. Function 1: To match the input information with the COI of the elderly, and at that time, to select information applicable to COI Function 2: In the above information, information of a particularly bad state (information of high urgency) is selected.

In this study, proposed system compares the COI for each patient in charge which each worker preset in advance with the input information. Furthermore, by picking up information which is worse in the corresponding information, it is possible to preferentially browse highly urgent information which needs to be coped with. The following example is given as an example of emergency information detection in this research.

<Example of COI setting>: "Body temperature is over 37.5 ° C or higher", "Body temperature is below 35 ° C", "Blood pressure is higher than 140 mmHg", "When the amount of feces does not come out", "Amount of urine is small Case " Information is notified when the shared information input to the

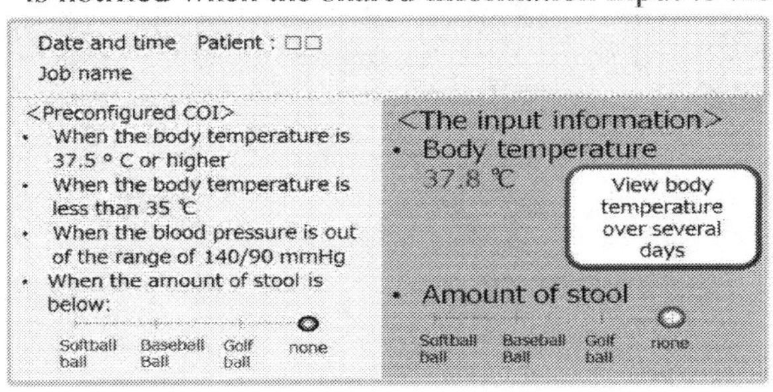

Fig. 5 Example of display of Notification Information

system satisfies the above-described COI setting condition. In that case, the COI set by himself and information to be notified at this time are displayed in advance. (FIG. 5)

4.3 Information Notifying Timing

In this research, we will consider and define the timing of notifying information according to interest conditions to each occupation based on hearings. (Table 1) Basically, in case of emergency and before visit) For example, the definitions of emergency notifications are as follows: (1) Visiting doctors and visiting nurses are able to provide medical care; (2) Care managers are in a position to summarize patient care plans So, care manager can define emergency. Because the care helper does not perform medical procedures, we decided that the timing of the notification to helper is just before visiting the patient 's home. Notification in "Before visiting" refers to information only made by matching with the user's COI. So, emergency information detection mentioned in 4.1 is not performed in the case of helper.

Table 1 Timing of Information notification

Visiting Doctor	Visiting Nurse	Care Manager	Helper
Emergency Timing and Timing before visit	Emergency Timing and Timing before visit	Emergency Timing and Timing before visit	Timing before visit

4.4 Issue Sending Function

The issue sending is based on the fact that the participants who noticed abnormality of the elderly. It is work with the following operation: (1) urge the corresponding care workers to call attention, (2) send caution points on the next countermeasure associated with the process performed by the care worker

The issue sending is usually carried out at home medical care / nursing care.

However, in the past, since it was done in an analog form, there was a problem that information is not sufficiently transmitted. The function of the issue sending in this proposal is to ensure information transmission.

In this research, we incorporate the issue sending function into a part of the information sharing function. The built-in the issue sending function has a kind of workflow system function. Care worker who noticed abnormality of elderly persons will submit anomaly contents via the workflow system to other care workers who will take necessary measures. The system successively and reliably transmits abnormality information to related care workers in a predetermined procedure.

The result and further correspondence of the involved participants are carried out via the system, and the flow of processing is automatically visualized on the shared bulletin board. In this manner, not only the care participants who sent the anomalies, but also the flow of correspondence to the abnormality are displayed to all related care participants. Therefore, there is no leakage in responding to elderly anomalies

At the same time, care worker who sent abnormality can grasp how far the correspondence process is progressing through the system bulletin board. Therefore, if the progress of the corresponding processing is not smooth, the care worker who sent the abnormality can respond further by other means. Such correspondence makes it possible to respond to the abnormality of the elderly and surely.

5. EXPERIMENT

5.1 Outline of Experiment

When this system notifies information to each worker, it is necessary to verify how to minimize necessary information and make it the optimum amount of information, so we will conduct comparative experiments on the amount of information. In the verification experiment, data close to information shared by each worker on the actual site was created based on hearings and use it as input data.

In order to clarify the effect of the proposed method, we conducted information notification simulation with the following three types of notification methods. After that, the amount of information notified to each worker was compared to verify the effect of the proposed method.

(x) <Current status method> "Notify all information" (Notification of all information of patients in charge of each worker)

(Y) <Simple method using only COI > (Notified according to the set COI)

(z) <Proposed method> " method with COI + Emergency information detection" (Information notified of urgency is notified in advance with information set COI)

Two reasons for selecting (X) and (Y) as comparison targets with the proposed method are shown below. (X) is to compare the current situation with the proposed method assuming that the method of notifying all the entered information of the patient in charge of each occupation is the information notification way in the current information sharing system. (Y) is selected to verify how useful the method of notifying urgent information among the information included in COI by comparison of the case where only COI is set and also to verify the proposed method is useful for the situation where information is over there.

The input data was prepared assuming a case where four occupations of a visiting doctor, a visiting nurse, a care manager and a care helper carry out the care of one home patient for two weeks. For visiting medical care simulation, scenarios such as nursing care records, etc. were created based on the hearing results. Also, COI preset by each worker was also created based on hearings. (The first part is shown in Table 2) The way of extracting the amount of information to be notified is the following; that is when two items of "body temperature" and "blood pressure" are included in one notification, the sum of all notification information is taken. In this case, 2 notification items is counted.

Table 2 Setting up COI for Experiment

Job category	Example of COI
Visiting Doctor	● Body temperature is less than 38C ● blood pressure is less than 140/80mmHg ● Stool
Visiting nurse	● Body temperature is less than 37.5C ● blood pressure is less than 140/80mmHg ● Inoculum moisture content is less than half of glass

As for the transfer function of the abnormality, we attempted the case where the helper noticed abnormally as an example

First of all, the helper asked the visiting nurse to seek a response. Depending on the circumstances, nurses coped with themselves or, in some cases, obtained comprehension from doctors and took action. For necessary treatment medicine, the visiting nurse asked a visiting pharmacy to order. After that, in cooperation with a helper, the visiting nurse observed the course after treatment, confirm recovery of abnormality

5.2 Experiment Result

The results of the above three types of information notification simulation are shown in Table 2.
In comparing the number of notifications of the proposed method (Z) with reference to the number of notifications of the current state method of (X), the average amount of information reduction was 83%. (See Table 3) In addition, the average number of notifications of (Z) is reduced by about 44% compared with (Y).

6. DISCUSSION

The proposed method exerts a large effect on information overload due to a significant reduction of less interesting information, because filtering is performed. The result is assumed before experiment.

Table 3 Number of information notified to each occupations

	Current method	Proposed method(1) (With COI)	Proposed method(1) (With COI + Emergent information)
Visiting Doctor	617	197	107
Visiting nurse	617	313	155
Care Manager	617	171	118
Care Helper	617	74	44
Average	617	188.8	106

From Table3, it is considered that the number of notifications of the proposed method is reduced by about 83% compared with the current method, and because important information in emergency is taken into consideration, it is considered that there is never too little information for each occupation . If you feel that the amount of information to be notified is small, each job category can respond by changing COI to your favorite condition.
In addition, the following opinions were received from the doctor in charge after the experiment.
1) Since the amount of information to be noticed is small, we can concentrate on grasping the situation, and the situation of the elderly can be grasped accurately.
2) Since there are multiple COIs, understanding of the disease condition is progressed because it was

possible to examine while comparing multiple measured value.

In addition, as percentage of information reduction by introducing COI, the proportion of reduction has increased in the order of visiting nurse, visiting doctor, care helper, care manager. In the occupation with a large proportion of information reduction,,

Table 4 Comparison of Information Notification number for three method

	Current method	Proposed method(1) (With COI)	Proposed method(1) (With COI + Emergent information)
Visiting Doctor	a	0.32a	0.17a
Visiting nurse	b	0.31b	0.25b
Care Manager	c	0.28c	0.19c
Care Helper	d	0.12d	0.07d
Average	e	0.31e	0.17e

items with detailed conditions were set by many COI. Although there are differences depending on how to create scenarios, it can be said that the more prominent information reduction can be realized when the proposed system sets more detailed COIs.

Depending on the situation, COI can be changed from a remote location, so care workers did not feel so much burdened with regard to COI setting. Actually, some doctors changed the COI according to the situation and verified the difference in reaction.

3) In the scenario used in this experiment, the flow of transforming issues was a relatively simple. For this reason, the flow of information delivery was very easy to understand for subjects who were involved in medical care workers. And the responsiveness of each participant was smooth. In some cases, responding to abnormalities in elderly people may branch on the way. In considering this case, it became clear that it is possible to respond to the case by adding a rule base to the assignment function, because we tried to modify the function during the experiment

7. CONCLUSION

In this research, it is possible to notify Push notification of highly urgent information by using COI (interest condition) of each worker against the problem of information overload among engagers of different occupations in home care nursing care site.

We propose an emergency specialized information sharing system that balances information sharing and inputs that workers do not incur a heavy burden on conventional work. From the verification experiments, it was confirmed that only necessary information can be reported when the degree of urgency is high, so the proposed method is effective

In this experiment, verification using one scenario was carried out. In the future, we will proceed with verification using various scenarios more suited to the site.

ACKNOWLEDGEMENTS

This research was subsidized by JSPS Grant-in-Aid for Scientific Research 16K00429

REFERENCES

Cabinet Office 2016 "Heisei era 28 year old society white paper

Ministry of Health, Labor and Welfare 2017 "Toward Building Regional Comprehensive Care System"

Takashi Yoshino, Rie Yamamoto, Masayuki Irie, Kunio Nakai : 2016 “Patient Information Sharing System among Multi-professional Healthcare Providers for Cooperating Home Medical Care”, IPSJ SIG Technical Report, Vol.2016-GN-99, No.24, p.1-6

Naoki Nakamura, Masaharu Nakayama, Teiji Tominaga, Takuo Suganuma, and Norio Shiratori 2016: “Development and Management of EHR system in Miyagi Prefecture”, IPSJ SIG Technical Report, Vol.2016-GN-97, No.3 pp.1-5 (in Japanese)

P.J.Denning 2006 : “Infoglut”, Communications of the ACM

Luis Carriço 2009, Groupware: Design, Implementation, and Use: Proceedings of 15th International Workshop, Peso da Régua, Douro, Portugal, September

Author Index